HOW TO DO PRIMARY CARE RESEARCH

WONCA Family Medicine

About the Series

The WONCA Family Medicine series is a collection of books written by worldwide experts and practitioners of family medicine, in collaboration with The World Organization of Family Doctors (WONCA).

WONCA is a not-for-profit organization and was founded in 1972 by member organizations in 18 countries. It now has 118 Member Organizations in 131 countries and territories with membership of about 500,000 family doctors and more than 90 percent of the world's population.

Primary Health Care around the World: Recommendations for International Policy and Development
Chris Van Weel, Amanda Howe

Family Practice in the Eastern Mediterranean Region: Universal Health Coverage and Quality Primary Care
Hassan Salah, Michael Kidd

Every Doctor: Healthier Doctors = Healthier Patients
Leanne Rowe, Michael Kidd

How to Do Primary Care Research
Felicity Goodyear-Smith, Bob Mash

The Contribution of Family Medicine to Improving Health Systems: A Guidebook from the World Organization of Family Doctors
Michael Kidd

International Perspectives on Primary Care Research
Felicity Goodyear-Smith, Bob Mash

Family Medicine: The Classic Papers
Michael Kidd, Iona Heath, Amanda Howe

For more information about this series, please visit https://www.crcpress.com/WONCA-Family-Medicine/book-series/WONCA

HOW TO DO PRIMARY CARE RESEARCH

EDITED BY

Felicity Goodyear-Smith, MBChB, MD, FRNZCGP (Dist)

Department of General Practice and Primary Health Care,
University of Auckland, Auckland, New Zealand

Bob Mash, MBChB, PhD, FRCGP (UK), FCFP (SA)

Division of Family Medicine and Primary Care,
Stellenbosch University, Tygerberg, South Africa

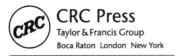

CRC Press
Taylor & Francis Group
Boca Raton London New York

CRC Press is an imprint of the
Taylor & Francis Group, an **informa** business

CRC Press
Taylor & Francis Group
6000 Broken Sound Parkway NW, Suite 300
Boca Raton, FL 33487-2742

© 2019 by Taylor & Francis Group, LLC
CRC Press is an imprint of Taylor & Francis Group, an Informa business

No claim to original U.S. Government works

Printed on acid-free paper
Printed by CPI Group (UK) Ltd, Croydon CR0 4YY

International Standard Book Number-13: 978-1-138-49958-4 (Paperback)
978-1-138-49959-1 (Hardback)

Visit the Taylor & Francis Web site at
http://www.taylorandfrancis.com

and the CRC Press Web site at
http://www.crcpress.com

Contents

SECTION III   Preliminary steps to doing primary care research

SECTION IV   Methods and techniques for doing primary care research

SECTION V   How to disseminate your research

SECTION VI   Building research capacity

Foreword

Research is fundamental to the quality clinical care people working in primary care who cater to our patients and our communities every single day. As health professionals, we are trained to deliver health care based on science and knowledge, on the evidence gained from clinical research, on the wisdom shared by our teachers and colleagues, and on the insights we gain each day from our own work with our individual patients.

Therefore, how do you become a primary care researcher? Research starts with being curious, with asking questions, with noticing things that others have not noticed, with wondering why things are the way they are, and how they could be better. In primary care our clinics and our communities are the source of our new research ideas – if you like, our laboratories. Our work with our patients allows us to gain insights and to think about human existence, health and disease every single day. Each of us has the capacity to become involved in primary care research. All it takes to start is curiosity and commitment.

I am convinced that every person working in primary care around the world needs to be involved in research. As clinicians we need the skills to search the research literature for the evidence we need to provide the best care we can to our patients and our communities. Involvement in clinical audits and quality improvement activities allows us to gain insights into our own practice and into the health issues facing our patients. Many of us become involved in other peoples' research through completion of surveys or involvement in studies. And the most fortunate of us get to conduct our own research, seeking to improve medical knowledge and lead the exploration of the boundaries of clinical medicine. Our involvement in research also provides us with the skills to adapt to the changes that inevitably take place as clinical practice evolves throughout our careers.

This book provides valuable advice to everyone interested in getting started as a researcher. What are the first steps to becoming a researcher? What areas of primary care excite you and stir your passions? What specific problems or challenges would you like to tackle? How can you make discoveries which can support the development of primary care in your own practice, in your own country and at a global level? And how can you share your findings, through publications, presentations and advocacy to influence changes in health policy and practice?

There are also many lessons here for seasoned researchers, with advice and wisdom shared by some of the great primary care researchers of our age.

Now is a great time to be a primary care researcher. Nations around the world are seeking to strengthen primary care as a way to move towards universal health coverage, ensuring that quality health care is available to every person in every community in every country of the world. If we are going to achieve universal health coverage, health for all people, then we are going to need research to support strong primary care, to guide developments in primary care, and to assist our advocacy efforts for much needed investment and growth in access to primary care. Research will support us to advocate for the role of primary care as the foundation of health service delivery in each of our countries. Research will support us to advocate about the benefits to our communities of strengthened primary care and the need for greater investment in research that addresses primary care challenges. Research will support us to advocate for family practice and other primary care settings as the ideal research locations to generate the evidence needed for the delivery of health care for the twenty-first century.

We are facing great global health challenges and primary care holds many of the answers. There are questions we can answer, that others cannot, about the prevention and management of chronic disease and mental health and comorbidity, the challenges of complexity and uncertainty, the ethical issues affecting health care, the contributions of integrated primary care services to the care of older people, the need to ensure equitable access to health care especially for those who are vulnerable and marginalised, and the need to tackle the social determinants of health and illness.

Enjoy reading about how to do primary care research, but don't stop there. Use this wonderful new book as your inspiration and guide to get started on your own research. I look forward to hearing about your discoveries.

Professor Michael Kidd AM
President, World Organization of Family Doctors (2013–2016)
Chair, Department of Family and Community Medicine, The University of Toronto, Canada
Senior Innovation Fellow, Institute for Health System Solutions and Virtual Care, Women's College Hospital, Canada
Professorial Fellow, Murdoch Children's Research Institute, Australia
Honorary Professor of Global Primary Care, Southgate Institute for Health, Society and Equity, Flinders University, Australia

Editors

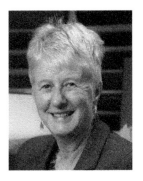

Felicity Goodyear-Smith is a general practitioner and academic head of the Department of General Practice and Primary Health Care, University of Auckland, Auckland, New Zealand. She and Professor Bob Mash co-edited the companion book to this current title: *International Perspectives in Primary Care Research*, CRC Press, 2016. She is Chair of the WONCA (world family doctors) Working Party on Research, and both books have been written on behalf of WONCA. She also chairs the International Committee of the North American Primary Care Research Group. Felicity was the founding editor-in-chief of the *Journal of Primary Health Care*. She has published over 200 peer-reviewed papers as well as a number of books and book chapters.

Felicity is passionate about the importance of research underpinning clinical practice in primary care. As well as her own research projects and those of her graduate students, she is actively engaged in research capacity-building globally, especially in low- and middle-income countries. This current book is particularly for emerging researchers, written as a 'how to' guide to conducting primary care research.

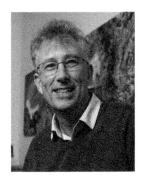

Bob Mash graduated from The University of Edinburgh and trained as a general practitioner in Scotland before emigrating to South Africa in 1991. He worked in the townships outside Cape Town with community health workers, providing community based primary care in the final days of the apartheid era. Following the onset of democracy, he worked for 10 years in the public sector, providing primary care in Khayelitsha. During this period, he worked with Stellenbosch University to create the first learning opportunities in family medicine and primary care for undergraduate medical students. Subsequently, he also developed a new online master's degree programme for the training of family physicians.

He obtained his PhD on mental disorders in primary care in 2002 and has now published over 150 articles in peer reviewed scientific journals. He is currently the head of Family and Emergency Medicine at Stellenbosch

University and responsible for research activities and training at both master's and doctoral levels. He is the editor-in-chief of the *African Journal of Primary Health Care & Family Medicine* and is a rated researcher with the National Research Foundation. He is a founding member of the Chronic Diseases Initiative for Africa (a network of researchers) and an active leader within the Primary Care and Family Medicine Education (Primafamed) Network, a group of departments of family medicine in sub-Saharan Africa. He is currently the President of the South African Academy of Family Physicians.

Contributors

Penelope Abbott, MBBS Hons, MPH, FRACGP
Department of General Practice
Western Sydney University
Sydney, Australia

Lauren Ball, PhD
Menzies Health Institute Queensland
Griffith University
Gold Coast Campus
Gold Coast, Australia

Katelyn Barnes, PhD, MNutrDiet, BAppSci, APD
Menzies Health Institute Queensland
Griffith University
Gold Coast Campus
Gold Coast, Australia

Gillian Bartlett-Esquilant, PhD
Family Medicine
McGill University
Montreal, Canada

Christopher Barton, PhD, MMedSc, BSc
Department of General Practice
Monash University
Melbourne, Australia

Jackie Crowe
Department of Academic Family
 Medicine
University of Saskatchewan
Saskatoon, Canada

Paresh Dawda, MB BS DRCOG DFRSH FRACGP FRCGP (UK)
Faculty of Health
University of Canberra
Canberra, Australia

Kevin Dew, PhD
School of Social and Cultural
 Studies
Victoria University of Wellington
Wellington, New Zealand

Miriam Dickinson, PhD
Family Medicine
University of Colorado Anschutz
 Medical Campus
Aurora, Colorado

Anthony Dowell, FRNZCGP
Department of Primary Health Care
 and General Practice
University of Otago
Wellington, New Zealand

Daniel J. Exeter, BA, MA (Hons), PhD
Section of Epidemiology and
 Biostatistics
School of Population Health
University of Auckland
Auckland, New Zealand

Tom Fahey, MB BCh, MSc, MD, MFPH, FRCGP
Department of General
    Practice and HRB Centre for
    Primary Care Research
Royal College of Surgeons in Ireland
    Medical School
Dublin, Ireland

Raquel Gómez Bravo, MD
Expert in Mental Health in
    Primary Care
Institute for Health and Behaviour
Research Unit INSIDE
University of Luxembourg
Luxembourg

Felicity Goodyear-Smith, MBChB, MD, FRNZCGP (Dist)
Department of General Practice and
    Primary Health Care
University of Auckland
Auckland, New Zealand

Trish Greenhalgh, MD, FMedSci
Nuffield Department of Primary
    Care Health Sciences
University of Oxford
Oxford, England

Elizabeth Halcomb, RN BN (Hons) PhD FCNA
School of Nursing
University of Wollongong
New South Wales, Australia

Sally Hall, RN, Grad Cert Clin Man
Rural Clinical School
College of Health and Medicine
Australian National University
Canberra, Australia

Willie Hamilton, BSc (hons), MBChB, MD, FRCP, FRCGP
Institute of Health Service Research
University of Exeter Medical School
Exeter, England

Amanda Howe, OBE, FRCGP, MA, MEd, MD
Norwich Medical School
University of East Anglia
Norwich, United Kingdom

Nasreen Jessani, BSc (Canada), MSPH (USA), DrPH (USA)
Center for Evidence Based Health Care
Department of Global Health
Stellenbosch University
Cape Town, South Africa
and
Department of International Health
Johns Hopkins Bloomberg School of
    Public Health
Baltimore, Maryland

Andrew W. Knight, MBBS, MMedSci (clinepid) FRACGP FAICD
The Fairfield GP Unit
University of New South Wales and
    the South Western Sydney Local
    Health District
Liverpool, Australia

Liliana Laranjo, MD, MPH, PhD
Australian Institute of Health
    Innovation
Macquarie University
Liverpool, Australia

Siaw-Teng Liaw, MBBS, PhD, FRACGP, FACMI, FACHI, MIAHSI
General Practice Unit
School of Public Health and
    Community Medicine
University of New South Wales
Sydney, Australia

Charilaos Lygidakis, MD
Institute for Health and Behaviour
Research Unit INSIDE
University of Luxembourg
Luxembourg

**Amanda Lyons, BSocSci (UNSW)
M of Bioethics (Monash)**
Member of Royal Australian College
  of General Practitioners
Research and Evaluation Ethics and
  Committee
Sydney, Australia

**Ann C. Macaulay, CM,
MD, FGFP**
Department of Family Medicine
McGill University
Montreal, Canada

**Lindsay Macdonald, BN, MA
(Applied)**
Department of Primary
  Health Care and
  General Practice
University of Otago
Wellington, New Zealand

**Bunmi Malau-Aduli, BSc, MSc,
GradtCertMgt, GradCertULT,
PhD**
College of Medicine and Dentistry
James Cook University
Townsville, Australia

**Bob Mash, MBChB, PhD, FRCGP
(UK), FCFP (SA)**
Division of Family Medicine and
  Primary Care
Stellenbosch University
Tygerberg, South Africa

**Sherina Mohd Sidik, MBBS,
MMED (Family Medicine), PhD**
Department of Psychiatry
Universiti Putra Malaysia
Serdang, Malaysia

**Celeste Naude, PhD, RD (SA),
RD (UK)**
Centre for Evidence-Based Health
  Care
Division of Epidemiology and
  Biostatistics
Stellenbosch University
Cape Town, South Africa

Ana Luísa Neves, MD, MSc, PhD
Centre for Health Policy
Institute of Global Health
  Innovation
Imperial College London
London, United Kingdom
and
Centre for Health Technology and
  Services Research
Department of Community
  Medicine, Information
  and Health Decision Sciences
University of Porto
Porto, Portugal

Liesl Nicol, PhD
Centre for Evidence-based
  Health Care
Department of Global Health
Stellenbosch University
Cape Town, South Africa

**William R. Phillips, MD, MPH,
FAAFP**
Department of Family Medicine
University of Washington
Seattle, Washington

Luís Pinho-Costa, MD
Gondomar Health Centres' Cluster
Gondomar, Portugal

Robyn Preston, BA(DevS) (Hons),
PGCertDisasRefugHlth, GCertEd,
MHSc (HealthProm), PhD
General Practice and Rural Medicine
College of Medicine and Dentistry
and
Division of Tropical Health and
    Medicine
and
Anton Breinl Research Centre for
    Health Systems Strengthening
James Cook University
Townsville, Australia

Robert Price, BSc (hons)
MBChB (hons) MSc FRCA
Department of Anaesthetics
Royal Devon and Exeter Hospital
    NHS Foundation Trust
Exeter, England

Sarah Price, BSc(hons) PhD
University of Exeter Medical School
Exeter, United Kingdom

Norma Rabbitskin, BN, RN
Community Health and Primary
    Care/Home and Community
    Care Program
Sturgeon Lake Health Centre
Sturgeon Lake First Nation
Sturgeon Lake, Canada

Vivian R. Ramsden, RN, BSN, MS,
PhD, MCFP (Hon.)
Department of Academic Family
    Medicine
University of Saskatchewan
Saskatoon, Canada

Robin Ray, BEd, MHSc, PhD
College of Medicine and Dentistry
Anton Breinl Research Centre
    for Health Systems Strengthening
James Cook University
Townsville, Australia

Danielle Rolfe, PhD
School of Epidemiology and Public
    Health
University of Ottawa
Ottawa, Canada

Grant Russell, MBBS FRACGP
MFM PhD
Southern Academic Primary Care
    Research Unit
Department of General Practice
Monash University
Melbourne, Australia

Lena Sanci, MBBS, PhD, FRACGP
Department of General Practice
University of Melbourne
Victoria, Australia

Tibor Schuster, PhD
Family Medicine
McGill University
Montreal, Canada

Eric K. Shaw, PhD
Department of Community Medicine
Mercer University School of Medicine
Savannah, Georgia

Lauren Siegmann, B.A (Melb),
PgG Assessment and Evaluation
(Melb), PgC Applied Statistics
(Swinburne)
College of Medicine and Dentistry
James Cook University
Townsville, Australia

Richard Stevens, BA MSc PhD
Nuffield Department of Primary
  Care Health Sciences
University of Oxford
Oxford, England

**Maria Stubbe, DipTESL,
NZDipTch, PhD**
Department of Primary Health Care
  and General Practice
University of Otago
Wellington, New Zealand

**Elizabeth Sturgiss, FRACGP
FHEA B.Med MPH MForensMed**
Academic Unit of General
  Practice
Australian National University
Canberra, Australian Capital
  Territory, Australia

**Chun Wah Michael Tam,
BSc(Med), MBBS, MMH(GP),
FRACGP**
Discipline of General Practice
University of Sydney
and
General Practice Unit
South Western Sydney Local Health
  District
Ingham Institute of Applied
  Medical Research
Sydney, Australia

**Judy Taylor, BA, DipSocWk,
MSW, PhD**
College of Medicine and Dentistry
Anton Breinl Research Centre for
  Health Systems Strengthening
James Cook University
Townsville, Australia

**David R. Thomas, BA, MA, PhD,
FNZPsS**
Social and Community Health
University of Auckland
Auckland, New Zealand

**Carissa van den Berk-Clark, PhD,
MSW**
Department of Family and
  Community Medicine
Saint Louis University
St. Louis, Missouri

**Chris van Weel, MD, PhD, (hon)
FRCGP (UK), (hon) FRACGP (Aus)**
Department of Primary and
  Community Care
Radboud University
Nijmegen, the Netherlands
and
Department of Health Services
  Research and Policy
Australian National University
Canberra, Australia

**Katherine E. Walesby, MRes,
MBBS, MRCP (UK)**
Alzheimer Scotland Dementia
  Research Centre and Centre for
  Cognitive Ageing and Cognitive
  Epidemiology
University of Edinburgh
Edinburgh, Scotland

**Emma Wallace, MBBAOBch,
BMedSci, PhD, MICGP**
Department of General Practice and
  HRB Centre for Primary Care
  Research
Royal College of Surgeons in Ireland
  Medical School
Dublin, Ireland

Katharine A. Wallis, MBChB,
PhD, MBHL, Dip Obst, FRNZCGP
Department of General Practice and
Primary Health Care
University of Auckland
Auckland, New Zealand

Valerie A. Wright-St. Clair,
PhD, MPH, DipProfEthics,
DipBusStudies (Health
management), DipOccTherapy
School of Clinical Sciences
Auckland University of Technology
Auckland, New Zealand

Taryn Young, MBCHB, FCPHM,
MMED, PhD
Centre for Evidence-based Health
Care
Division of Epidemiology and
Biostatistics
Stellenbosch University
and
Cochrane South Africa
South African Medical Research
Council
Cape Town, South Africa

SECTION I

Introduction

CHAPTER 1

What makes research primary care research?

Felicity Goodyear-Smith and Bob Mash

This book is an initiative of the WONCA (World Organisation of Family Doctors) Working Party on Primary Care Research and a companion to *International Perspectives on Primary Care Research*, which made the case for why primary care research is essential to building effective primary health care systems.[1]

There are many articles and books on how to conduct medical and other health research. However, traditionally, the majority of health research has been either biomedical or hospital focused. Since the 1970s, family medicine/general practice has developed as an academic discipline, with a growing recognition of the need for research that answers questions important to primary care. Research informs clinical practice, organisation of primary care services and teaching, and developing its own body of research is the hallmark of a maturing academic discipline. Such research should happen in the primary care context, either within the community itself or population at risk or within facilities where people come seeking health care. Evidence generated within the primary-care context is more likely to be relevant and applicable. Unfortunately, much of the evidence applied to the primary-care context is generated in other settings such as the tertiary hospital.

Effective primary health care is the foundation on which successful health systems are built. Countries with strong primary health care systems have better outcomes, increased patient satisfaction, less hospitalisation and lower costs. Such primary health care systems can also contribute to enhanced equity in society. Primary care is the first level of contact that patients and their families have with the health system. In comparison to episodic, hospital-based, secondary care, primary care offers accessible, coordinated and comprehensive services to all people over their lifetime and can include health promotion, prevention and management of both acute and chronic conditions, as well as basic rehabilitation.[2] It is often characterised by its acceptability and affordability to the whole population and its ability to address needs on an ongoing basis. It can range from maternal and neonatal to end-of-life and palliative-care services, and it may be delivered by a variety of practitioners as well as family physicians/general practitioners, including nurses, pharmacists and community workers, often working in teams. Health systems vary considerably between countries, and the services provided are context specific, depending on the population's needs, with a wide range of different health professionals delivering care. What is provided also depends on a number of other factors, including economics, political commitment to primary health care and the available health workforce.

Along with variation in health systems, the terminology used in different countries also varies. Vocationally trained doctors providing first-line care are called general practitioners (GPs) in countries such as the United Kingdom, The Netherlands, Australia and New Zealand. However, in other countries, such as South Africa and Malaysia, GPs do not have advanced training, and the family physician is the doctor with specialised family medicine training. In the United States, a GP is a hospital-based general physician practising internal medicine.[3] In this book, we have chosen to retain the terms used by our individual authors, rather than attempting uniformity and risking changing meaning.

The focus of this book is primary care research. As noted in *International Perspectives on Primary Care Research*, the terms 'primary care' and 'primary health care' are often considered synonymous.[1] However, primary care generally refers to first-line, facility-based services delivered to patients and their families, whereas primary health care is a broader concept, including both individual primary care and also population-based public health services.[4] It involves more than the health sector alone and requires inter-sectorial collaboration, active community engagement and a commitment to social justice to address health inequities.

In contrast, secondary care refers to the second tier of health services, provided by specialists in hospital settings,[5] although in low- and middle-income countries, secondary care at rural and district hospitals may be provided by family physicians or GPs, which further blurs the boundaries. However, just like the terms GP and family physician, primary care and primary health care have different shades of meaning in different parts of the world, with no consistent single and simple definition.[6] While the central aim is to address research issues facing front-line doctors, nurses, community pharmacists and many other health practitioners, there is no hard line between primary care and primary health care, and many of the approaches and methods outlined will be just as relevant to those conducting public health and community-based service delivery research. Ultimately, primary care research is research relevant to primary care practitioners and academics.

Primary care implies comprehensive personal care over time.[7] It deals not only with the presenting complaint, but also ongoing physical, emotional and social issues and the opportunity to address risky health behaviours to prevent the development of disease and promote health. A component is communication and the importance of the relationships between health providers and patients and their families. It is eclectic by nature, and similarly, primary care research employs a wide range of diverse approaches and methodologies. It was an early adopter of mixed methods, combining quantitative and qualitative research to add the narrative to the numbers, to answer the questions of how and why.[8]

Primary care research may be conducted by a wide variety of disciplines and is often interdisciplinary. As outlined in *International Perspectives on Primary Care Research*,[1] the general typology of primary care research includes basic research (examines the methods used to conduct research in primary care), clinical research (clinical diagnosis and treatment), health-services research (delivery of care and organisation of services), health-systems research (large-scale economic and political factors that impact primary care) and educational research (for both students and practitioners).

Many core professionals such as family doctors and primary care nurses have limited capacity to conduct or participate in primary care research. This is particularly true in low- and middle-income countries. Over the last 50 years, the growth in the number of academic departments of general practice, family medicine and primary care has linked research to the requirements of undergraduate and postgraduate training. The number of established researchers, however, in many parts of the world remains small. Governmental commitment to universal coverage and primary health care systems may also influence the provision of funding for primary care research. The emergence of many research networks in different regions has promoted collaboration between researchers and practitioners, resulting in robust and meaningful research.

This book is written as a practical guide, particularly for new and emerging researchers, providing the necessary tools and frameworks on how to conduct the various steps involved in designing, conducting and disseminating robust research. It provides guidance on how to choose and define your question and design and implement your methods, as well as how to report on your results or findings. While it is not the definitive text on specific methodologies, it covers a range of common quantitative and qualitative methods with useful tips and guides, and it points you in the direction of freely available online resources when more in-depth knowledge is required.

REFERENCES

1. Goodyear-Smith F, Mash B, editors. *International Perspectives on Primary Care Research*. London: CRC Press; 2016.
2. Organisation for Economic Co-operation and Development. *Caring for Quality in Health: Lessons Learnt from 15 Reviews of Health Care Quality*. Paris, France: OECD; 2017. p. 62.
3. American Board of General Practice. Welcome to the Board. *Secondary Welcome to the Board* 2013. http://www.abgp.org/.
4. Muldoon LK, Hogg WE, Levitt M. Primary care (PC) and primary health care (PHC). What is the difference? *Can J Public Health* 2006;97(5):409–11.
5. International Conference on Primary Health Care. *Declaration of Alma-Ata*. Alma-Ata, USSR: WHO; 1978.
6. Amisi J, Downing R. Primary care research: Does it defy definition? *Prim Health Care Res Dev* 2017;18(6):523–26.
7. Jones R. Primary care research: Ends and means. *Fam Pract* 2000;17(1):1–4.
8. Goodyear-Smith F. Practising alchemy: The transmutation of evidence into best health care. *Fam Pract* 2011;28(2):123–7.

CHAPTER 2

Ontology and epistemology, methodology and method, and research paradigms

Eric K. Shaw

The year was 1999, or so Thomas Anderson and much of humanity thought. Anderson is a computer programmer living a double life under the hacker alias 'Neo'. He thinks he is living a normal existence, going through the motions of his typical mundane routines; he thinks he frequently goes outside and experiences the warmth of the sun and the smells of a vibrant city. In reality, though, the year is 2199 and the world has been ravaged by sentient machines. Neo and most of humanity are enslaved – encased in liquid-filled pods with cables connected to their bodies, providing electrochemical energy to the machines. Their minds are imprisoned in a virtual reality – a computer simulation called the Matrix.

While in the 'normal' world of 1999, Neo is contacted by members of an underground resistance who have figured out how to hack into the Matrix and unplug the enslaved humans so that they too could join the rebellion and fight back against the hostile machines. Morpheus, a messianic figure within the resistance, presents Neo with a life-changing option: Swallow a red pill that will allow him to learn the truth about the Matrix so that he may fight against the machines, or swallow a blue pill that will return him to his old life – that of blissful ignorance as an enslaved body while the machines decimate their world. This, of course, is the set up for the popular film *The Matrix* (and the entire trilogy). Lest I spoil the storyline for those unaware, I'll refrain from describing which pill Neo chooses and what happens to humanity!

ONTOLOGY AND EPISTEMOLOGY

Why am I introducing a chapter about primary care research with an action-packed 'sci-fi' movie? The answer is that *The Matrix* prompts us to confront two fundamental philosophical questions that also undergird virtually every research endeavour: The ontological question of 'what is the nature of reality?' (or, more simply, 'what is real?') and the epistemological question of 'how do we know what is real?' These are, in fact, classic questions which have generated philosophical debates for thousands of years and *The Matrix* is but one example from popular culture where these questions are explicitly manifested within the plot.

In *The Matrix*, the ontological question of 'what is real' is perplexing. The enslaved humans' minds are being tricked into believing that they are, in fact, walking down a street, driving a car to work, eating delicious foods and developing relationships with family and friends. So what counts as real? Is a real thing something that has an objective quality? That exists independently of being perceived? Or is a thing real only because we (human beings) perceive, define and construct it as such? Such questions form the basis for the materialism/idealism framework.[1] Materialism posits that a thing is real because it is rooted in or constituted by an objective, material (physical) nature. Idealism posits that a thing is real because it is rooted in peoples' *ideas*. Using a simplistic example, if you hear someone claim 'what is real doesn't matter... perception is reality!', s/he is drawing upon the essence of the idealists' standpoint: Whatever thing we are observing, experiencing or studying is only real because we (human beings) have perceived and defined it as such and have an agreed-upon understanding of what that thing is. Primary care researchers (and all kinds of researchers) may be unwittingly, but undoubtedly, making certain assumptions about what counts as real in terms of this material/ideal dualism in the ways in which they approach a line of inquiry, formulate a research question, collect data and interpret results.

The epistemological issue in *The Matrix* is also relevant for primary care researchers. Clearly, the enslaved humans do not know that they are not living in the 'real' world that has been decimated by the machines. But as viewers of the movie, we do know what is real. How? Precisely because we are external viewers, situated outside of the story, watching the plot unfold, fully aware of both the real and the artificial worlds. We are in a *privileged position of knowing*. Can primary care researchers ever be in a privileged position of knowing (akin to watching a movie)? Debates on this question abound, and researchers have approached this issue through various paradigmatic stances, some of which are presented in this chapter. Arguments can be made that, following strict study-design protocols, researchers are attempting to conduct research in a privileged position. Yet, there are always potential confounding variables, or biases, or simply study-design constraints that limit one's ability to make knowledge claims that are real or true in all cases, across all contexts and through all historical time periods. I will 'tip my hand' and argue that, unlike the moviegoer, the researcher is an interconnected part of the research process regardless of the type of study. Try as we may to control for confounders, to select representative samples, to set up comparable experimental and control groups or to elicit rich qualitative stories, we are operating within the world (and therefore conducting a study) only as we know it.

This epistemological issue is framed by Guba and Lincoln as, 'What is the nature of the relationship between the would-be knower and what can be known?'[2(p108)] This question can be addressed using the emic versus etic positions. Although numerous variations and definitions have proliferated,[3] an 'etic viewpoint studies behaviour as from outside of a particular system', while the 'emic viewpoint results from studying behaviour as from inside the system'.[4(p37)] Thus, a researcher taking an emic approach will attempt to be 'close to' his/her subjects and tries to understand what is real by 'look[ing] at things through the eyes of members of the culture being studied'.[5(p100)] A researcher taking an etic approach attempts to maintain distance from his/her subjects by relying on or focusing upon the 'structures and criteria developed outside the culture as a framework for studying the culture'.[5(p100)]

Given that the emic/etic epistemological framework is rooted in the study of human behaviour which may not apply to all primary care research endeavours, what can primary care researchers glean from this dualism? Researchers taking an etic approach use various research methods and tools which are designed to minimise the effects of their own personal biases, preferences or values on the knowledge that is discovered or achieved through their research endeavour. One example would be a double-blind, randomised controlled trial in which the researcher maintains 'distance' by staying completely unaware of which study group receives an experimental drug and which group receives a placebo. Another example is a physician–researcher asking subjects to rate their pain on a quantitative pain scale. Such a tool, in effect, creates some distance between researcher and subject by turning a deeply personal and individualised experience into an 'objective', translatable and comparable number. In contrast, a central premise from the emic position is that the researcher must interact 'closely' with one's research subjects in order to gain an in-depth, insider's understanding. The potential influence of the researcher on what is being researched is readily acknowledged and, thus, becomes part of the research process. This notion of distance and interaction between the researcher and object being researched thus has a profound impact on the research methods that are chosen and employed.

METHODOLOGY AND METHOD

Although the terms research 'methodology' and 'method' are often used interchangeably, an important distinction must be made clear. Methodology refers to philosophies that guide how knowledge should be discovered or achieved; research methods are the specific data-gathering techniques. Methodology involves '…the description, the explanation, and the justification… of methods, and not the methods themselves'.[6] A description of a project's research methods in a journal publication (or other medium) provides the audience with a practical understanding of how subjects were identified, selected and/or sampled, and how data was collected, managed and analysed. However the aim of a project's methodology is to 'throw light on (the project's methods) limitations and resources, clarifying their presuppositions and consequences… to help (the audience) to understand, in the broadest possible terms, not the products of scientific inquiry, but the process itself'.[6] How these complex research concepts (ontology, epistemology, methodology and method) influence, relate to or shape each other is debatable, and there is no clear-cut, agreed-upon answer.

A map of these connections (Figure 2.1) shows that a researcher's ontological and epistemological beliefs are ever present, interconnected and cover the entire research endeavour. As Grix put it, 'Researchers' differing ontological and epistemological positions often lead to different research approaches towards the same phenomenon'.[7(p64)]

Consider the following hypothetical example:

A primary care researcher is interested in studying pain. An impetus includes witnessing first-hand family members who have suffered with chronic pain and struggled with use of opioid pain medications. The researcher identifies a critical gap in the literature regarding the use of amitriptyline for pain regulation and aims to gain a better understanding of the complex pathophysiological contributors underlying a patient's pain to inform development of a comprehensive evidence-based management plan.

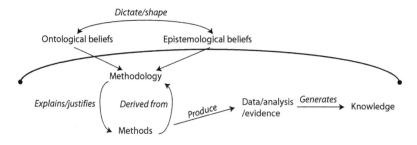

FIGURE 2.1 Dynamic relationship between ontology, epistemology, methodology, methods and knowledge.

One underpinning ontological assumption evident in the way this study is framed is that the physical nature of pain results from a complex combination of objective, measurable factors. A second assumption is about what it means to be in pain (e.g. a debilitating and negative experience). As such, finding an effective treatment plan is deemed worthwhile for research inquiry.

Another researcher is interested in understanding peoples' experiences with pain. An impetus for this study comes from reading the novel 'Fifty Shades of Grey', which depicts explicitly erotic scenes involving bondage/discipline, dominance/submission and sadism/masochism.[8] Here, the notion is about people defining painful experiences as pleasurable. Pain pathways are being stimulated in their bodies and yet those participating in these sexual practices do not seek immediate attention at the emergency room nor pain medications from their primary care physician. This study aims to understand the context and subjective definitions of a pain experience and the implications on peoples' health and health care. The ontological assumption about the nature of reality – 'pain' – is rooted in what people think (idealism) about it. This is not to deny nor downplay the existence of the physical pain pathways in the body, but the assumption is that how humans interpret, define and construct meanings of those painful experiences is important and deemed worthwhile for research. For this study, pain is not an objective thing 'out there' to be discovered. Rather, the assumption is that pain cannot be known without investigating what these painful sensations actually mean for people, and thus, there may be multiple realities of pain (including pain as a traumatising event and as a pleasurable experience).

The essential, underlying premise of each study – one rooted in and driven by a material/objective basis and, the other, an ideal/subjective basis – dictates and shapes additional beliefs and subsequent next steps for conducting the study, analysing data and ultimately generating knowledge.

Returning to Figure 2.1, one can mentally walk through a logical progression of decision points for these two different studies of pain. In study #1 ('pain pathways'), the researcher would likely take an etic epistemological approach to maintain 'distance' between self and the subjects, to minimise any personal values or biases in understanding what this objective pain pathway 'looks like' and to determine how a particular treatment plan may provide effective pain relief. This epistemological approach lends itself to finding common elements that would be applicable to all (or some defined groupings of) humans. The researcher would then develop, in a synergistic process, the methodological grounds and the practical research methods for the study. There are many possible paths. A logical study design based on these ontological and epistemological beliefs could include a quantitative-based, randomised controlled trial wherein pain reduction is based on a validated pain-assessment instrument.

In contrast, for study #2 ('pain as pleasure'), the researcher would likely take an emic epistemological approach to get 'inside' the subjects' heads and attempt to see their understanding of pain through their eyes and in their own words. Such an approach lends itself to identifying themes or patterns in how people experience pain as pleasure, but acknowledges that there is no single 'truth' that must be discovered; rather, defining pain as pleasure may be based on multiple foundations or exhibited in various ways. These assumptions, then, directly influence the development of the methodology and research methods. Again, although there are numerous methods for this approach, trying to understand the thought processes for how someone perceives and defines certain painful experiences as pleasurable may be well-suited with a qualitative-based, in-depth-interview study design.

RESEARCH PARADIGMS

'A paradigm is a model or framework for observation and understanding, which shapes both what we see and how we understand it'[9(p33)] and includes each of the core concepts of ontology, epistemology, methodology and methods.[10] Once researchers can identify and label their particular epistemological, ontological, and methodological premises, they can better understand the perspectives and research decisions of others who are operating from a different paradigm. 'Stepping outside' of one's dominant paradigm can open up new ways of 'seeing and explaining things'.[9]

The sheer number of different paradigms and their associated labels – some of which are used differently in different texts – can easily lead to confusion and frustration. However, there are particular paradigms that may be of value to primary care researchers. While certainly not a comprehensive list or explication, there are variations in how particular research paradigms approach the ontological and epistemological questions and how their methodologies and methods are tied to these positions.

Research paradigms have not developed in a vacuum. They arise out of tensions faced from their own inherent limitations and through points of contention with other paradigms. The fragmentation and proliferation of research paradigms means that not only are there numerous paradigms, but within particular paradigms, there are numerous branches and offshoots based on ever-more refined tensions and disagreements. Moreover, as Lincoln and Guba contend, '...the various paradigms are beginning to "interbreed" such that two theorists previously thought to be in irreconcilable conflict may now appear, under a different theoretical rubric, to be informing one another's arguments'.[11(p164)] It is important not to stake a claim (e.g. 'I am/my work definitely falls within the positivist paradigm!') but rather to gain insights into a paradigm that resonates with one's ontological and epistemological assumptions, while acknowledging inherent tensions and limitations within any given paradigm. One may then gain greater appreciation for research based on a 'radically different' paradigm. Moreover, one may drift towards another paradigm in order to strengthen one's research endeavour. While certain movements between paradigms may be less likely or more challenging than other movements, there may be good reason and real benefits 'to blend elements of one paradigm into another, so that one is engaging in research that represents the best of both worldviews'.[11(p169)]

Positivism

Positivism entails the view that research can only be conducted by means of observable material things. The positivist's ontological position can be labelled 'realism'. This maintains 'that objects have a (material) existence independent of the knower'.[12(p7)] Knowledge is obtained through sensory experience. The epistemological position is 'objectivism', which maintains that 'the researcher and the researched are independent entities'.[10(p10)] Using *The Matrix* analogy, a strict positivist maintains that the researcher is like the moviegoer who can study something objectively and discover what is 'real' or 'true'. Objectivism assumes that one can discover knowledge in a value-free way. The relationship and 'distance' between the researcher and researched bears an etic approach. A positivist methodology is typically directed at identifying causes which influence outcomes and generating probabilistic generalisations and explaining relationships.[13(p19)] Within this paradigm, common methods reflect practical efforts to maintain 'distance' between the researcher and researched. Typically, such methods generate quantitative data and include standardised tests, closed-ended questionnaires and descriptions of phenomena using standardised observation tools.[14(p34)] 'Research is deemed good if its results are due to the independent variable (internal validity), can be generalised/transferred to other populations or situations (external validity), and different researchers can record the same data in the same way and arrive at the same conclusions (replicable and reliable).'[10(p11)]

Interpretivism

In contrast, interpretivism takes a very different ontological stance by viewing reality as a social construct. That is, the evidence one obtains from a research endeavour must be understood as merely the outcome of the interpretative activities of individual humans. Facts generated from such research are rooted in, and based on, the ideas (perceptions, definitions, interpretations) that humans have of a particular thing in question. The interpretivists' ontological position can be labelled 'relativism'. This assumes reality is subjective and differs from person to person.[2(p110)] That we have common realities and agreed-upon definitions means that we have co-constructed reality as a normal negotiation process to make sense of the world. Interpretivist epistemology is 'subjectivism' – it holds that the world does not exist independently of the researcher's knowledge of it.[7(p83)] Operating with this assumption, the researcher seeks to understand these subjective realities of individuals and gain insights into the negotiated outcomes of individuals' interpretations.[13] A second epistemological assumption is that the researcher is also engaged in interpreting 'what is going on' as s/he is seeking to understand a reality from the subjects' viewpoints. Contrary to positivism, any accounts, descriptions or analyses of one's data cannot be factually described, free of one's own subjective interpretations. The researcher does not hold a privileged place (like a moviegoer) 'outside' of whatever reality s/he is researching but rather is, metaphorically speaking, part of the movie as well. Given these philosophical foundations, an interpretivist methodology is designed to understand reality from individuals' perspectives as well as the historical and cultural contexts which people inhabit.[15(p8)] Particular methods derived from these ontological, epistemological and methodological assumptions include those that allow a researcher to 'get close to' a subject, including in-depth interviews, focus groups and open-ended observations. Such methods typically generate qualitative data, wherein rich descriptions elucidate 'answers' to a research question, and commonly, thematic analyses induced from the data generate abstract/ conceptual/theoretical insights.

Post-positivism

This paradigm reflects a concrete example of 'movement' from an existing, established paradigm (positivism) towards other ontological and epistemological assumptions based on inherent tensions within and criticisms of a paradigm. Like positivism, post-positivism maintains an assumption about the nature of reality – it has a material existence independent of our thinking about it that can be measured and studied. A critical difference between them lies in their epistemological assumptions: Unlike positivism, post-positivism assumes that reality can never be fully apprehended, only approximated.[16(p22)] Within the post-positivist paradigm, it is assumed that all empirical observation is fallible and influenced by one's values, worldviews or biases. Researchers operating within a post-positivist paradigm may take either an etic or emic approach to investigation. Moreover, post-positivist methodology moves away from a strict positivist approach by conducting research in natural settings, seeking to determine purposes and meanings people ascribe to their actions and using qualitative methods to do so.[2] There is an aim to discover and verify theories and create new knowledge that (presumably) gets as close to objectivity and understanding reality as possible.[17] Theories that survive the process of intense peer scrutiny and that build on new knowledge are likened to species that survive in the evolutionary struggle. It is posited that knowledge evolves by natural selection through a process of variation, selection and retention.[18]

Critical paradigm

This paradigm shares the ontological position of positivism ('realism') but extends this view by emphasising the role of power relations or power structures that shape and mould reality.[19] What counts as knowledge is determined by the social and positional power of those who advocate for it.[12(p27)] The critical paradigm assumes that what is studied is constituted by material, objective things and that a given (material) reality has been shaped by 'social, political, cultural, economic, ethnic, and gender factors'.[2(p110)] Epistemologically, assumptions within the critical paradigm are similar to interpretivism ('subjectivism'). That is, researchers do not come to research as a *tabula rasa* – a blank slate. Research interests are influenced by culture, race, gender and location.[20(p5)] The critical paradigm emphasises knowledge creation through research as a means to expose injustice address social ills of exclusion, oppression and marginalisation and engage in social action.[10,21]

Transformative emancipatory paradigm

This paradigm bears similarities to the critical paradigm in its emphasis on issues of social justice and marginalised people,[15(p9)] an awareness of power differentials in the research context, and a research action agenda that seeks to address the effects of oppression and discrimination through social action.[22(p159)] Ontologically, this paradigm moves away from the critical paradigm's material view of reality towards that of an ideal reality. Like the critical paradigm, this paradigm makes an epistemological assumption regarding the importance of a close link between the researcher and participants and the impact of social and historical factors in this relationship.[22(p141)] Researchers who explicitly frame their research within this paradigm may use quantitative, qualitative, or mixed methods. Contextual and historical factors must be considered, with sensitivity to issues of power that can affect social justice and equity.[22(p142)] How a particular research question is framed and the goal of the research may determine methods used. As a methodological principle, this paradigm emphasises that research participants must be involved throughout the research process, including the initial research idea generation/identification process, the study design, the collection and analysis of data and any dissemination efforts.[22(p142)]

CONCLUDING REMARKS

In this chapter, I have presented the philosophical underpinnings of research: The ontological question of 'what is real?' and the epistemological question of 'how do we know what is real?'. Two contrasting positions – materialism and idealism – pose 'answers' to the ontological question. For the epistemological question, I have explored the emic versus etic positions. Presenting these dichotomies in this way should not be taken to mean that each one is a clear-cut, exclusive position into which any researcher must 'fit'. Indeed, the various paradigms (which include a scaffolding of 'answers' to the ontological and epistemological questions as well as attendant research methods) that have been developed over time reflect the fact that each 'answer' has its own tensions and limitations. Thus, researchers have 'drifted towards', for example, a contrasting ontological position or developed a new paradigm offshoot based on ever-more refined tensions and disagreements between contrasting positions and methods.

As I elaborated in this chapter, a researcher's ontological and epistemological beliefs are ever present, interconnected and cover the entire research endeavour. Importantly, one's standpoint has implications for the practical aspects of a research project (e.g. from sampling strategies, to data collection tools, to analytic operations, etc.). In a simplified form, Table 2.1 highlights some key comparisons across the paradigms of positivism, interpretivism and critical-emancipatory. (Note: This last column reflects in itself the 'interbreeding' of paradigms.) The practical implications of taking a positivist approach to a research study include (typically) developing a testable hypothesis that is set by the researcher prior to data collection; using quantitative testing and measuring tools that allow one to 'know' or better understand some objective, material thing that exists 'out there' and using statistical analyses in such a way that allows one to generalise the study findings to a larger population. Operating within an interpretivist framework, one would be more inclined to use qualitative data collection strategies as a way to explore salient issues directly from study participants. Unlike a study designed to generalise the findings, what is learned from a study conducted within the interpretivist framework may be transferable to other contexts. Finally, for the critical-emancipatory framework, a notable distinction lies with the role of the subject/participant. Here, the entire research process – from origination of the research question to the choice of methods to dissemination efforts (typically) involves joint, participatory actions.

Perhaps one could argue, 'I just want to jump into a research project that is going to make a difference for my patients/community of learners/(fill in the blank)… I don't need to attend to all of these abstract, philosophical concerns'. It may be that some research projects are not designed with these numerous –ologies and –isms or paradigms explicitly in mind. However it can be argued that *they are there*. When researchers identify questions deemed worthy of research and spell out research questions/objectives/aims/hypotheses, they make assumptions about what is real and how one can know what is real. Answers to these questions fundamentally shape the succession of steps for designing and carrying out a study as well as the interpretations of data and conclusions that are made.

TABLE 2.1 Comparison of methodological implications of different research paradigms

	Positivism	Interpretivism	Critical-emancipatory
Relationship with research 'reality'	Testing Measuring	Exploring Interpreting Constructing	Changing Creating Transforming
View of researched person	Object to be studied and measured	Subject to be understood and interpreted by researcher	Participant in the research
View of truth	Correspondence to external facts	Coherence within the data	Consensus of each person's learning
Research process	Predominantly quantitative measurements	Predominantly qualitative interpretations	Participatory using both qualitative and quantitative techniques
Research question	Fixed hypothesis. Set by researcher	Open-ended hypothesis. Set by researcher.	Negotiated in dialogue with participants as part of the research process
Implementation of results	Recommendations made for action by people other than researcher	Insights offered for use by other people	Findings implemented as part of the research process and the implementation studied
Concept of methodological objectivity	Generalisability	Transferability	Transferability
Concepts of reliability and validity	Standardisation and control of bias, chance and confounding factors. Statistical analysis	Credibility Dependability Confirmability Transferability	Practical application Alignment with purpose Ownership Group process Documentation Reflectivity Knowledge construction

Source: Adapted from Mash B. The development of distance education for general practitioners on common mental disorders through participatory action research [Phd thesis]. Cape Town: Stellenbosch University; 2002.

Referring back to *The Matrix*, primary care researchers have a choice. Take the blue pill: Jump into a research endeavour blissfully ignorant of one's ontological and epistemological assumptions and how these shape key research decisions. Take the red pill: Identify one's ontological and epistemological assumptions; identify and draw on existing paradigm(s) that resonate with these starting points; acknowledge the tensions and limitations inherent to one's particular paradigmatic approach and make these elements of the research process explicit as a means to guide the methodology, methods and knowledge creation. Choose wisely!

REFERENCES

1. Walsh D. Idealism/materialism. In: Jenks C, editor. *Core Sociological Dichotomies.* Thousand Oaks, CA: SAGE Publications; 1998. p. 179–207.
2. Guba EG, Lincoln YS. Competing paradigms in qualitative research. In: Denzin NK, Lincoln YS, editors. *Handbook of Qualitative Research.* Thousand Oaks, CA: SAGE Publications; 1994. p. 105–17.
3. Headland TN. A dialogue between Kenneth Pike and Marvin Harris on emics and etics. In: Headland T, Pike K, Harris M, editors. *Emics and Etics: The Insider/Outsider Debate.* Newbury Park, CA: SAGE Publications; 1990. p. 13–27.
4. Pike K. *Language in Relations to a Unified Theory of Human Behavior,* 2nd revised ed. The Hague: Mouton & Co.; 1954/1967. p. 37–72.
5. Willis JW. *Foundations of Qualitative Research: Interpretive and Critical Approaches.* Thousand Oaks, CA: SAGE Publications; 2007.
6. Kaplan A. *The Conduct of Inquiry: Methodology for Behavioral Science.* San Francisco: Chandler; 1964.
7. Grix J. *The Foundations of Research.* London: Palgrave Macmillan; 2004.
8. James, EL. *Fifty Shades of Grey.* New York: Vintage Books; 2012.
9. Babbie E. *The Practice of Social Research,* 10th ed. Belmont, CA: Wadsworth/Thomson Learning; 2004.
10. Scotland J. Exploring the philosophical underpinnings of research: Relating ontology and epistemology to the methodology and methods of the scientific, interpretive, and critical research paradigms. *Eng Lang Teach J* 2012;5(9):9–16.
11. Lincoln YS, Guba EG. Paradigmatic controversies, contradictions, and emerging confluences. In: Denzin NK, Lincoln YS, editors. *Handbook of Qualitative Research,* 2nd ed. Thousand Oaks, CA: Sage Publications; 2000. p. 163–88.
12. Cohen L, Manion L, Morrison K. *Research Methods in Education,* 6th ed. London: Routledge; 2007.
13. Johnson T, Dandeker C, Ashworth C. *The Structure of Social Theory.* London: MacMillan; 1984.
14. Pring R. *Philosophy of Educational Research.* London: Continuum; 2000.
15. Creswell JW. *Research Design: Qualitative, Quantitative, and Mixed Methods Approaches,* 2nd ed. Thousand Oaks, CA: Sage Publications; 2003.
16. Guba EG. The alternative paradigm dialog. In: Guba EG, editor. *The Paradigm Dialog.* Newbury Park, CA: Sage Publications; 1990. p. 17–30.
17. Denzin NK, Lincoln YS. The discipline and practice of qualitative research. In: Denzin NK, Lincoln YS, editors. *Handbook of Qualitative Research,* 2nd ed. Thousand Oaks, CA: Sage Publications; 2000. p. 1–28.
18. Popper KR. *Objective Knowledge: An Evolutionary Approach.* Oxford: Clarendon Press; 1972.
19. Frowe I. Language and educational research. *J Phil Educ* 2001;35(2):175–86.
20. Siegel H. Epistemological diversity and educational research: Much ado about nothing much? *Educ Res* 2006;35(2):3–12.
21. Ceci C, Limacher LH, McLeod DL. Language and power: Ascribing legitimacy to interpretive research. *Qual Hlth Res* 2002;12(5):713–20.
22. Mertens DM. Mixed methods and the politics of human research: The transformative-emancipatory perspective. In: Tashakkori A, Teddlie C, editors. *Handbook of Mixed Methods in Social and Behavioral Research.* Thousand Oaks, CA: Sage Publications; 2003. p. 135–64.
23. Mash B. *The development of distance education for general practitioners on common mental disorders through participatory action research [Phd thesis].* Cape Town: Stellenbosch University; 2002.

CHAPTER 3

How to choose your topic and define your research question

William R. Phillips

The primary care perspective is unique and makes special contributions to both patient care and research. It encounters different patients and problems, in deeper contexts, across broader responsibilities and over longer periods. Primary care researchers ask different questions and answer them in different ways.[1] This scope creates great opportunities for the researcher but can also present challenges in choosing among many interesting areas of study and focusing specific research questions. As in clinical practice, primary care team members can play many roles in research. Choosing the topic and refining the research question are among the most important and exciting contributions to conducting research and improving care. (See Box 3.1 at the end of this chapter for a list of online resources for researchers.)

This chapter aims to help the researcher choose a topic and define a research question to reach four essential goals:

1. Ask a question that is researchable.
2. Design a study that is doable.
3. Produce results that are publishable.
4. Create a sustainable programme of inquiry.

Research, like care, is a human enterprise and—at its best—should serve personal, team and community goals. Questions that help motivate the work and organise the study often start with big questions. What is your grand agenda? What outcome do you want? What do you want to improve or change? More practical issues also lead to legitimate questions. Whom do you want to work with? What methods do you want to learn? What activity do you want to do? For example, do you want to interview patients, review research reports, analyse data sets, conduct surveys or facilitate focus groups?

These larger questions and many of the day-to-day choices that researchers must make can be guided by development of a professional mission statement. This is a paragraph describing one's durable values and short, medium and long-term goals. It is a living document that begins with a values clarification exercise and evolves over time in response to discussions with mentors, growth in expertise and focus on interests. The professional mission statement is best crafted in parallel with a personal mission statement. Together, they can serve as a compass to help the researcher navigate career decisions, multiple opportunities and competing demands. On the quest for key questions, this compass can guide the researcher on the journey to investigate familiar landscapes, explore new territories and reach distant horizons.

Research requires balancing personal and professional goals with those of the research team, patient care team, patients and community. As the process progresses, the interests of other stakeholders, sponsors and funders deserve attention.

The life of the research question cycles through five phases that will serve as the outline for this chapter: find, refine, define, design and align (Table 3.1).

FIND

To find your question, first draw inspiration from your work, your patients and your reading. Research questions flow from the problems we see and the questions that arise every day in caring for our patients, teaching our trainees and improving our practice systems. As outlined in the introduction, primary care research questions may address the basic tools needed for research, clinical questions, health service and system related questions or educational issues.

In the clinic, what questions arise that have no answer or at least no answer applicable to primary care? What decisions are you called upon to make that do not rest on solid evidence? What questions do your patients ask that you find most difficult to answer? What dilemmas do you face in the complex work of taking care of real people with real problems?

What questions arise as you read the medical literature, news reports or social media? To explore a specific topic, go directly to systematic reviews or clinical guidelines to learn what identified knowledge gaps require further research. Most published research studies identify unanswered questions that need further research in the discussion section. Browse clinical question services to learn what is known—and not known—to inform clinical decisions.

In your practice or health care system, what problems and frustrations do you face? What challenges stimulate reflection? What issues lead to questionable assumptions or heated arguments among your colleagues? What

TABLE 3.1 Life cycle of a research question

Find	Identify problems or questions from patient care, teaching, reading, research, practice organisation.
	Elicit problems or questions from patients, communities, colleagues, managers, networks.
	Find existing data or research programmes that you could use or join.
	Consider why your problem needs to be addressed in a primary care setting and how it fits into the typology of primary care research (see page 5, Chapter 1).
Refine	Review literature and answer three key questions: What is known? What knowledge gaps exist? What gap will this study fill?
	Focus the specific question and articulate it in researchable form.
Define	Define each key word in the question.
	Consider using the PICOTT model to build a specific answerable question.
	Consider the need to identify secondary questions that are closely related to and aligned with the primary question (can also be expressed as aim and objectives).
Design	Use the research question(s) to determine the appropriate research methods and study design(s).
	Outline the key issues regarding the setting, selection of participants, any interventions, data collection and data analysis.
	If necessary, design methods for each secondary question in the study.
	Review FINER criteria to assess success of the study plan.
Align	Before finalising the proposal, check again:
	• Does this study have social value? So what? Who cares? Why?
	• Does this study have scientific value? Will this study fill a critical gap in knowledge to help improve patient care, learning, research or policy?
	• How does this research leverage what is special about primary care?
	• How well does the proposed work align with the needs of all involved?

questions do the local decision makers need guidance on? The team meeting and the office break room can suggest potential research questions.

Try keeping a daily log of new questions, doubtful answers and recurrent frustrations. Nurture reflection in your practice and teaching. When drawn from the world of primary care practice, even little questions can drive valuable research. Remember, 'It ain't what you don't know that gets you into trouble, it is what you know for sure just ain't so.'[2]

Research is organised curiosity.[3] Different people view the same problem through different lenses and see research questions in different ways. In primary care, researchers often view research topics through the three lenses of patients/populations, problems or processes.[4] For example, three researchers might be interested in learning more about how primary care clinicians prescribe antibiotics to treat otitis media in children. Using the patient/population lens, one researcher envisions a study to help improve language development in young children. Another researcher uses the problem lens to see a study on reducing unnecessary use of antibiotics. A third researcher using the process lens may see otitis media as an opportunity to study shared decision making. With insight into one's preferred lens, the researcher can find direction and motivation to pursue personal passions. Mentorship and team discussions can nurture this process to help focus research questions.

If you are fortunate to work in a research network, encourage colleagues to pursue these strategies and share their questions. Practice-based research networks can collect a wealth of questions that arise from patients, problems and practices. The perspectives and experiences of primary care clinicians often raise new questions or frame familiar questions in new ways. Build mechanisms into your network to stimulate, collect and discuss these questions. In community-based networks, patients, family and community members can all contribute to the process of exploring problems and generating potential research questions.

Many new researchers, particularly trainees, may be directed to one or a few options, based upon the current research of their supervisor or research group. Although the dream of the independent investigator is to explore one's own evolving interests, there is a time and place for learning and practising the required skills with available data, structured studies and expert guidance. Investigators can make great contributions working with questions defined by others, including practitioners, networks, agencies and health care systems. Research done under contract usually comes with specified questions. Even when working with someone else's questions, researchers can usually find or create some part of the project that fits their interests and can become their own. Be creative in looking for these opportunities, and be transparent in negotiating a study plan that meets diverse needs.

Important clinical and population health questions often have only partial answers based on data that are not directly applicable to primary care. Valuable questions can be found within major published studies, often by focusing on a subgroup that was not identified or studied in the original research. Minority, rural and vulnerable populations are of special interest in primary care research but are too often excluded or underrepresented in mainstream medical research. Useful studies can be done by taking a large study done in one population and replicating it in a more-focused subpopulation, using similar design and methods.

Most biomedical research is done in tertiary academic health centres, hospitals and referral populations and does not adequately represent primary care, where most of the patients obtain most of the care for most problems most of the time. This creates opportunities and obligations for primary care research to collect data in community settings and practices.

REFINE

The breadth, depth and duration of primary care present the researcher with a wealth of important problems begging for good answers. To move from problem to answer requires care in articulating and refining the research question.

Moving from a general interest or clinical problem to a researchable question and successful study is an exciting challenge, particularly if the idea arises from clinicians, decision makers, networks or community groups. Including the group in the process helps build momentum for the study and helps assure that the results will be applicable to the setting that generated the question. There is power in partnerships combining the clinical wisdom of the practitioner with the methodologic expertise of the researcher.

Some important but simple questions can be stated as disprovable hypotheses. Other questions, particularly early in the process, cannot be reduced so easily and call for descriptive research. Many intriguing questions that arise in primary care are difficult to capture and characterise. Often, pilot studies and qualitative methods are the best first steps to understand fundamental problems, organise overarching concerns or develop the vocabulary needed to refine the question.

With a topic on the drawing table, the team must first ask several questions. What is currently known? What do we need to know? How will this study fill an important gap? This requires review of the scientific literature and appropriate theoretical models. This may come easier to researchers in more limited specialties, but the work is critical if primary care research is to meet the needs of our scientific, clinical and policy communities. For many novice researchers, the knowledge gap may be small or quite contextual in that similar work may have been conducted elsewhere but not in your specific context.

Having narrowed down the topic to identify the question you want to answer in order to contribute to filling an important knowledge gap, the question must be fully defined.

DEFINE

One framework for defining your research question is to apply the PICOTT model from evidence-based medicine, originally developed to guide medical literature searches.[5,6] Researchers can frame and define their question by applying the same elements: (1) patient, problem or population; (2) intervention or exposure; (3) comparison or context; (4) outcomes, (5) type of question and (6) type of study (Table 3.2).

Finding and focusing a valuable research question often leads to other good questions. Some of these will need to be set aside, perhaps to become studies of their own. Questions can sometimes be strategically lined up in a series or pursued by teams in parallel. Formal research proposals and grant applications often identify one main research question or aim, which might have one to three secondary questions or objectives. Each must be carefully

TABLE 3.2 PICOTT model for formulating clinical questions

P	**Patient, Population or Problem** What patients or population are of interest? What problem do they have? What are the key characteristics, inclusion and exclusion criteria?
I	**Intervention, Exposure, Prognostic Factor** What intervention to test? What risk factor, exposure or prognostic factor to examine?
C	**Comparison** What are the main alternatives to the intervention, etc.?
O	**Outcome** What to measure, improve or affect? What outcome is the desired goal of the intervention?
T	**Type of Question** Examples: diagnosis, risk factors, prognosis, therapy, natural history, prevention, harms
T	**Type of Study** Systematic review, RCT, cohort study, case control, qualitative

Source: Adapted from Haynes B. *J Clin Epidemiol* 2006;59:881–6; Straus SE et al. *Evidence-Based Medicine: How to Practice and Teach It.* 4th ed. Edinburgh: Churchill Livingstone, 2010 and others.

defined and supported by a detailed plan for data collection and analysis. Avoid the temptation to cover too much ground. Include only questions that support the principal question, fit within the resources and advance the central mission of the research.

Successful research demands careful attention to articulating the question, defining its terms and mapping its scope. The choice of words is also important in terms of the implications for the design of the research. The research question is expressed in the form of a question, while the aim of the research will usually be very similar but conveyed as a statement. Words such as 'measure' or 'evaluate' will imply research in a positivist research paradigm; words such as 'explore' or 'interpret' will imply an interpretivist paradigm and words such as 'how to …' may imply a more critical-emancipatory paradigm (see Chapter 2). Define—in writing—every key term in the question.

DESIGN

With a question now down on paper in some detail, design your study around your question. The research question determines the research methods and study design. Outline what the key issues would be in terms of the setting, selection of participants, any interventions, data collection and analysis. Researchers can assess the potential success of the proposed study applying the FINER criteria: feasible, interesting, novel, ethical and relevant.[7,8] (Table 3.3)

TABLE 3.3 FINER criteria for study success

FEASIBLE	Adequate number of subjects
	Adequate technical expertise
	Affordable in time and money
	Manageable in scope
	How risky is success of the project?
INTERESTING	Interesting to you, practitioners and community
	Interesting to other researchers
	Interesting to funding agencies
	What journal will publish this study?
	Will the results be a contribution, no matter what you find?
	Will it lead to subsequent research questions?
NOVEL	Confirms, refutes or extends previous findings
	Addresses a clearly defined knowledge gap
	New population or patient group
	New application of intervention
	Addresses question from a primary care perspective
ETHICAL	Fair selection of participants
	Risks, benefits and risk/benefit ratio
	Informed consent
	Respect for participants, confidentiality and privacy
	Need for independent review and permissions
RELEVANT	To communities or patients
	To clinical practice and patient care
	To health policy
	To education and training
	To future research
	So what? Who cares? Why?

Source: Adapted from Cummings SR et al. Chapter 2: Conceiving the research question and developing the study plan. In: Hulley SB et al (Eds.). *Designing Clinical Research*, 4th Ed., pp. 14-22. Philadelphia, PA: Wolters Kluwer – Lippincott Williams and Wilkin, 2013.

This tool can also be used to compare the potential success of different topics or research questions that you may be considering.

ALIGN

You have now nurtured the inquiry from a general topic born of clinical and community needs into a specific researchable question with an outline of the appropriate methods and study design. Before finalising the proposal, return to the beginning of the cycle to ask four fundamental categories of questions:

- Does this study have social value? So what? Who cares? Why?
- Does this study have scientific value? Will this study fill a critical gap in knowledge to help improve patient care, learning, research or policy?

- How does this research leverage what is special about primary care?
- How well does the proposed work align with the needs of all involved?

Answering these questions requires continuing active engagement with the clinical teams, networks, decision makers, community and funders. This is the same engagement that empowers the commitment, momentum and teamwork necessary for the successful completion of your study and eventual implementation of any intervention.

Following these steps through the life cycle of the research question can help manage the most-common challenges that new primary care researchers encounter:

- Identifying an engaging project
- Assessing what is known and what is needed
- Focusing on an answerable research question
- Selecting appropriate research methods and study designs
- Keeping the project within a feasible scope
- Staying on the path of the original mission
- Producing results that meet the needs of an identified audience

---

BOX 3.1   LINKS TO ONLINE RESOURCES

- Phillips WR, Chen F, Neogi T, Sheth A. Organizing curiosity into realistic research, STFM Resource Library; 2012. http://resourcelibrary.stfm. org/viewdocument/organizing-curiosity-into-realistic
- University of Alberta Clinical Research Consortium. Research Question Development Guide. http://acrc.albertainnovates.ca/public/download/ documents/26
- National Library of Medicine, NIH. PubMed via PICO online search tools:
  - PICO A http://pubmedhh.nlm.nih.gov/nlm/picostudy/pico3.html
  - PICO B http://pubmedhh.nlm.nih.gov/nlm/picostudy/pico2.html
- McMaster University Health Sciences Library. Resources for Evidence-Based Practice: Forming Questions. http://hsl.mcmaster.libguides. com/c.php?g=306765&p=2044787
- Ohio Literacy Resource Center. Leadership Development Institute: Personal Mission Statement. literacy.kent.edu/Oasis/Leadership/ mission.htm

All web sites accessed 30 June 2017.

ACKNOWLEDGEMENT

I thank Allison M. Cole, MD, MPH, for her thoughtful comments on this work.

Conflicting and Competing Interests: No conflicting and competing interests to disclose in connection with this work.

Funding Statement: None. Dr Phillips was supported by the Theodore J. Phillips Endowed Professorship in Family Medicine.

REFERENCES

1. McWhinney I. William Pickles lecture 1996. The importance of being different. *Br J Gen Pract* 1996;46:433–36.
2. Shaw H. *Everybody's Friend, or; Josh Billing's Encyclopedia and Proverbial Philosophy of Wit and Humor.* Hartford, Conn, USA: American Publishing Co, 1874.
3. Eimerl T. Organized curiosity: A practical approach to the problem keeping records for research purposes in general practice. *J Coll Gen Pract* 1960;3:246–52.
4. Phillips WR. Pursuing personal passion: Learner-centered research mentoring. *Fam Med* 2018;50:41–6.
5. Haynes B. Forming research questions. *J Clin Epidemiol* 2006;59:881–6.
6. Straus SE, Glaziou P, Richardson WS, Haynes RB. *Evidence-Based Medicine: How to Practice and Teach It.* 4th ed. Edinburgh: Churchill Livingstone, 2010.
7. Cummings SR, Browner WS, Hulley SB. Chapter 2: Conceiving the research question and developing the study plan. In: Hulley SB, Cummings SR, Browner WS, Grady DG, Newman TB (Eds.). *Designing Clinical Research*, 4th Ed., pp. 14–22. Philadelphia, PA: Wolters Kluwer – Lippincott Williams and Wilkin, 2013.
8. Farrugia P, Petrisor B, Farrokhyar F et al. Research questions, hypotheses and objectives. *Can J Surg* 2010;53:278–81.

SECTION II

Innovative approaches to primary care research

CHAPTER 4

Interdisciplinary research approaches in primary care

Trish Greenhalgh

WHAT ISN'T INTERDISCIPLINARY RESEARCH?

Too often, the term 'interdisciplinary research' is used as rather lazy shorthand for a study that collects and combines both qualitative and quantitative data (also known as 'mixed methods' research). But the term 'interdisciplinary' means more than that.

It is crucial to understand that 'qualitative research' is not a discipline and neither is 'quantitative research'. A study that collects only quantitative data could be interdisciplinary and likewise for qualitative data. A study that collects both qualitative and quantitative may *not* be interdisciplinary.

Box 4.1 shows an example of what interdisciplinary research *isn't*. I've used a fictional example so as not to cause offence, but I regularly see this kind of study in grant proposals or journal articles.

The reason why this research is *not* interdisciplinary is that the researcher is looking at all aspects of the problem through the same lens. He has been trained in a single discipline – clinical epidemiology – and knows how important it is to take a systematic sample, use randomised trial designs wherever possible and assess the efficacy of interventions using predefined outcome measures. In his limited thinking-through of the qualitative element, John presumably believes that the data on women's experiences of the 'complex intervention' will help him explain the programme's success or failure. Missing from this study is a serious engagement with the cultural–historical context these Somali women find themselves in (which might have come from involving an

---

BOX 4.1   HOW NOT TO DO 'INTERDISCIPLINARY' RESEARCH

John, a well-meaning primary care doctor on his first academic placement, was interested in domestic violence in Somali immigrants. He had been trained in clinical epidemiology, so he planned to recruit a sample of women from general practice and administer a questionnaire to them to document the kind of domestic violence they experienced, the frequency and severity of the abuse both now and at two-year time points in the past and their views on the causes. These quantitative data, once aggregated, would provide a useful overview of the incidence, natural history and severity of domestic violence in his target population. John then planned to develop a complex intervention to improve the women's self-efficacy. This would be delivered by trained bilingual assistants in a randomised trial design. A qualitative phase (interviews) would capture free text data on the women's experience of the intervention. The efficacy of the intervention would be measured using a closed-item self-efficacy questionnaire and also a repeat assessment of frequency and severity of self-reported domestic abuse.

---

anthropologist and/or an expert in migration studies), interest in the women's subjective experience of domestic violence (for which expertise in narrative and phenomenology would be useful), openness to what those experiences mean (the choice of self-efficacy as a key construct *before* gaining a rich picture of what the problem is and how it plays out is putting the cart before the horse) or a reflection on the appropriateness (or otherwise) of a white male physician researcher undertaking a study of domestic violence in the power-charged context of a GP surgery.

Fictional John perhaps believes that by 'picking and mixing' his methodologies, he will get more than the sum of the parts – yet his resulting study plan reads as naïve, paternalistic and unrigorous. Rowland calls this approach 'non-disciplinarity' and cites Struppa who has described such attempts at interdisciplinarity as 'entropic'.[1] By 'entropic' is meant a tendency towards increasing disorderliness and an erosion of what makes individual disciplines distinctive from one another. Entropic non-disciplinarity is identifiable by the absence of critical reflection about the differing and conflicting knowledge bases of the primary disciplines on which it draws.

WHAT IS (GOOD) INTERDISCIPLINARY RESEARCH?

A discipline is typically viewed as 'a branch of knowledge' or 'a field of study'. Scholars within a discipline share a set of core assumptions, values, approaches and techniques, though – importantly – much scholarly activity within disciplines serves to challenge and redefine these core elements (indeed, one definition of a discipline is 'a forum for engaging in disagreements'[2]).

Broadly speaking, there are two (arguably) legitimate approaches to interdisciplinary research: Collaboration and contestation. Let me describe these in turn before describing an example of how interdisciplinary research might be *done* in a primary care setting.

'Interdisciplinarity as collaboration' refers to a situation in which two or more disciplines with complementary knowledge, skills, methodological expertise and/or technical resources join forces to address a 'grand challenge'. An example is the International Human Genome Project, for which the underpinning disciplines embraced statistics, computer science and molecular genetics. The key challenges of such large-scale collaborative research are often practical, relating, for example, to allocation of roles and responsibilities, governance of budgeting and project management across institutions and attribution of intellectual copyright. Interdisciplinary endeavour in such circumstances is often (though not always) oriented to (1) raising large amounts of funding and (2) generating innovations with economic as well as intellectual potential. High-quality collaborative research would generally be recognised by significant scale and scope and by tangible outputs that can be traced directly to the collaboration (typically, scientific and/or technological breakthroughs).

'Interdisciplinarity as contestation' focuses on drawing out, and learning from, the conceptual, theoretical and methodological differences between disciplines.[3] Not only is contestation between disciplines a fundamental and time-honoured purpose of academic inquiry, but this process of deliberation and debate *between* disciplines is essential for transferring ideas, challenging assumptions and stimulating the creative imagination – and also for guarding against the fragmentation and commodification of knowledge and its appropriation by discipline-specific interest groups.[3,4]

High-quality interdisciplinary contestation would be characterised by a level of critical engagement by all parties on an important issue that would not otherwise have been achieved. One example of contestation is the vigorous debates that have been held about the building of dams in India, to which scholars from many disciplines (e.g. engineering,[5] economics,[6] ecology,[7] development studies,[8] sociology,[9] literature and drama[10] and political philosophy[11]) have contributed. Arguably (and without assigning a value to any particular contribution), something was gained when scholars from different disciplinary backgrounds re-examined their assumptions and reflected on the significance of their findings in the light of what those from *other* disciplines had proposed. Note that 'success' in this example cannot be measured by any simple metric of 'consensus' or 'collaboration' (or by the number or size of dams built).

EXAMPLE OF INTERDISCIPLINARY RESEARCH: THE HepFREE STUDY

The HepFREE study (based in inner London, UK) was established to address the very high level of untreated chronic viral hepatitis (B and C) in some minority ethnic groups. Pilot studies had shown that few people from such groups accepted an invitation for screening, yet modern treatment regimens mean that early detection and treatment saves lives and reduces transmission.

HepFREE had five aims: (1) to build links with the communities most severely affected by hepatitis B and C, (2) to gain a rich understanding of people's understandings of the causes and natural history of these diseases and the reasons why they were reluctant to participate in screening, (3) to design a screening programme that was culturally congruent and practically feasible in inner-city family practice, including a cost-effectiveness study, (4) to undertake a randomised controlled trial of a screen-and-treat intervention and (if successful) (5) to work with national policymakers to scale this up into a national screen-and-treat programme.

Chronic viral hepatitis was common in a number of immigrant ethnic groups in inner-city London (e.g. Chinese, Romany, Pakistani) who had not assimilated closely into mainstream society and who were relatively under-researched anthropologically. Gaining access to these communities, establishing a relationship of trust and cooperation and building the partnerships needed to sustain the work over several years was not going to be easy.

Like the fictitious example in Box 4.1, the HepFREE study used a number of different research methods, both qualitative and quantitative. Unlike that example, the mixed methods approach used in HepFREE rested on several different underpinning disciplines and even on different philosophical positions about the nature of knowledge (see Section 'Ontology and Epistemology', Chapter 2). As is typical with health-services research, there was a basic science component (which drew on the pathophysiology of blood-borne hepatitis and some exciting new pharmacological therapies), a trial component (a cluster randomised trial with the general practice as the unit of analysis) and a policy-development component (to inform and influence the national hepatitis screening programme – ongoing[18]).

But before the trial could even begin, there was a qualitative systematic review component to identify and synthesise a huge and inchoate literature on barriers to screening in ethnic groups with blood-borne hepatitis,[12] and a partnership-building component with local community groups, based on the principles of community-based participatory research.[13] We used an adaptive 'key informant interview' methodology for the dual purpose of gaining data *from* and building partnerships *with* key contacts in our target communities.[14] There was then a training component (to convey the principles of nondirective qualitative research to community advocates and voluntary-sector staff) on the grounds that immigrants with limited English express very different views when interviewed by members of their own community compared with white British researchers working through professional translators.[15] Finally, there was a two-pronged qualitative component (focus groups conducted in community centres by trained members of their own community) and interviews with local general practitioners to explore the feasibility of proposed screening approaches.[16]

To undertake the preliminary qualitative work, we appointed two qualitative researchers – an anthropologist (with similar ethnic background to one of the targeted groups) and an applied sociologist who had extensive experience undertaking community-based participatory research with a different 'hard-to-reach' group in a different setting.[17] Their skill included gaining access, developing dialogue and respecting where the different participating communities were coming from.

Interdisciplinarity in the HepFREE study often played out as a more-or-less productive tension (and even, occasionally, misunderstandings and conflict) as qualitative researchers who were committed to developing genuine power-sharing relationships with 'hard-to-reach' communities worked with triallists who were committed to obtaining the right sort of stratified sample to test their hypotheses about alternative approaches to screening. Philosophically, *dialogue with a community* sits awkwardly with *doing research on a population sample*. But whilst the process of working across disciplines sometimes felt more difficult than working within a single-discipline silo, the research that resulted was more than the sum of the parts: On the one hand, it was characterised by a high degree of participation from traditionally under-researched communities; but on the other hand, a high-quality randomised controlled trial became possible with interventions and endpoints that reflected those communities' priorities.

DRAFT QUESTIONS TO GUIDE CRITICAL APPRAISAL OF INTERDISCIPLINARY RESEARCH

Given the many forms and interpretations of the terms 'interdisciplinary', a single, prescriptive framework for guiding or appraising such research would be impossible (though some people have attempted to produce such frameworks). The following questions might guide assessment.

First, what is the nature of the claim to interdisciplinarity? In other words, is this submission collaboration, contestation or would it better classified as 'entropy'?

Second, within its category, what is the extent and quality of the interdisciplinary effort? For example, if 'collaboration', what is the evidence for synergy between disciplines? To what extent does the outcome truly demonstrate something unachievable by a single discipline? If 'contestation', what is the evidence of critical and reflexive interdisciplinary engagement, resulting in new framings of the issue and/or significant revisiting of assumptions? What are the direct outputs and to what extent have they been generated or enhanced through the input of more than one discipline? What are the indirect outcomes (in terms of researchers examining their disciplinary assumptions and gaining new insights) and to what extent (if at all) can they be measured? If the work is considered 'entropic', how is this categorisation justified? What is the evidence that the mix of disciplinary contributions was eclectic and unscholarly?

Third, how might this piece of research have been done differently? What would have made it better or worse? In reflecting on their study, have the authors distinguished between limitations that are inherent to the topic taken on and those that were potentially remediable?

HOW CAN RESEARCH INSTITUTIONS SUPPORT INTERDISCIPLINARY RESEARCH?

As the HepFREE example illustrates, interdisciplinary research may be particularly helpful when working with underserved communities on questions that span the social and cultural determinants of health and illness and which seek to identify and overcome barriers to accessing health care. But such research is not easy, and universities are not traditionally designed to promote it. Those who lead research institutes may like to consider how to create a research environment that supports the development of high-quality interdisciplinary research. Such environments are often implicitly rather than explicitly defined, but might include such things as (1) a strong and efficient infrastructure for management and governance of large, multi-centre research (collaboration); (2) a supportive and enabling culture for interdisciplinary discussion and debate (contestation); (3) active and mature partnerships with service or commercial organisations (applied research); (4) studentships and fellowships which cross disciplinary or organisational boundaries and (5) human resource practices that reward interdisciplinary research (e.g. including such work as a criterion for promotion).

In conclusion, before you embark upon interdisciplinary research, remember what it is not. It is not 'pick and mix'. It is not 'mixed methods' for the sake of mixing methods. It is not a bit of qualitative tinsel tied around a quantitative study. And remember what it is: It involves collaboration between disciplines to achieve a large and ambitious project requiring, for example, computational, statistical and epidemiological input and/or contestation between disciplines to produce creative tensions, contrasting framings and a re-examining of assumptions about the topic being researched.

REFERENCES

1. Struppa D. The nature of interdisciplinarity. *J Assoc Gen Liberal Stud* 2002;30(1):97–105.
2. Star SL. Infrastructure and ethnographic practice: Working on the fringes. *Scand J Info Syst* 2002;14(2):6.
3. Rowland S. *The Enquiring University: Compliance and Contestation in Higher Education.* Buckingham: Open University Press; 2006.
4. Nussbaum M. *Not for Profit: Why Democracy Needs the Humanities.* Princeton: Princeton University Press; 2010.
5. Tortajada C. Dams: An essential component of development. *J Hydrol Eng* 2014;20(1):A4014005.
6. Baruah S. Whose river is it anyway? *Econ Polit Wkly* 2012;47(29):41.
7. Shah SH, Gibson RB. Large dam development in India: Sustainability criteria for the assessment of critical river basin infrastructure. *Int J River Basin Manag* 2013;11(1):33–53.
8. Klingensmith D. *'One Valley and a Thousand': Dams, Nationalism, and Development.* USA: Oxford University Press; 2007.
9. Arora V. 'They are All Set to Dam (n) Our Future': Contested Development through Hydel Power in Democratic Sikkim. *Sociol Bull* 2009;58(1):94–114.
10. Roy A. The Greater Common Good. In: *Frontline.* Vol 16, Issue 11, May. 22 - June 04, 1999. Available at http://web.cecs.pdx.edu/~sheard/course/Design&Society/Readings/Narmada/greatercommongood.pdf.
11. Cochran J, Ray I. Equity reexamined: A study of community-based rainwater harvesting in Rajasthan, India. *World Dev* 2009;37(2):435–44.
12. Owiti JA, Greenhalgh T, Sweeney L et al. Illness perceptions and explanatory models of viral hepatitis B & C among immigrants and refugees: A narrative systematic review. *BMC Public Health* 2015;15(1):151.
13. Jagosh J, Macaulay AC, Pluye P et al. Uncovering the benefits of participatory research: Implications of a realist review for health research and practice. *The Milbank Quarterly* 2012;90(2):311–46.
14. Jagosh J, Bush PL, Salsberg J et al. A realist evaluation of community-based participatory research: Partnership synergy, trust building and related ripple effects. *BMC Public Health* 2015;15:725.
15. Greenhalgh T, Robb N, Scambler G. Communicative and strategic action in interpreted consultations in primary health care: A Habermasian perspective. *Soc Sci Med (1982)* 2006;63(5):1170–87.
16. Sweeney L, Owiti JA, Beharry A et al. Informing the design of a national screening and treatment programme for chronic viral hepatitis in primary care: Qualitative study of at-risk immigrant communities and healthcare professionals. *BMC Health Serv Res* 2015;15(1):97.
17. Sweeney L, Owens C, Malone K. Communication and interpretation of emotional distress within the friendships of young Irish men prior to suicide: A qualitative study. *Health Soc Care Community* 2015;23(2):150–58.
18. Foster GR on behalf of the HepFREE study team. Chronic viral hepatitis in ethnic minorities. Strategies to prevent the predicted increase in mortality. Final report. NIHR Journals Library (Health Services and Delivery Research), under review.

CHAPTER 5

Combining quantitative and qualitative methods

Elizabeth Halcomb

Primary care settings are becoming increasingly complex, as they strive to manage growing multimorbidity and acuity amongst their patient populations and navigate both systems change and evolving workforce trends. As the environment in which primary care professionals work becomes more complex, so too do the problems presenting to health care researchers.[1] To address increasingly complex research problems, researchers must seek innovative methods which capture the multidimensional nature of the phenomena that they investigate.[2,3] Mixed methods research is one approach to address complex health issues. This approach provides deeper insight into these complex problems than would be achieved if either quantitative or qualitative methods were used alone.[4,5] However, mixed methods research is more than simply combining quantitative or qualitative techniques within a single study. Mixed methods research is driven by a number of key principles and may be underpinned by different methodological or philosophical considerations. This chapter provides an overview of the key considerations for undertaking mixed methods research in primary care.

UNDERSTANDING MIXED METHODS RESEARCH

Mixed methods research combines both qualitative and quantitative features within a single study.[3,6] The concept of 'combining' is a key element, as mixed methods research is more than simply conducting two pieces of data collection. Rather qualitative and quantitative elements are integrated to provide more comprehensive insight into the phenomenon under investigation.[1,7] As such, mixed methods research maximises the various strengths of each type of research, while compensating for their relative weaknesses.[8,9] Mixed methods research may also incorporate an interdisciplinary approach but is not necessarily interdisciplinary (see Chapter 4).

Just because you can undertake a mixed methods investigation, doesn't mean that you should. The choice of methods should logically flow from the specific research question(s) that the researcher is setting out to answer. The scope of the question should also consider the researchers' skills and experience, the timeline and available resources to ensure that the proposed project is achievable.[10] It may be difficult for a novice researcher to master a variety of methods at the same time. A mixed methods approach should only be chosen when the central research question or main aim of the study is best addressed through multiple objectives that necessitate a variety of different methods in order to achieve them.[4,5] For example, a trial which measures the effect of a primary care intervention on a health outcome might overlook factors that affect individuals in the intervention group (such as the time burden of intervention or discomfort). The addition of qualitative data collection to explore the experiences of intervention participants adds significant insights to the evaluation of the intervention. The common rationale for using mixed methods research is summarised in Box 5.1.

BOX 5.1   RATIONALE FOR UNDERTAKING MIXED METHODS RESEARCH[6,11–13]

- *Corroboration*: Exploring a single phenomenon in which the results of one method are used to corroborate the findings of another.
- *Complementarity*: The one set of findings elaborate, enhance or clarify the findings from another approach.
  - *Process*: Outcomes provided by quantitative data whilst processes are explored by qualitative data.
  - *Unexpected results*: A second method is used to explain surprising results obtained from one method.
  - *Confirmation*: Hypotheses generated from qualitative findings are tested by quantitative methods.
- *Development*: The results of one method inform the other method.
  - *Instrument development*: A quantitative instrument is designed based on qualitative results and then tested via quantitative investigation.
  - *Sampling*: One method facilitates sampling for the second approach (e.g. survey identifies individuals with certain characteristics who can be targeted to participate in interviews).
- *Initiation*: One method is employed to explore the paradoxes and contradictions that have been observed in the findings from another method.
- *Expansion*: The study's depth and breadth is expanded by employing different methods within the data collection.

MIXED METHODS DESIGNS

Qualitative and quantitative elements can be integrated in a mixed methods study at various points of the research process. The researcher can be guided in the development of a mixed methods study by the various mixed methods research designs. Box 5.2 outlines four key mixed methods design characteristics.[3] Table 5.1 gives examples of how these characteristics are employed in the various mixed methods designs and primary care studies.

BOX 5.2   CHARACTERISTICS OF MIXED METHODS DESIGNS[3]

- *Interaction between qualitative and quantitative elements*: Does one dataset inform the other? Are the datasets gathered independently?
- *Sequence of data collection*: Are qualitative and quantitative data collected simultaneously/concurrently or sequentially?
- *Priority*: Are qualitative and quantitative data given equal priority? Which dataset is prioritised?
- *Timing of integration*: When are qualitative and quantitative data integrated?

INTEGRATING QUALITATIVE AND QUANTITATIVE ELEMENTS

One of the most important, but often poorly executed, aspects of mixed methods research is the integration of the qualitative and quantitative elements.[7,12,24] While four distinct approaches have emerged from the literature to describe the various integration strategies, these are not mutually exclusive and each study may use one or a combination of these (Table 5.2).[7,25] The choice of integration methods should be congruent with both the design (Table 5.1) and purpose of the study (Box 5.1). Understanding which integration method is appropriate to your specific project and incorporating this within the research plan is important to ensure that study quality is optimised.

DEMONSTRATING RIGOUR

Although the combination of qualitative and quantitative aspects within a single study may enhance validity, there is still a need to demonstrate rigour.[31] There is yet to be clear agreement as to how best to demonstrate rigour in mixed methods investigations.[32] However, most agree that mixed methods studies should employ criteria relevant to quantitative and qualitative studies, as well as those specific to mixed methods research.[3,33] The investigator needs to demonstrate a clear rationale for the methodological choices in the study that allows the reader to follow the decision-making process throughout the research process.[31]

TABLE 5.1 Mixed methods designs

Research design	Sequence	Interaction	Priority	Example
Concurrent (parallel/ convergent)	Qualitative and quantitative collected together	Collected independently	Equal	Administration of the Patient Enablement and Satisfaction Survey was combined with interviews with staff and practice patients to explore relationships between general practice and nurse consultation characteristics, and the levels of patient satisfaction and enablement.[14]
Sequential explanatory	Quantitative → qualitative	Qualitative data explains quantitative data	Quantitative dominant	A national online survey of experienced nurses who had transitioned from acute care to primary health care employment was undertaken. Following the survey, interviews were undertaken to explain and explore the survey data in more detail.[15–17]
Sequential exploratory	Qualitative → quantitative	Quantitative data builds on qualitative data	Qualitative dominant	Focus groups were conducted with older family carers to identify factors that affect the quality of life of older family carers. These data generated items for inclusion in a dementia caregiving– and age-specific tool. The tool was then tested on 182 family carers and construct validity and internal consistency established.[18]
Embedded (nested)	Quantitative within qualitative or qualitative within quantitative	Complementary research question is answered by embedded data	Either dominant	A before-and-after pilot study was conducted of a general practice nurse-led intervention to improve blood pressure control amongst those with uncontrolled hypertension. The impact of the intervention on outcomes such as blood pressure, adherence to treatment, body mass index and weight was reported.[19] Subsequently, a series of interviews which investigated participating nurses', doctors' and consumers' experiences of the trial was undertaken.[20] These interview data explore how the intervention was implemented and the barriers and facilitators to the intervention delivery.
Multistage/ Multiphase	Combinations of exploratory, explanatory sequential and concurrent approaches			A systematic approach, based on the Medical Research Council framework, was used to develop an intervention to reduce polypharmacology in older people in primary care.[21,22] The next phase of the study tested the intervention in a feasibility study.[23] It is intended that the findings from this study will inform a randomised controlled trial to formally test the intervention's effectiveness.

TABLE 5.2 Integration approaches

Approach	Description	Example
Merging	Concurrent collection of qualitative and quantitative data and independent analysis. Integration occurs during interpretation.	In a study to explore the perceived impact of PTSD among veterans on their parenting, participants first completed a focus group or individual interview.[26] Directly after this, they completed a survey tool which incorporated several standardised self-report measures. The data were therefore only integrated during the reporting phase.
Building	Findings from one data collection inform the second data collection.	Qualitative data were used to inform the development of 38 items about COPD patient experience.[27] These items are to be further tested to reduce the item number and establish reliability and validity.
Connection	The second approach is built upon the findings of the first approach via sampling.	Young adult cancer survivors were surveyed about their treatment and follow-up care experience, as well as the barriers to accessing care.[28] The second phase was a series of interviews with a subset of survey respondents to explore their experiences and survey findings.
Embedding	Data collection and analysis are linked at multiple points. Often involves some combination of connecting, building or merging.	Cluster randomised controlled trial to test the effectiveness of a practice nurse smoking cessation intervention.[29] Qualitative interviews with patients, nurses and general practitioners. Trial participants evaluated the interventions' implementation, feasibility and acceptability.[30]

Source: Zhang W, Creswell J. *Med Care* 2013;51(8):e51–7; Fetters MD et al. *Health Serv Res* 2013;48(6pt2):2134–56.

CONCLUSION

Mixed methods research provides a strategy for health care researchers to gain a deeper understanding of complex issues in primary care than could be achieved via either quantitative or qualitative methods alone. This deeper insight can help researchers to explore the range of complex problems faced in primary care practice. However, the use of mixed methods requires careful consideration of the rationale for this methodological decision, the specific design used and the way in which the quantitative and qualitative aspects will be integrated (Box 5.3).

BOX 5.3 ADDITIONAL RESOURCES

Creswell JW, Klassen AC, Plano Clark VL, Smith KC. 2011. Best practices for mixed methods research in the health sciences. *Bethesda (Maryland): National Institutes of Health*, 2013, pp. 541–545.

Creswell JW. 2013. 'Steps in Conducting a Scholarly Mixed Methods Study'. DBER Speaker Series. 48. http://digitalcommons.unl.edu/dberspeakers/48.

Wisdom J., Creswell JW. 2013. Mixed Methods: Integrating Quantitative and Qualitative Data Collection and Analysis While Studying Patient-Centered Medical Home Models. AHRQ Publication No: 13-0028-EF Retrieved from https://pcmh.ahrq.gov/page/mixed-methods-integrating-quantitative-and-qualitative-data-collection-and-analysis-while.

REFERENCES

1. Glogowska M. Paradigms, pragmatism and possibilities: Mixed methods research in speech and language therapy. *Int J Lang Commun Disord* 2011;46(3):251–60.
2. Andrew S, Halcomb EJ. Mixed methods research is an effective method of enquiry for working with families and communities. *Adv Contemp Nurs* 2006;23(2):145–53.
3. Creswell JW, Plano Clark VL. *Designing and Conducting Mixed Methods Research*, 2nd ed. Thousand Oaks, California: Sage Publicaitons; 2011.
4. Andrew S, Halcomb EJ. Mixed method research. In: Borbasi S, Jackson D, editors. *Navigating the Maze of Research: Enhancing Nursing & Midwifery Practice*, 3rd ed. Marrickville, New South Wales: Elsevier; 2012. p. 147–66.
5. Simons L, Lathlean J. Mixed methods. In: Gerrish K, Lacey A, editors. *The Research Process in Nursing*, 6th ed. London: Wiley-Blackwell; 2010. p. 331–42.
6. Wisdom JP, Cavaleri MA, Onwuegbuzie AJ et al. Methodological reporting in qualitative, quantitative, and mixed methods health services research articles. *Health Ser Res* 2012;47(2):721–45.
7. Zhang W, Creswell J. The use of 'mixing' procedure of mixed methods in health services research. *Med Care* 2013;51(8):e51–7.
8. Scammon DL, Tomoaia-Cotisel A, Day RL et al. Connecting the dots and merging meaning: Using mixed methods to study primary care delivery transformation. *Health Ser Res* 2013;48(6pt2):2181–207.
9. Andrew S, Halcomb EJ, editors. *Mixed Methods Research for Nursing and the Health Sciences*. London; England: Wiley-Blackwell; 2009.
10. Halcomb EJ, Andrew S. Practical considerations for higher degree research students undertaking mixed methods projects. *Int J Mult Res Approaches* 2009;3(2):153–62.
11. Greene JC, Caracelli VJ and Graham WF. Toward a conceptual framework for mixed-method evaluation designs. *Edu Eval Policy Anal* 1989;11:255–74.
12. Bryman A. Integrating quantitative and qualitative research: How is it done? *Qual Res* 2006;6(1):97–113.
13. Halcomb EJ, Hickman L. Mixed methods research. *Nurs Stand* 2015;29(32):42–48.
14. Desborough J, Bagheri N, Banfield M et al. The impact of general practice nursing care on patient satisfaction and enablement in Australia: A mixed methods study. *Int J Nurs Stud* 2016;64:108–19.

15. Ashley C, Brown A, Halcomb E, Peters K. Registered nurses transitioning from acute care to primary healthcare employment: A qualitative insight into nurses' experiences. *J Clin Nurs* 2018;27(3–4): 661–8.
16. Ashley C, Halcomb E, Brown A, Peters K. Experiences of registered nurses transitioning from employment in acute care to primary health care – quantitative findings from a mixed methods study. *J Clin Nurs* 2018;27(1–2):355–62.
17. Ashley C, Halcomb E, Brown A, Peters, K. Exploring the reasons why nurses transition from acute care to primary health care: A mixed methods study. *Applied Nursing Research* 2017;38:83–7.
18. Oliveira DC, Vass C, Aubeeluck A. The development and validation of the Dementia Quality of Life Scale for Older Family Carers (DQoL-OC). *Aging Ment Health* 2017:1–8.
19. Zwar N, Hermitz O, Halcomb E et al. Improving blood pressure control in general practice: Quantitative evaluation of the ImPress intervention. *Aust Fam Physician* 2017;46(5):306–11.
20. Stephen C, Hermitz O, McInnes S, Halcomb EJ, Zwar N. Feasability and acceptability of a nurse-led hypertension management intervention in general practice. *Collegian 2018*;25(1): 33–8.
21. Cadogan CA, Ryan C, Francis JJ et al. Improving appropriate polypharmacy for older people in primary care: Selecting components of an evidence-based intervention to target prescribing and dispensing. *Implementation Sci* 2015;10(1):161.
22. Cadogan CA, Ryan C, Francis JJ et al. Development of an intervention to improve appropriate polypharmacy in older people in primary care using a theory-based method. *BMC Health Serv Res* 2016;16(1):661.
23. Cadogan CA, Ryan C, Gormley GJ et al. A feasibility study of a theory-based intervention to improve appropriate polypharmacy for older people in primary care. *Pilot Feasibility Stud* 2017;4(1):23.
24. Andrew S, Salamonson Y, Halcomb EJ. Integrating mixed methods data analysis using NVivo©: An example examining attrition and persistence of nursing students. *Int J Mult Res Approaches* 2008;2(1):36–43.
25. Fetters MD, Curry LA, Creswell JW. Achieving integration in mixed methods designs– principles and practices. *Health Serv Res* 2013;48(6pt2):2134–56.
26. Sherman MD, Gress Smith JL, Straits-Troster K et al. Veterans' perceptions of the impact of PTSD on their parenting and children. *Psychol Serv* 2016;13(4):401–10.
27. Walker S, Andrew S, Hodson M et al. Stage 1 development of a patient-reported experience measure (PREM) for chronic obstructive pulmonary disease (COPD). *NPJ Prim Care Respir Med* 2017;27:47.
28. Berg CJ, Stratton E, Esiashvili N et al. Young adult cancer survivors' experience with cancer treatment and follow-up care and perceptions of barriers to engaging in recommended care. *J Cancer Educ* 2016;31(3):430–42.
29. Zwar NA, Richmond RL, Halcomb EJ et al. Quit in general practice: A cluster randomized trial of enhanced in-practice support for smoking cessation. *Fam Pract* 2015;32(2):173–80.
30. Halcomb E, Furler J, Hermitz O et al. Process evaluation of a practice nurse-led smoking cessation trial in Australian general practice: Views of general practitioners and practice nurses. *Fam Pract* 2015;32(4):468–73.
31. Lavelle E, Vuk J, Barber C. Twelve tips for getting started using mixed methods in medical education research. *Med Teach* 2013;35(4):272–76.
32. Brown KM, Elliott SJ, Leatherdale ST et al. Searching for rigour in the reporting of mixed methods population health research: A methodological review. *Health Educ Res* 2015;30(6):811–39.
33. Halcomb EJ. Appraising mixed methods research. In: P. Liamputtong (Ed.), *Handbook of Research Methods in Health Social Sciences*. Singapore: Springer, 2018.

CHAPTER 6

Authentic engagement, co-creation and action research

Vivian R. Ramsden, Jackie Crowe, Norma Rabbitskin, Danielle Rolfe and Ann C. Macaulay

BACKGROUND

Primary health care, as defined by the World Health Organization (WHO) in 1978, is essential health care; based on practical, scientifically sound and socially acceptable methods and technology; universally accessible to all in the community through their full participation; at an affordable cost and geared towards self-reliance and self-determination.[1] Primary health care shifts the emphasis of health care to the people themselves and their needs, reinforcing and strengthening their own capacity to shape their lives. Thus, as a strategy, primary health care focuses on individual and community strengths (assets) and opportunities for change (needs); maximises the involvement of the community; includes all relevant sectors but avoids duplication of services and uses only health technologies that are accessible, acceptable, affordable and appropriate.[2,3]

Primary health care research may also involve strategies to engage individuals, organisations and communities in identifying and addressing locally relevant issues that impact health and wellness. In Canada, a framework for engaging individuals/patients, organisations and/or communities is outlined in Chapter 9 of the Tri-Council Policy Statement: Ethical Conduct for Research Involving Humans.[4] This was specifically developed for research projects involving First Nations, Inuit and Métis peoples (Indigenous peoples) and their communities as they are to have a role in shaping and co-creating all research that affects them. However, this is extremely relevant to all research partnerships, because it goes on to indicate that respect should be given to the autonomy of individuals/patients, organisations and/or communities to decide whether or not they will participate in research. (See Box 6.1 for a template for engagement with these communities.)

The purpose of this chapter is to encourage primary care researchers to consider this framework as they engage individuals/patients, organisations and/or communities. Ensuring that engagement is both welcome and authentic is particularly relevant for working with and in communities and developing other global health initiatives, and within the context of Canada's relatively new Strategy for Patient Oriented Research that implores health researchers to engage patients as equal partners in all aspects of the research process. Primary health care professionals are well placed to engage with individuals/patients and communities as they have already adopted the WHO's philosophy of promoting patient/community self-reliance and self-determination.[5]

Thus, in reading this chapter, it is important to recognise that worldwide, depending on the country and the discipline, there is a complex range of terminology describing research partnerships, including authentic engagement, community-partnered participatory research, participatory research, participatory health research, action research, community-based participatory research and co-design. However, a common component found in all is that the end users of the research product engage in the research process.[3,6]

METHODS

The engagement of individuals/patients, organisations and/or communities has become increasingly important in all aspects of the research process. Research that is co-created with individuals/patients, organisations and/or communities is designed to improve health and well-being and to minimise health disparities.[7] This partnership approach to research equitably involves individuals/patients, organisations and/or communities *and* researchers in all aspects of the research process, and all partners contribute expertise and share decision making and ownership.[8-10] In addition, research that is co-created is utilised to study and address community-identified issues through a collaborative and empowering action-oriented process that builds on strengths and assets of individuals/patients, organisations and the community.[11,12]

Research that is co-created takes time, patience, energy and commitment. Building with and on the aspirations of individuals/patients, organisations and/or communities enhances capacity and sustains the changes made at all levels. Capacity, in this case, is defined as strengthening people's capacity to determine their own values and priorities and to organise themselves to act on these.[13] Thus, building capacity is the process of reflection, leadership, inspiration, adaptation and search for greater coherence between the purpose, governance and activities. This fosters the building of communication through the processes of negotiation, relationship building, conflict resolution and improvement in the ability of each of the partners to celebrate their diversity while building on strengths. In collaborative action research, the community members are considered to be experts in their lived experience and about their community.[14]

Authentic engagement and co-creation have been utilised to study and address individual/patient, organisation and/or community-identified issues which build on strengths rather than deficits.[11,12] Transformative action research encompasses a high level of participation, transformative learning and facilitation.[15,16] It requires true collaboration where power and empowerment are shared horizontally. Thus, researchers utilising this method engage with individuals/patients, organisations and/or communities, which is reflected in the process, methods, results and interpretation.[15,17] Learning and research are done together and are iterative as new insights are gained and implemented.[13,18] Systematic reviews, using realist evaluation, have documented the significant benefits of authentic engagement of partnering with communities: shaping the scope and direction of research, developing programmes and implementing research protocols, interpreting and disseminating research findings, building capacity, generating systemic changes and developing new unanticipated projects and activities.[19] In addition, the partnership synergy produces ripple effects in which successes from early stages form the basis for the next undertaking.[20,21]

Research that is co-created brings the best and the latest technology for design and measurement to the strengths, challenges and opportunities for change. In addition, authentic engagement and co-creation of research integrated with action research allows for an immediate change/transformation of the purpose, values, feelings and meanings that have been uncritically assimilated from others into our lives (academic, workplace, recreational) to gaining greater personal control over our lives as socially responsible, clear-thinking decision makers.[22,23]

Guiding values need to be negotiated initially and then further developed over time by the members of the research team. The guiding values could include respect for ourselves and others, building trust in relationships, responsibility and accountability of the individual and the community, freedom of the individual, kindness and compassion, patience, humility, transparency and inclusiveness.[2,10,24]

RESULTS AND DISCUSSION

The theoretical constructs of community action for health are based on the principle that the knowledge and skills of individuals/patients, organisations and communities are strengths which contribute to enhancing health and well-being.[18] Developing capacity through participation can best be achieved by building on and strengthening existing knowledge and expertise. Authentic engagement must be real, not just doing what has always been done: *making decisions for* and then indicating that the individual was noncompliant because they did not do what they were told to do. Thus, analysis by local people is an essential part of community action for health, and the role of health care practitioners and researchers should be to work with individuals/patients, organisations and/or communities in ways that are meaningful to them (patient-centred). This is research *with* individuals/patients, organisations and communities, not research *on* or *for* or *about* others.

The goal is to build meaningful programmes; thus, the research team must find ways to learn about the health needs of individuals/patients, organisations and communities and to work with them to enhance their health and well-being.

The following tools have been developed over time to identify authentic engagement, co-creation and action research within practice.

Practical tips: Authentic engagement, co-creation and action research

Working *with* individuals/patients, organisations and/or communities to develop equitable partnerships broadens the base of perceptions and expectations that powerfully influence assumptions that structure the way we engage in research and interpret the results/findings.[25] (See Examples 6.1 and 6.2.)

EXAMPLE 6.1

The personal impact that participatory research has had on me and my relationships is briefly outlined in this narrative. As a community member, I began working with the Department of Academic Family Medicine at the University of Saskatchewan in 1998–1999 on a research project that was to engage the five core communities where I grew up in a community health survey. Through this process of coming together, working on questions and sharing the decision making, I learned that we all had valuable thoughts and ideas to contribute to the project and that this would be key in the outcomes of the relationships that would evolve from working with the communities, outcomes that brought about positive changes such as the Green Light Program. The Green Light Program is about celebrating smoke-free homes rather than focusing on asking people to stop smoking. Thus, I learned that I too have had an impact on changing the way we work with communities by ensuring transparency in the research process through building relationships, as well as sharing responsibilities and information about healthy choices that lead to sustainable change.

The relationship that I have with the researcher has led to addressing my own health concerns, including my journey to stop smoking. She was always supportive and non-judgemental; she has never nagged me to stop; she was always there to say, 'How can I support you? What do you need?'. Of the many times I chose to stop, the language and support never changed. It helped me to feel in control and that it was in fact my choice to stop smoking. I think that for me to stop smoking after 35 years was a miracle/a choice, but when I was ready, it would happen. I have now been smoke-free for three years.

EXAMPLE 6.2

The experience with authentic engagement, co-creation and action research has been very empowering. Working at the community level, delivering services to the best of our abilities has always been the priority. With increasing health mobility and a shift in health trends, our community needed to look at more innovative ways to be responsive to the needs of the people. Research has provided the vehicle to affect change and advocate for policy changes for the community with the community. The highlight of this experience for our community was having an opportunity to provide input into the design of the research questions based on the questions that our community wanted to know and based on the health literacy level of the community. Knowledge exists in the community, and it is by allowing the people an opportunity to tell their stories and give directions on the research being undertaken that true healing is achieved. Thus, participatory health research has been empowering for the community. To effect small changes, whether at the individual and/or community level, is this ultimate success. This experience has been inspiring and life altering for our people.

BOX 6.1   TEMPLATE FOR ENGAGEMENT WITH INDIVIDUALS/PATIENTS, ORGANISATIONS AND/ OR COMMUNITIES IN RESEARCH[15,26]

Co-creating/co-designing/co-developing a grant/proposal

Introduction/Research Questions

- Co-create a set of values that will describe how the team will work together.
- Co-create a conceptual framework using participatory principles.
- Identify and engage individuals/patients as early as possible in order to build sustainable relationships, which will maximise the input and impact.

- Provide support, encouragement and recognition for individuals/patients, organisations and communities by recognising them as experts and members of the research team.
- Co-create, using the principles of consensus, the purpose, objectives and questions to be asked and data collection methods to be used in the grant.

Methods
- Be clear on the roles and responsibilities for each member of the research team; determine these together so that each member of the team contributes what they do best.
- Ensure a trusting and positive work environment by providing structural supports, e.g. honorariums, food, childcare, bus tickets/taxis.
- Provide relevant training for all members of the research team.[4]
- Co-create/co-develop a document that describes what is going to be undertaken in this grant/proposal and by whom, and have every member of the team critique it so that the research process is transparent.
- Develop a Data Sharing Agreement (written or oral) so that everyone is aware of the principles of Ownership, Control, Access and Possession (OCAP)[27] which enable self-determination over all research. This was developed for First Nations in Canada to make decisions regarding what research will be done, for what purpose information or data will be used, where the information will be physically stored and who will have access. The document is extremely relevant for all other partnerships 'working with individuals, patients, organisations and communities'.[27]
- Reflect on the results and process.
- Return data to individuals/patients, organisations and/or communities for interpretation, decision making and identification of new questions before external dissemination.
- Identify insights, prioritise actions to be taken and subsequently disseminate the results, first at the level of the individuals/patients, organisations and/or communities and then in ways that are meaningful to all members of the research team.

Knowledge Translation
- Funding needs to be built into the grant/proposal to ensure that co-creation/co-development of how best to share the results is clearly identified in the grant/proposal.
- In addition, the individuals/patients need to be able to travel to present at some if not all of the conferences with researchers, as well as being able to determine where the data should be presented and to whom.
- Particular attention needs to be paid to including individuals/patients in dissemination activities, including publications, which provides an obvious description of authentic engagement on the research continuum. It also minimises the risk of potential stigmatisation of individuals/patients, organisations and/or communities.

Authentic engagement

When considering whether or not authentic engagement with individuals/ patients in research is being undertaken or described, consider the following questions:[28,29]

1. Are individuals/patients, organisations and/or communities equitably involved in all appropriate aspects of designing the proposal?
2. Is there co-production of the processes to be used during and throughout the research proposed?
3. Are individuals/patients named as Investigators (provide a description of past collaborations with the individual/patient, organisations and/or community) and/or members of the Leadership Team?
4. How are individuals/patients, organisations and/or communities involved in analysis and interpretation of results, dissemination of findings through presentations and as co-authors?
5. How is mutual learning to be fostered?
6. Are individuals/patients, organisations and/or communities involved with the review process?

Criteria

1. Given that authentic engagement is about the development of a sustainable and enduring relationship over time, individuals/patients, organisations and/or communities should be seen as being involved in the research and in all aspects of designing the proposal, including the development of meaningful questions; co-production of the processes to be used during and throughout the project; being named as investigators and/or members of the leadership team; being engaged in the analysis and interpretation of findings/results; and dissemination of findings/results through presentations; as well as being co-authors.

   All aforementioned aspects should be in place if a proposal is to be considered for funding.
2. The ways that the individuals/patients, organisations and/or communities will be included in the various aspects of knowledge translation and dissemination need to be negotiated and agreed to when developing the proposal/design of the project and should address presentations, as well as publication of manuscripts, book chapters and books.
3. Letters of support from the individuals/patients, organisations and/or communities should clearly describe why they value the research; the relationship that they have with the research team; the origin of the research question(s)/study topic; the role of the individual/patient, organisation and/ or community in defining the goals, objectives and research question(s);

and plans for interpretation of findings and ongoing participation including dissemination, which should include the significance of the research from the perspective of the individual/patient, organisation and/or community and how the results will be used.

4. The research team should describe meetings and other events convened to engage individuals/patients, organisations and/or communities in the planning of the research, including the guidance offered by individuals/ patients, organisations and/or communities on all aspects of the research being planned, designed, implemented and evaluated.

5. Within the presentations and manuscripts, the following aspects need to be clearly described: The relationship with the research team; the origin of the research question/study topic; the role of the individual/patient, organisation and/or community in defining the goals, objectives and research question(s), as well as their role(s) in data collection, interpretation of the findings/results and the summary/conclusions.

CONCLUSIONS

We have highlighted the various aspects of applying authentic engagement, co-creation and action research in answering meaningful questions with individuals/patients, organisations and/or communities.

Those of us participating in this approach to research find it stimulating, rewarding and exciting to be part of the process and also to experience both the expected outcomes and, frequently additional and unexpected outcomes that ripple out or arise from the authentic engagement or research experience.[20,21]

REFERENCES

1. World Health Organization, UNICEF. *Alma-Ata 1978: Primary Health Care.* Geneva, Switzerland: World Health Organization; 1978.
2. Ramsden VR, McKay S, Crowe J. The pursuit of excellence: Engaging the community in participatory health research. *Glob Health Promot.* December 2010;17(4):32–42.
3. Jones L, Wells K. Strategies for academic and clinician engagement in community-participatory partnered research. *JAMA.* 24 January 2007;297(4):407–10.
4. Canadian Institutes of Health Research, Natural Sciences and Engineering Research Council of Canada and Social Sciences and Humanities Research Council of Canada. Chapter 9 of the Tri-Council Policy Statement: Ethical Conduct for Research Involving Humans. [Internet] December 2014 [cited 30 June 2017]. Available from: http://www.pre.ethics.gc.ca/eng/policy-politique/initiatives/tcps2-eptc2/chapter9-chapitre9/.
5. Macaulay AC. Promoting participatory research by family physicians. *Ann Fam Med.* November-December 2007;5(6):557–60.
6. Goodyear-Smith F. Collective enquiry and reflective action in research: Toward a clarification of the terminology. *Fam Pract.* 1 June 2017;34(3):268–71.
7. Israel BA, Eng E, Schulz AJ, Parker EA. *Methods in Community-Based Participatory Research for Health.* San Francisco, CA: Jossey-Bass; 2005.

8. Israel BA, Schulz AJ, Parker EA, Becker AB. Review of community-based research: Assessing partnership approaches to improve public health. *Annu Rev Public Health* 1998;19(5):173–202.

9. Israel BA, Schulz AJ, Parker EA, Becker AB, Allen A, Guzman JR. Critical issues in developing and following community-based participatory research principles. In: Minkler M, Wallerstein N, editors. *Community-Based Participatory Research for Health*. San Francisco, CA: Jossey-Bass; 2003. p. 56–73.

10. Allen ML, Salsberg J, Knot M et al. Engaging with communities, engaging with patients: Amendment to the NAPCRG 1998 Policy Statement on Responsible Research With Communities. *Fam Pract*. 1 June 2017;34(3):313–21.

11. Minkler M, Vasquez VB, Warner JR, Steussey H, Facente S. Sowing the seeds for sustainable change: A community-based participatory research partnership for health promotion in Indiana, USA and its aftermath. *Health Promot Int*. December 2006;21(4):293–300.

12. Wallerstein N, Duran B. Using community-based participatory research to address health disparities. *Health Promot Pract* 2006;7(3):312–23.

13. Eade D, Williams S. *The Oxfam Handbook of Development and Relief*. Oxford, UK: Oxfam; 1995.

14. Fetterman D, Wandersman A. *Empowerment Evaluation Principles in Practice*. New York, NY: Guildford Press; 2005.

15. Ramsden VR; Integrated Primary Health Care Research Team. Learning with the community: Evolution to transformative action research. *Can Fam Physician* 2003;49(2): 195–7, 200–2.

16. Ramsden V, Vilis E, White H. Facilitation as a vehicle for change. In: Government of Newfoundland and Labrador, Barrett J, Hogg W, Ramsden V, White H, editors. *Guiding Facilitation in the Canadian Context: Enhancing Primary Health Care*. St. John's, NL: Department of Health & Community Services, Government of Newfoundland and Labrador; 2006. p. 20–7.

17. Martin R, Chan R, Torikka L, Granger-Brown A, Ramsden V. Health fostered by research. *Can Fam Physician*. February 2008;54(2):244–5.

18. World Health Organization. Community involvement in health development: A review of the concept and practice. In: Kahssay H, Oakley P, editors. Geneva, Switzerland: World Health Organization; 1999, vol. 5, p.160.

19. Jagosh J, Macaulay AC, Pluye P et al. Uncovering the benefits of participatory research: Implications of a realist review for health research and practice. *Milbank Q*. June 2012;90(2):311–46.

20. Jagosh J, Bush PB, Salsberg J, Macaulay AC, Greenhalgh T, Wong G, Cargo M, Green LW, Herbert CP, Pluye P. A realist evaluation of community-based participatory research: Partnership synergy, trust building and related ripple effects. *BMC Public Health*. 30 July 2015;15:725.

21. Trickett EJ, Beehler S. Participatory action research and impact: An ecological ripples perspective. *Educ Action Res* 2017;25(3):1–16.

22. Mezirow J and Associates. *Fostering Critical Reflection in Adulthood: A Guide to Transformational and Emancipatory Learning*. San Francisco, CA: Jossey-Bass; 1990.

23. Mezirow J and Associates. *Learning as Transformation: Critical Perspectives on a Theory in Progress*. San Francisco, CA: Jossey-Bass; 2000.

24. Canadian Institutes of Health Research. Strategy for Patient-Oriented Research: Patient Engagement Framework. [Internet] January 2014 [cited 26 June 2017]. Available from: http://www.cihr-irsc.gc.ca/e/documents/spor_framework-en.pdf. Date accessed 26 June 2017.

25. Macaulay AC. Participatory research: What is the history? Has the purpose changed? *Fam Pract*. 1 June 2017;34(3):256–8.

26. Shen S, Doyle-Thomas KA, Beesley L, Karmali A, Williams L, Tanel N, McPherson AC. How and why should we engage parents as co-researchers in health research? A scoping review of current practices. *Health Expect.* 2017;20(4):543–54. DOI: 10.1111/hex.12490. Epub 12 Aug 2016.

27. National Aboriginal Health Organization. OCAP (Ownership, Control, Access and Possession). [Internet] 2007 [cited 30 June 2017]. Available from: http://cahr.uvic.ca/nearbc/documents/2009/FNC-OCAP.pdf.

28. Ramsden VR, Salsberg J, Herbert CP, Westfall JM, LeMaster J, Macaulay AC. Patient- and community-oriented research: How is authentic engagement identified in grant applications? *Can Fam Physician.* January 2017;63(1):74–6.

29. Ramsden VR, Rabbitskin N, Westfall JM, Felzien M, Braden J, Sand J. Is knowledge translation without patient or community engagement flawed? *Fam Pract.* 1 June 2017;34(3):259–61.

CHAPTER 7

Development and use of primary care research networks

Emma Wallace and Tom Fahey

INTRODUCTION

Internationally, several types of primary care research networks exist with varying principal functions, but all aim to improve the quality of primary care by building a setting-appropriate evidence base. There are global differences in the stages of development and implementation of these networks, with some of the most well-developed in countries such as the UK and the Netherlands.[1] In general, primary care research networks can be subdivided into sentinel practice networks, practice-based clinical research networks, networks contributing data to routine databases and specific condition/purpose networks.

SENTINEL PRACTICE RESEARCH NETWORKS

Sentinel practices focus on infectious disease reporting (e.g. influenza). An example is the Australian Sentinel Practices Research Network (ASPREN) which is a network of general practitioners who report deidentified information on influenza-like illness and other conditions seen in general practice (http://www.aspren.com.au/).[2] This network was originally developed by the Royal Australian College of General Practitioners in 1991 but is currently funded by the Commonwealth's Department of Health and managed through a General Practitioner (GP) academic department at The University of Adelaide.[2] In Ireland, the Disease Surveillance Sentinel Practice Network Project is led by the Irish College of General Practitioners in collaboration with the Health Protection Surveillance Centre and the National Virus Reference Laboratory. The project involves running an electronic surveillance network for certain infectious diseases in the community and involves 60 sentinel GP practices spread throughout the country.[3] A recent review of 50 years of infections surveillance in the UK highlighted the importance of nationally representative data to monitor and inform the national influenza vaccination programme.[4]

PRACTICE-BASED RESEARCH NETWORKS

GP practice-based research networks are usually formal collaborations between participating practices and academic institutions. These networks aim to increase the number of clinicians participating in research and also to examine factors that may make research participation more favourable.[5,6] Clinicians who have a positive experience of research participation, in theory, are more likely to utilise research findings and more likely to take part in future research, thus building capacity.[7]

In England, the National Institute for Health Research (NIHR) Clinical Research Network (CRN) enables patients and health care professionals across England to participate in clinical research studies within the National Health Service (NHS) (https://www.nihr.ac.uk/about-us/how-we-are-managed/managing-centres/crn/). The NIHR CRN Coordinating Centre manages the CRN on behalf of the Department of Health. This comprises 15 local clinical research networks and provides the infrastructure that enables high-quality clinical research to be undertaken throughout the networks. The NIHR network was established following the closure of the Medical Research Council (MRC) General Practice Research framework and Clinical Trials Unit in 2012 because of changes in how research activity was funded.[8]

In 2012, the Canadian Institutes of Health Research (CIHR) launched the Roadmap Signature Initiative to fund research that supports the delivery of high-quality community-based primary health care across Canada (http://www.cihr-irsc.gc.ca/e/44079.html). As part of this initiative, the pan-Canadian Strategy for Patient-Oriented Research (SPOR) Network in Primary and Integrated Health Care was developed. This comprises a network of networks that builds on regional networks in community-based primary health care. It aims to facilitate the integration of research, policy and practice, initially focusing on complex care (http://www.cihr-irsc.gc.ca/e/49554.html).

RESEARCH NETWORKS CONTRIBUTING DATA TO ROUTINE DATASETS

Other primary care networks focus on contributing primary care data to routine datasets. In the UK, the Clinical Practice Research Datalink (CPRD) was developed in 1987 as a governmental, not-for-profit research service, jointly funded by the NHS NIHR and the Medicines and Health care products Regulatory Agency (MHRA), which is part of the Department of Health (https://www.cprd.com).[9] The primary care database contains anonymised, longitudinal medical records of patients registered with contributing UK primary care practices. There are currently 22 million patient lives in the CPRD primary care database, representative of the general UK population in terms of age, sex and ethnicity.[10] Recorded data includes patient demographics, clinical symptoms and signs, investigations, medical diagnoses, prescriptions and referrals to secondary care. CPRD can also provide linkage with datasets from secondary care, disease-specific cohorts and mortality records.[11]

Another UK example is the Health Improvement Network Database (THIN) which is a primary care electronic medical record (EMR) data resource covering more than 3.7 million active patients.[12] These patients are representative of the UK population and available data includes medical diagnoses, clinical symptoms, prescriptions and investigations. There are also two UK routine databases linked to UK academic institutions: (1) QResearch, a collaboration with the University of Nottingham, which includes 754 general practices and over 13 million patients (http://www.qresearch.org/), and (2) ResearchOne, a collaboration with the University of Leeds, comprising 30 million research records (http://www.researchone.org/).

In the Netherlands, the Dutch Institute for Health Services Research (NIVEL) Primary Care database (https://www.nivel.nl/en/dossier/nivel-primary-care-database) comprises more than 500 general practices with 1.6 million patients (accounting for 10% of the total Dutch population).[13] Their aim is to carry out high quality research which has a demonstrable impact upon society. Available data includes medical diagnoses, consultations, prescriptions, referrals, investigations and claims. In 2016, an independent international review committee rated the scientific quality and societal relevance of NIVEL's research very highly.[14]

The Canadian Primary Care Sentinel Surveillance Network (CPCSSN) is a primary care research initiative which commenced in 2008 under the College of Family Physicians of Canada with funding from the Public Health Agency of Canada (http://cpcssn.ca/).[1] This network consists of 10 practice-based research networks associated with academic departments of family medicine and pools anonymised electronic medical record data on eight chronic medical conditions. There are 400 family physicians enrolled currently.

Another example is the Australian Bettering the Evaluation and Care of Health (BEACH) programme which collected routine data including GP characteristics, patient demographics, medical diagnoses, prescriptions, investigations and referrals to secondary care (http://sydney.edu.au/medicine/fmrc/beach/).[15] As of 2016, the BEACH programme's funding was withdrawn and therefore data collection has ceased. The BEACH database currently includes about 1.78 million GP-patient encounter records. It used a cross-sectional, paper-based data-collection system developed and validated over 30 years at the University of Sydney.[15]

RESEARCH NETWORKS WITH A SPECIFIC PURPOSE

Finally, research networks can be developed for a specific purpose such as prescribing investigation or for named conditions. In Australia, MedicineInsight is a quality improvement programme focused on prescribing data developed and managed by the National Prescribing Service MedicineWise with funding from the Department of Health (https://www.nps.org.au/medicine-insight). MedicineInsight allows GPs to examine their own patterns of prescribing and compare these with other GPs in their practice. These can be benchmarked at local, regional and national levels. Participating practices are offered customised quality-improvement activities that support alignment with best practice and identify key areas for improvement as well as continuous professional development (CPD) points. In the UK, approximately 1,400 GPs with an interest in contraception participated in the Royal College of General Practitioners (RCGP) Oral Contraception cohort study, which examined long-term mortality risk in women taking oral contraceptives and reported that there was no increased mortality risk for oral contraception users compared to never users.[16]

International networks have also been developed, with the GRACE-09 study (Genomics to combat Resistance against Antibiotics in Community-acquired LRTI in Europe) being a good example.[17] This collaboration has resulted in multiple studies including a multi-centre randomised controlled trial which recruited from six European countries and included a total of 246 practices and 4,264 patients. This study reported that internet training achieved important reductions in antibiotic prescribing for respiratory-tract infections across language and cultural boundaries.[17]

DEVELOPING A PRACTICE-BASED RESEARCH NETWORK

Existing research networks offer a great opportunity for primary care researchers to access good quality data for their particular project. This is invaluable in facilitating timely research completion and facilitating larger scale projects in primary care. To develop a practice-based research network *de novo* requires careful planning and consideration of relevant issues. It is important to be clear on the vision for and envisaged function of the network.

An example of a recently developed network is the Stellenbosch University Family Physician Research Network (SUFFREN) in South Africa. A workshop was conducted in Stellenbosch University in August 2017 to facilitate discussion between relevant stakeholders, including family physicians and academics. This workshop resulted in the development of a framework for

BOX 7.1   KEY ISSUES IN DEVELOPING A PRACTICE-BASED RESEARCH NETWORK

Roles and responsibilities

It was agreed that family physicians would be responsible for the identification and prioritisation of research questions, data collection and help in disseminating findings, while the academic partners would be responsible for developing the research protocol, ethical approval, data cleaning and analysis and writing of the report/research article. It was also agreed that coordination and communication of meetings was to be facilitated by administrative staff in the academic department.

1. *Types of research questions and methods*: This activity involved a research-question prioritisation exercise using a variety of research methodologies, e.g. quality improvement for disease specific, patient-centred and health service-related issues, effectiveness of diagnostic and therapeutic interventions and long-term monitoring of health outcomes. The framework included examples of good research questions and the appropriate methodology to answer specific research questions.
2. *Data management and ethical considerations*: This process included consideration as to data collection methods locally and data storage, cleaning and analysis. It was decided that data storage, cleaning and analysis should be the responsibility of the academic institution.
3. *Dissemination of results*: A summary of how results could be disseminated to practitioners, policymakers and other stakeholders was discussed and summarised.

the design and anticipated implementation of the network. The framework focused on defining the vision and mission statement of the network, intended participants and stakeholder involvement. Other key issues considered in developing the network are summarised in Box 7.1. This network is currently in its early stages with approximately 20 practices participating.

IMPACT OF PRIMARY CARE NETWORK RESEARCH

In terms of examining the overall quality of care, a recent NIHR primary care network study, published in *The Lancet*, examined over one million consultations in English primary care.[18] This study reported a substantial increase in practice consultation rates, average consultation duration and total patient-facing clinical workload over the period 2007–2014.[18] This type of research is crucial in workforce and health care delivery planning. Another example is a time-series analysis of the impact of the UK pay for performance scheme, published in *The New England Journal of Medicine*, which demonstrated that the quality of care for asthma and diabetes improved in the short term, with no change in heart disease outcomes.[19] However, once targets were reached, the improvement in the quality of care for patients with these conditions slowed and the quality of care declined for two conditions that had not been linked to incentives.[19]

Primary care research networks are also important in examining pharmaco-epidemiology and the safety of prescribing. Longitudinal electronic databases such as the UK CPRD provide detailed patient and practice level data essential for examining trends in prescribing, the use of newer agents and the risks associated with medication use.[20–23] This type of data is also very useful in examining clinical symptoms and signs associated with cancer diagnosis in primary care and has been utilised to examine diagnostic features of colorectal cancer and leukaemia.[24–26] Another area where primary care research networks have proved impactful is in developing and validating prognostic models across different clinical domains, including cardiovascular disease, diabetes and cancer.[27–29] These tools are valuable in clinical practice as they use patient level information to calculate the probability of experiencing the outcome(s) of interest. This facilitates informed shared decision making for patients when deciding upon a particular treatment of management option.

Countries with well-developed research networks, such as the UK and Netherlands, are amongst the best performers internationally in terms of primary care research output and citation impact.[30] In addition, primary care research can effectively address national health policy priorities, such as multimorbidity, appropriate prescribing and infectious disease and contribute to both clinical guidelines and government health policy.[31]

CONCLUSION

In summary, the development and implementation of primary care research networks has huge potential in informing primary care delivery and patient outcomes with high-quality, setting-appropriate evidence. Capacity building can include the development and implementation of sentinel practices, clinical practice research networks, specific-purpose networks or networks contributing to electronic longitudinal databases. Well-developed research networks are impactful in terms of primary care research output and contribution to health care policy and clinical guidelines.

REFERENCES

1. Peckham S, Hutchison B. Developing primary care: The contribution of primary care research networks. *Health Policy = Politiques de Sante* 2012;8(2):56–70 [published online: 24 August 2013].
2. ASPREN. The National GP Disease Surveillance Network. Available at: http://www.aspren.com.au/. Date accessed: 9 September 2017.

3. Irish College of General Practitioners (ICGP). Annual Report 2016 (January – December). ICGP, Dublin, May 2017. Available at: https://www.icgp.ie/speck/properties/asset/asset.cfm?type=LibraryAsset&id=AF31070A%2DFF81%2D351A%2DE26838172 4AF521D&property=asset&revision=tip&disposition=attachment&app=icgp&filena me=Annual%5FReport%5F2016%2Epdf. Date accessed: 9 September 2017.

4. de Lusignan S, Correa A, Smith GE et al. RCGP Research and Surveillance Centre: 50 years' surveillance of influenza, infections, and respiratory conditions. *Br J Gen Pract* 2017;67(663):440–41. [published online: 1 October 2017].

5. Hoffmann AE, Leege EK, Plane MB et al. Clinician and staff perspectives on participating in practice-based research (PBR): A report from the Wisconsin Research and Education Network (WREN). *J Am Board Fam Med* 2015;28(5):639–48. [published online: 12 September 2015].

6. Cadwallader JS, Lebeau JP, Lasserre E et al. Patient and professional attitudes towards research in general practice: The RepR qualitative study. *BMC Fam Pract* 2014;15:136. [published online: 23 July 2014].

7. Mold JW, Aspy CB, Smith PD et al. Leveraging practice-based research networks to accelerate implementation and diffusion of chronic kidney disease guidelines in primary care practices: A prospective cohort study. *Implementation Sci* 2014;9:169. [published online: 25 November 2014].

8. Medical Research Council (MRC). Clinical Trials Unit. Available from: http://www.ctu.mrc.ac.uk/news/2012/general_practice_research_unit_to_close_290312. Date accessed: 9 September 2017.

9. Medicines and Healthcare Products Regulatory Agency CPRD. https://www.cprd.com/home/.

10. Jick SS, Kaye JA, Vasilakis-Scaramozza C et al. Validity of the general practice research database. *Pharmacotherapy* 2003;23:686–9.

11. Boggon R, Staa TP, Chapman M, Gallagher AM, Hammad TA, Richards MA. Cancer recording and mortality in the general practice research database and linked cancer registries. *Pharmacoepidemiol Drug Safety* 2013;22(2):168–75.

12. Lewis JD, Schinnar R, Bilker WB et al. Validation studies of the health improvement network (THIN) database for pharmacoepidemiology research. *Pharmacoepidemiol Drug Saf* 2007;16:393–401.

13. NIVEL Primary Care Database (NIVEL Zorgregistraties eerste lijn). Netherlands institute for health services research. 2017. Available from: www.nivel.nl/en/dossier/nivel-primary-care-database. Date accessed: 4 September 2017.

14. Research assessment of the Netherlands institute for health services research (NIVEL) 2010–2015. Available from: https://www.nivel.nl/sites/default/files/bestanden/NIVEL_assessment_report_2016.pdf. Date accessed: 4 September 2017.

15. Britt H, Miller GC. The BEACH program: An update. *Aust Fam Physician* 2015; 44(6):411–14.

16. Hannaford PC, Iversen L, Macfarlane TV et al. Mortality among contraceptive pill users: Cohort evidence from Royal College of General Practitioners' Oral Contraception Study. *BMJ (Clinical research ed)* 2010;340:c927. [published online: 13 March 2010]

17. Little P, Stuart B, Francis N, Douglas E, Tonkin-Crine S, Anthierens S. Effects of internet-based training on antibiotic prescribing rates for acute respiratory-tract infections: A multinational, cluster, randomised, factorial, controlled trial. *Lancet* 2013;382:1175–82.

18. Hobbs FDR, Bankhead C, Mukhtar T et al. Clinical workload in UK primary care: A retrospective analysis of 100 million consultations in England, 2007–2014. *Lancet* 2016;387(10035):2323–30. [published online: 10 April 2016].

19. Campbell SM, Reeves D, Kontopantelis E et al. Effects of pay for performance on the quality of primary care in England. *N Engl J Med* 2009;361(4):368–78. [published online: 25 July 2009].
20. Hulley S, Cummings S, Browner W et al. Chapter 2: Conceiving the research question. *Designing Clinical Research*. Philadelphia, PA: Wolters Kluwer–Lippincott Williams and Wilkins 2013.
21. Straus S, Glaziou P, Richardson W et al. *Evidence-Based Medicine: How to Practice and Teach It*. 4th ed. Edinburgh: Churchill Livingstone 2010.
22. Farrugia P, Petrisor B, Farrokhyar F et al. Research questions, hypotheses and objectives. *Can J Surg* 2010;53:278–81.
23. Haynes B. Forming research questions. *J Clin Epidemiol* 2006;59:881–86.
24. Mounce LTA, Price S, Valderas JM et al. Comorbid conditions delay diagnosis of colorectal cancer: A cohort study using electronic primary care records. *Br J Cancer* 2017;116(12):1536–43. [published online: 12 May 2017].
25. Stapley SA, Rubin GP, Alsina D et al. Clinical features of bowel disease in patients aged <50 years in primary care: A large case-control study. *Br J Gen Pract* 2017;67(658):e33 6–e44. [published online: 30 March 2017].
26. Shephard EA, Neal RD, Rose PW et al. Symptoms of adult chronic and acute leukaemia before diagnosis: Large primary care case-control studies using electronic records. *Br J Gen Pract* 2016;66(644):e182–8. [published online: 27 February 2016].
27. Hippisley-Cox J, Coupland C, Brindle P. Development and validation of QRISK3 risk prediction algorithms to estimate future risk of cardiovascular disease: Prospective cohort study. *BMJ (Clinical research ed)* 2017;357:j2099. [published online: 26 May 2017].
28. Hippisley-Cox J, Coupland C. Development and validation of risk prediction Equations to estimate future risk of blindness and lower limb amputation in patients with diabetes: Cohort study. *BMJ (Clinical research ed)* 2015;351:h5441. [published online: 13 November 2015].
29. Hippisley-Cox J, Coupland C. Development and validation of risk prediction equations to estimate survival in patients with colorectal cancer: Cohort study. *BMJ (Clinical research ed)* 2017;357:j2497. [published online: 18 June 2017].
30. Glanville J, Kendrick T, McNally R et al. Research output on primary care in Australia, Canada, Germany, the Netherlands, the United Kingdom, and the United States: Bibliometric analysis. *Br Med J* 2011;342:d1028.
31. Campbell J, Hobbs FD, Irish B et al. UK academic general practice and primary care. *BMJ (Clinical research ed)* 2015;351:h4164. [published online: 2 August 2015].

CHAPTER 8

Using big data in primary care research

Daniel J. Exeter and
Katherine E. Walesby

In this chapter, we discuss the characteristics, opportunities and pitfalls of big health data in the primary care context. 'Big data' is a current buzzword in health, which is particularly surprising given the widespread use of routine health datasets for research, policy and planning purposes. William Farr first used routine data in Victorian England and found some districts experienced better health than poor districts. Today, big data is an umbrella term encapsulating massive amounts of data from both traditional and more contemporary sources, data management systems and analytical techniques. The opportunities that big data offers primary health care are endless but require care to ensure these data are used appropriately.

Through the development of electronic health records (EHR), every interaction a patient has with the health care system is systematically recorded, giving physicians ready access to a wide range of data. The last time you visited your general practitioner (GP), your interactions may have included visiting the medical centre, the pharmacy (to collect several medications) and a community histology lab to give a blood sample testing different biomarkers. That one visit may easily have generated a dozen different sets of information – some structured using clinical codes, others unstructured – written notes in your EHR by the GP, additional notes from histology with results from the blood tests. Perhaps you needed an X-ray or MRI as part of the diagnosis. To ensure all this information is stored in a database about you, and not your sibling, wider family or an unrelated person with a similar name, these data require a unique identification code. Now multiply this by the few times a year you visit the doctor and again by the population for the region or country you live in. With this simple example, it is not surprising that health care is one of the major industries involved in discussions about big data.

WHAT DO WE MEAN BY 'BIG DATA'?

Surprisingly, there is no universal agreement on the meaning of big data. Herschel and Miori[1] refer to it as a 'phenomenon that is fundamentally changing what we know and do'. An alternative definition is the 'emerging use of rapidly collected complex data in such unprecedented quantities that terabytes, petabytes or even zettabytes of storage may be required.'[2] Unlike clinical trials or more traditional research designs, which can include highly selective patient groups, big-data research involves real people (patients) and their interaction with health care through their health, well-being and diseases. Box 8.1 outlines the '7 Vs' commonly used to describe big data.

DATA (LINKAGE) IS POWER

The real potential for big data to impact primary care (and health care more broadly) arises from data linkage, which may be defined as 'a merging that brings together information from two or more sources of data with the object of consolidating facts concerning an individual or an event that are not available in any separate record'.[3] There are two common approaches to link data, deterministic and probabilistic. Deterministic linkage requires a set of predefined rules to match data from two or more different sources. For example, data from two different sources would successfully merge if records both contain exactly the same patient identifier, surname, first name and sex information. By contrast, probabilistic approaches use statistical weights and

---

BOX 8.1 THE 7 Vs TO DESCRIBE BIG DATA

1. *Volume*: Size of the storage space required to store and analyse data.
2. *Velocity*: Speed at which those data are created and analysed.
3. *Variety*: Types of data sources available (routine health data, text, images, social media).
4. *Veracity*: Accuracy and credibility of data (were personal data and diagnoses entered correctly?).
5. *Variability*: Internal consistency of your data, (e.g. are your results reproducible with similar data for different periods?).
6. *Visualisation*: Use of novel techniques to communicate the patterns that would otherwise be lost in massive tables of data.
7. *Value*: Costs required to undertake big-data analysis should pay dividends for your organisation and their patients.

threshold cut-points to determine the likelihood that records in different datasets match. See Harron et al. for a thorough discussion of data linkage.[4] Regardless of the method used, the quality of linkage can only ever be as good as the quality of underlying datasets.

Routinely collected health data require a unique personal identifier (UPI) to allow one dataset (e.g. pathology) to be linked with another (e.g. hospitalisations). Most countries have their own system of uniquely identifying the population using health services. New Zealand's National Health Index (NHI) provides each person who receives health care in New Zealand a unique number.[20] The Scottish equivalent is the Community Health Index (CHI)[21] which includes the person's date of birth and a unique identifier which includes the person's sex. Other countries use UPIs across health, administrative and social care data allowing multiple data sources to be easily linked.[5-7]

While record linkage and data analysis using the actual UPIs, such as the NHI and CHI numbers, is common practice in hospitals and within health boards for funding and planning purposes, it is imperative that these 'live' data are not released to researchers. Rather, many countries now have central data repositories that provide bona fide researchers access to deidentified data, mitigating the risk of identifying individuals with corresponding governance and data-security protocols.[8] Some countries also have a number of specific advisory groups (e.g. disability, ethnicity, public benefit) to ensure marginalised or indigenous populations are not further disadvantaged from inappropriate use of big data.

BIG DATA FROM A SMALL ISLAND: NEW ZEALAND'S INTEGRATED DATA INFRASTRUCTURE

The Integrated Data Infrastructure (IDI) is the New Zealand government's big-data repository containing data routinely collected by the government's tax, social development, health, education, immigration/visa and justice agencies, as well as significant national surveys (census, health) and some nongovernment organisation's data.[9] Maintained within a 'data safe haven' under restrictions by Statistics NZ, the IDI uses birth and death, immigration visa and tax data to probabilistically assign every person who has lived in NZ a unique identifier, referred to as the 'IDI spine'. Users are given access to selected datasets based on their research aims, and data from different providers link together using the unique ID. The IDI can therefore 'enrich' health studies by linking easily with other administrative data, producing research that has direct and indirect influences on primary care. Current IDI projects include exploring relationships between occupation, mental health problems, intentional self-harm and suicide; estimating the national prevalence of dementia; estimating the cost of cardiovascular disease on the primary health care system; and determining the employment and income effects of major chronic and acute health conditions.[22]

WHAT CONTRIBUTIONS CAN BIG DATA MAKE TO HEALTH CARE?

Big-data research in health care allows researchers to gather (anonymised) information on daily patient health care interactions. The potential to influence health policy and service design is substantial if we know who uses our health care services, for what reasons, what length of time and with which outcomes. Such information is vital for planning services. For example, establishing how many individuals have hypertension or are smokers can help tailor public health education and disease prevention and improve health care by targeting variations across different geographical regions. Using near real-time epidemiological data, researchers may be able to harness big-data analytics, such as machine learning and neural networks to develop hypotheses for why variations in disease incidence and prevalence exist or to prevent the diffusion of disease.

Big-data research is complementary to, rather than a replacement for, traditional study designs. Being able to study health care interactions in a group of patients that are not the rarefied populations of clinical trials can provide valuable insight. For example, traditional research methods typically under-represent older people,[10] and yet we have a worldwide ageing population and increasing numbers of this important health-service user group with complex multimorbidity. Understanding and unravelling the complex health care interactions between primary and secondary care of this patient group is important. Fortunately, with anonymised big-data health records, we can better establish the health care needs of this vulnerable patient group.

Despite the clear benefits big data affords, there are some pitfalls to be aware of. Whilst it may seem a quick and easy alternative to traditional research, it equally needs meticulous planning (see Table 8.1). Careful consideration of limitations, which might not be significant at a small scale but could lead to wrong assumptions when applied at a population level, is required. Linking to and analysing routinely collected data can highlight reporting deficiencies, where diseases are recorded incorrectly or are missing. This could have significant implications for interpreting the national prevalence of a disease. Therefore, big-data users must consider validating information obtained from routinely collected data. Furthermore, even though health data are coded using the World Health Organization's (WHO) standardised method of coding diseases, there are several versions of the ICD-10 throughout the world.[11] Therefore, comparison of different years or countries may highlight the use of different International Classification of Diseases (ICD) versions. For example, the ICD-Australian Modification (ICD-AM) classifies dementia with Lewy bodies differently from the ICD version used in North America

TABLE 8.1 An example workflow for doing big health data research

Research phase	Step	Description
Before research begins	1	a. Define research questions b. Check the 7 Vs: Do you need big data? c. Check that you have the resources (hardware, software and research team) d. Identify data sources and seek advice from data custodians e. Establish public/stakeholder consultation f. Apply for ethical approval
Initiating research	2	a. What problem are you addressing? b. Why do you need big data and not traditional study designs? c. Why is the proposed research important? (public good as well as science) d. What datasets do you need? e. How will data be linked and by whom? f. What methods and analyses do you propose?
During research	3	a. Data safe-haven training (including Information Governance training) b. Define the population, demographics, exposures, outcomes c. Record and store outputs securely and in a systematic way (so code and data can be made available later if appropriate) d. Ensure confidentiality maintained and prepare for dissemination
After conducting research	4	a. Prepare the manuscript/report (RECORD statement) b. Feedback to stakeholders/data custodians/public c. Make data and/or code available for sharing (if appropriate)

and the UK. This subtle difference can be significant if attempts are made to compare country variations in specific diseases. When exploring geographical variations over time, analysts also need to harmonise their data to a common geographical boundary file,[12,13] as administrative boundaries change in response to population dynamics.

Whilst most big data are deidentified and anonymised, researchers must be aware that this does not mean that individuals *cannot* be identified. You must consider this in any big-data study design, working alongside data custodians to ensure that you report results at a geographical level that ensures anonymity. Most statistical agencies have disclosure rules that are designed to mitigate the identification of individuals in research. This varies between countries, some enshrine within a legal framework and others have a more pragmatic approach. What is paramount across all countries is that the researcher must be able to justify the need to access (anonymised) big data and state why conventional 'small data' would not be appropriate. For example, Statistics New Zealand considers applications in relation to the '5 safes' (safe people, projects, settings, data and output)[14] prior to allowing researchers access and will supress data in which there are less than 20 cases of a rare disease within

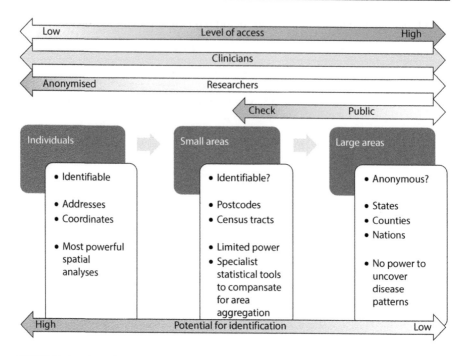

FIGURE 8.1 Level of access and potential for identification in big-data research. Reproduced with permission Exeter DJ et al. *Health Policy* 2014;114(1):88–96. [published online: 13 August 2013].[15]

a given geographical area. Data custodians should grant users access to data of different granularities according to their role as clinician, researcher or member of the public (see Figure 8.1).[15]

Big data research has several important terminologies to understand. These can be found in the glossary of terms (Table 8.2). Given the complexities of big data that have been outlined, new researchers must consider working with a multidisciplinary team to understand the data they are investigating. Including data custodians, who are familiar with the data sets, when you begin thinking about the research (i.e., grant writing) is highly recommended. Other considerations include the time, cost and access to facilities required to undertake big-data research securely. Time spent on specific training and accessing the data can be lengthy, and whilst big-data research is normally more cost efficient than similar large-scale epidemiological studies, the costs will vary between region and country and must not be underestimated. Most big-data research is now, or should be, carried out within a safe haven (or secure Data Lab). This is essential to ensure appropriate governance of the clinical (or otherwise highly sensitive) data. Creating this secure data environment requires money, and ensuring there is adequate digital capacity for back-ups of data storage creates additional set-up costs.

TABLE 8.2 Glossary of terms

Big-data research terminology

Routinely collected health data	Data collected as part of a patient's routine interactions with a health care system or service. It is not collected *a priori* for research but for the sole benefit of delivering health care to that individual.
Electronic health records (EHR)	This is the electronic storage of patient information, health care interactions and clinical reviews. Many health care systems introduced electronic paper trails in the 1980s.
Data linkage	Process of linking records from different sources that all relate to one individual and creating joined (linked) datasets.
Deterministic data linkage	Matching records using a set of predefined rules. Records successfully match when the data sources contain exactly the same patient identifier, surname, first name and sex information.
Probabilistic data linkage	The linkage of data using statistical weights and threshold cut-points to determine the likelihood that records with comparable data (e.g. patient identifier, surname, first name and sex details) relate to the same individual.
Unique personal identifier (UPI)	A unique identifier to link a record to an individual person. This may be in the form of an identifying number that includes the person's date of birth and/or a number that can only be used by that person in national records (e.g. CHI in Scotland or NHI in New Zealand).
Health informatics	Data linkage which creates large health datasets to understand and improve health care and diseases.
Data custodians	A person who has responsibility for institutional data.

REPORTING BIG-DATA RESEARCH IN PUBLICATIONS

The STROBE (strengthening the reporting of observational studies in epidemiology) Statement[16] is a proforma used to report observational epidemiological studies. In 2012, a team of international experts identified key gaps when using the STROBE Statement for reporting big-data research. These deficiencies meant that big-data research was being published without consistency, the ability to reproduce the results or transparency in how the data-linkage process was undertaken, which might produce inherent bias in data sets and interpretation. These gaps, in addition to the absence of a Medical Subject Heading (MeSH) term for routinely collected data, resulted in the RECORD (Reporting of studies conducted using observational routinely-collected health data) statement.[17] All researchers using big data should use these for reporting, and many publishers insist on their use.

BIG DATA AND THE PUBLIC: THE NEED FOR SOCIAL LICENCE

Not surprisingly, there is public concern around the use of patient information, access to patient data by third parties and the potential for commercialisation arising from research using these data. Social licence refers to not just the legal or ethical agreement to conduct research, but the *acceptance* of the proposed research by the local community and involved stakeholders.[18] NHS England's plans for care.data is a recent example of failing to obtain social licence. Care.data proposed to use primary care data for commissioning health care services, research and 'other' purposes. There are many reasons proposed relating to how the NHS failed to obtain social license; however, three critical points stand out: Firstly, the loss of the public's trust in the use of their data; secondly, concerns that general practitioners' traditional role and duties were in conflict with the proposal's aims; and thirdly, it was not seen by the general public as being in the public good.[18] This is important learning for those new to big data. It is your responsibility to check whether or not there is a Public Benefit and Privacy Panel, or equivalent, for health and social care research in your country. For example, in Scotland, researchers must complete a detailed application to justify their research proposal using routinely collected data[19] and in which they must also illustrate how they have engaged with the public to inform them of their work.

This chapter has described big data and its potential, and provided a list of considerations when using big data for conducting primary care research. There is an ever-growing list of institutes of Primary Care and Population Health that are using big health care data (such as the The Health Improvement Network, THIN, database)(REF) to understand health and disease and for conducting large-scale research studies. Big data can be extremely valuable for primary care research both now and in the future as electronic health care advances. Understanding how to harness big data to improve patient care, as well as the limitations, is vital.[23]

REFERENCES

1. Herschel R, Miori VM. Ethics & big data. *Technol Soc* 2017;49:31–36.
2. Groves P, Kayyali B, Knott D et al. *The 'Big Data' Revolution in Healthcare. Accelerating Value and Innovation*. New York: McKinsey & Company; 2013.
3. Organisation for Economic Co-operation and Development (OECD). Glossary of statistical terms. 2006. Available at: http://stats.oecd.org/glossary (Accessed 30 January 2018).
4. Harron K, Goldstein H, Dibben C. *Methodological Developments in Data Linkage*. London: John Wiley & Sons; 2015.
5. Furu K, Wettermark B, Andersen M et al. The Nordic countries as a cohort for pharmacoepidemiological research. *Basic & Clinical Pharmacol Toxicol* 2010;106(2):86–94. [published online: 8 December 2009].
6. Johannesdottir SA, Horvath-Puho E, Ehrenstein V et al. Existing data sources for clinical epidemiology: The Danish National Database of Reimbursed Prescriptions. *Clin Epidemiol* 2012;4:303–13. [published online: 4 December 2012].
7. Wyber R, Vaillancourt S, Perry W et al. Big data in global health: Improving health in low- and middle-income countries. *Bull World Health Organ* 2015;93(3):203–8. [published online: 15 March 2015].

8. Burton PR, Banner N, Elliot MJ et al. Policies and strategies to facilitate secondary use of research data in the health sciences. *Int J Epidemiol* 2017;46(6):1729–33. [published online: 13 October 2017].
9. Statistics New Zealand. Integrated Data Infrastructure. 2017. Available at: http://archive.stats.govt.nz/browse_for_stats/snapshots-of-nz/integrated-data-infrastructure.aspx (Accessed 6 February 2018).
10. McMurdo ME, Witham MD, Gillespie ND. Including older people in clinical research. *BMJ (Clinical research ed.)* 2005;331(7524):1036–7. [published online: 5 November 2005].
11. World Health Organization W. International Classifications of Diseases Version 10, ICD-10. Available at: http://apps.who.int/classifications/icd10/browse/2016/en (Accessed 14 June 2018).
12. Exeter DJ, Boyle PJ, Feng Z, Flowerdew R, Scheirloh N. The creation of 'consistent areas through time' (CATTs) in Scotland, 1981–2001. *Popul Trends* 2005;(119):28–36.
13. Norman P, Rees P, Boyle P. Achieving data compatibility over space and time: Creating consistent geographical zones. *Int J Popul Geography* 2003;9(5):365–86.
14. Statistics New Zealand. How we keep IDI and LBD data safe. Available at: http://archive.stats.govt.nz/browse_for_stats/snapshots-of-nz/integrated-data-infrastructure/keep-data-safe.aspx 2017 (Accessed 6 February 2018).
15. Exeter DJ, Rodgers S, Sabel CE. 'Whose data is it anyway?' The implications of putting small area-level health and social data online. *Health Policy* 2014;114(1):88–96. [published online: 13 August 2013].
16. von Elm E, Altman DG, Egger M et al. The Strengthening the Reporting of Observational Studies in Epidemiology (STROBE) statement: Guidelines for reporting observational studies. *Annals of Internal Medicine* 2007;147(8):573–7. [published online: 17 October 2007].
17. Benchimol EI, Smeeth L, Guttmann A et al. The REporting of studies Conducted using Observational Routinely-collected health Data (RECORD) statement. *PLOS Medicine* 2015;12(10):e1001885. [published online: 7 October 2015].
18. Carter P, Laurie GT, Dixon-Woods M. The social licence for research: Why care.data ran into trouble. *J Med Ethics* 2015;41(5):404–9. [published online: 27 January 2015].
19. Information Governance Scotland NHS. Public Benefit and Privacy Panel for Health and Social Care (http://www.informationgovernance.scot.nhs.uk/pbpphsc/) (Accessed 6 February 2018).
20. Ministry of Health. National Health Index Overview, 2018. Available at: http://www.health.govt.nz/our-work/health-identity/national-health-index/national-health-index-overview (Accessed 20 May 2018).
21. Information Statistics Division National Health Service - Scotland, 2018. Community Health Index. Available at: http://www.ndc.scot.nhs.uk/Dictionary-A-Z/Definitions/index.asp?Search=C&ID=128&Title=CHI%20Number (Accessed 20 May 2018).
22. Statistics New Zealand. How researchers are using the IDI, 2018. Available at: http://archive.stats.govt.nz/browse_for_stats/snapshots-of-nz/integrated-data-infrastructure/researchers-using-idi.aspx (Accessed 20 May 2018).
23. The Health Improvement Network (THIN) database. University College London, 2015. https://www.ucl.ac.uk/pcph/research-groups-themes/thin-pub/database.

CHAPTER 9

Conducting primary care research using social media

Charilaos Lygidakis,
Ana Luísa Neves, Liliana Laranjo
and Luís Pinho-Costa

Social media offers great potential in primary care research. Online platforms can be used to conduct experimental studies, facilitating the recruitment and retention of participants, as well as the delivery of the intervention. As patients are increasingly able to use information technology to help make informed decisions about their health care,[1,2] reports show that the use of social media for health-information seeking is not limited to the younger demographics anymore.[3] Notably, patients seem to be willing to share their health data in communities of peers, such as PatientsLikeMe, and actively engage with researchers.[4] Additionally, publicly available social media data can be used for secondary analysis purposes, potentially contributing to the monitoring of health topics and disease surveillance. Finally, social media tools can be used to outsource tasks (Box 9.1), streamline the management of research projects and facilitate team collaboration.

RECRUITMENT AND RETENTION OF STUDY PARTICIPANTS

Recruiting an adequate and representative sample and tackling attrition are two important determinants of the validity of study results. Social media facilitates access to a large group of people who are not limited by geographic boundaries. Depending on the desired sample, advertisements on social networks can be useful for recruitment, especially for those populations that are underserved and/or difficult to reach, such as geographically isolated

BOX 9.1 CASE STUDY: CROWDSOURCING

In February 2015, Stanford Medicine X—the academic conference on emerging technology and medicine—challenged all health care stakeholders to spark scholarly research activity in health care social media. Proposals should address one of the following questions:

- How is social media transforming health care?
- How is social media being used to innovate medical education?
- How did social media contribute to the preceding Medicine X conference?

Word of this research challenge soon reached a group of new and future family doctors from across the world who were interested in change management and innovation on a global level. The primary communication platform for the group was social media, most notably with regular tweetchats on Twitter under the hashtag #FMChangeMakers.

In response to this challenge, a tweetchat was organised as an open call to collaborative brainstorming, to leverage the crowd's judgment to filter and rank proposals and to recruit researchers for a working group. Thanks to multiple contributors, such a tweetchat and ensuing discussions on social media became the cornerstone of a research project where the selection of the theme and research question, researcher's recruitment, drafting and implementation of the research protocol and as dissemination of results/publication, were outsourced to 'an undefined (and generally large) network of people in the form of an open call', thereby meeting the definition of crowdsourcing. The research aimed to create and study an index of global reach for health care hashtags (and tweeters therein), focusing on the field of primary care and family medicine. Such research ended up being selected as one of the ten finalists of the Medicine X Research Challenge that year and led to a publication.[31]

people, adolescents and young adults, at-risk populations who find it less confrontational to engage online initially, minorities and shift workers.[5,6] Thanks to the tools provided by platforms such as Facebook and Google Adwords, potential participants can be effectively targeted depending on their demographic characteristics and interests. Advertisements can be paid or free, and their results can be monitored in real time to improve the targeting strategy. Furthermore, investigators can post messages in specific communities of users and collaborate with opinion leaders to increase the chance of identifying and recruiting appropriate participants.

To encourage participation throughout a study, maintain contact and limit losses to follow-up,[7,8] appropriate strategies should be put in place, aiming at establishing a relationship between researchers and participants.[9] These may include providing a direct line of communication with the investigators via private messaging, as well as sharing progress reports, important milestones and study outcomes with the participants.[8] Using mailing lists to send newsletters with rich multimedia content can also be an affordable and fast way of reaching out.

It is also crucial to comprehend the nuances of how the existing popular social networks, such as Facebook and Instagram, are employed by their users, so that investigators can capitalise on their high retention rates.[10] For instance, many users interact on social networks with people who they already know offline; applying positive peer-pressure techniques (e.g. publishing lists of achievements) can help with the engagement of participants who are familiar with each other.[10,11]

Information with low relevance to the individual's context and/or needs may have a limited effect.[12] Tailoring communication and limiting unnecessary messages are effective strategies to assimilate health-related information. Personalised feedback based on the patient's answers can result in more behavioural changes. Particular caution, however, may be needed to avoid possible contamination, and efforts to prevent the identification of study participants must be made, ensuring that a participant or a situation cannot be identified by the sum of the information shared.

DELIVERY OF HEALTH INTERVENTIONS
Behaviour-change interventions using social media

The growing burden of chronic disease highlights the urgency to optimise lifestyle behaviours. Although interventions to promote health behaviour change have shown efficacy, strategies to improve their dissemination and accessibility are critical to realise their full potential. Social media and other informatic interventions may be useful in addressing these issues.

Social media can be employed in behaviour-change interventions, such as those based on Social Cognitive Theory – one of the most commonly used behavioural change theories. According to SCT, 'an individual's knowledge acquisition can be directly related to observing others within the context of social interactions, experiences, and outside media influences'.[13,14] Systematic reviews evaluating the effects of social media (e.g. blogs, discussion boards, wikis) on health behaviour change and health promotion have shown promising results.[15,16]

One particular type of social-media tool increasingly being used in behaviour-change interventions is social networking sites (SNS).[17] SNSs are platforms that enable users to create their own personal profiles and build a network of connections with other users. So far, Facebook has been the most commonly used SNS in such interventions.[18–20] However, some studies are also using more-specific SNSs, sometimes designed for particular research purposes.[21,22]

General SNSs, like Facebook, present some advantages for the implementation of health interventions, compared with health-specific SNSs.[23] They are a part of the daily lives of millions of users worldwide, potentially facilitating the recruitment of participants and minimising problems of retention and lack of adherence to interventions.[17] Despite all the advantages and benefits of SNSs, it is important to consider the potential risks and unintended consequences of the use of social media in health interventions. One of the main concerns is the quality and validity of the information disseminated through them. A study of diabetes social networks has found a considerable variation in scientific validity of the information disseminated, as well as in the moderation and auditing of those discussions.[24] Another risk is that social media may be used for marketing purposes (e.g. tobacco, alcohol, direct-to-consumer advertisement of medications) or as public displays of unhealthy behaviour (e.g. pro-anorexia, self-injury, drug use).[25] Social media may have a negative psychological impact on individuals if used to propagate offensive, inappropriate or stigmatising content.

MENTAL HEALTH INTERVENTIONS

Cognitive behavioural therapy (CBT) is effective in the management and treatment of a variety of mental health problems, especially anxiety and depression. CBT can be delivered online, with very good results, including high adherence and effectiveness.[26,27] Such interventions can be widely accessible and convenient, turning them into a cost-effective alternative that is able to benefit a greater number of patients than is possible in traditional CBT.

Online CBT can be self-guided or supported by a clinician, and it may include reminders, access to lessons and educational content.[28] The role of health professionals can also be to actively encourage access to online CBT (known as 'facilitated access').[29] The involvement of the physician in such interventions has the potential to strengthen the therapeutic alliance between him/her and the patient, thus aiding the attainment of the goals of the therapy.[30]

SECONDARY ANALYSIS OF PUBLICLY AVAILABLE SOCIAL MEDIA DATA

Social media posts have a rich health care content. Monitoring infectious and noncommunicable diseases, as well as adverse drug reactions, is possible by analysing content from both official sources and informal communications (see Figure 9.1 on Ebola outbreaks as an example). If curated and analysed in a meaningful way, these data can be used to derive useful insights into patients' needs and expectations towards their health.

Seminal knowledge on emerging health topics can be provided by classic social media post metrics (identification of tweets with a higher number of retweets or replies or posts with a higher number of 'likes' on Facebook). The

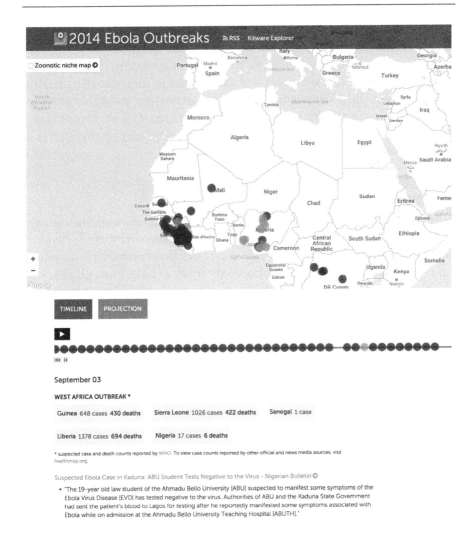

FIGURE 9.1 HealthMap crawls a wide range of sources in different languages, including reports and tweets, to monitor disease propagation, such as the 2014 Ebola outbreak.

global relevance of specific health care hashtags can also be ranked according to their global reach index, which incorporates the number of impressions, tweets, tweeters, user locations and user languages.[31]

Another approach to studying emerging health topics, as perceived by patients, is to map the content of posts into concepts or themes (e.g. thematic analysis). A systematic analysis of 2.5 million tweets has recently provided novel information on the most common themes that arise in the diabetes debate on Twitter.[32] This type of analysis also provides useful insights into the type of users that contribute to each theme, and can be used as a proxy measure of patient engagement in specific health topics. Notably, mapping the interaction between users using network analysis of social-media content generates relevant information regarding the identification of influential users and social hubs in disseminating health information.[32] This knowledge has implications for public health, as establishing partnerships with influential users, as well as encouraging interactions between different communities of users, can be effective as a health-promotion strategy.

SOCIAL CITATION, TEAM COLLABORATION AND PROJECT MANAGEMENT

Social citation tools can enhance the collaboration of teams working together on a joint manuscript or, generally, on a common project. In modern reference managers, such as Zotero and Mendeley, users can follow curated bibliographies, and establish their own groups and/or join others. Within these groups, it is possible to collect and share articles and other research-related outputs, such as data sets and drafts, and discuss with the fellow team members.

The inclusion of social-networking features in project-management tools can increase productivity and facilitate team collaboration and coordination, while maintaining the motivation of the study investigators and data collectors and supporting their operations throughout the project. Among the wide range of available platforms, two different, yet complementary, examples of collaborative tools are provided below: Trello and Slack.

Trello

Trello is a visual, flexible and agile tool that helps with keeping track of the tasks of a project and the assignments of the activities, while enabling communication with the team members. It features an easy-to-use user interface—one that you can be sure that all your team members will understand—and it is available both on desktop computers (on browsers) and as a mobile app.

With Trello, the project leader can create teams of co-workers (e.g. investigators and data collectors) and assign them to *boards*, which can be considered as virtual workspaces. Borrowing from Toyota's Kanban system, Trello provides a representation of the project's tasks as *cards*, which can be moved around the workspace, signifying the different dependences and steps that need to be completed. The cards can be classified into 'lists', which provide a visual way to categorise the activities and create a workflow. For instance, one very typical way of using this is to create lists with *To Do*, *Work in Progress* and *Done* tasks (Figure 9.2).

The cards provide a simple, yet flexible way to describe tasks (Figure 9.3). Each card can:

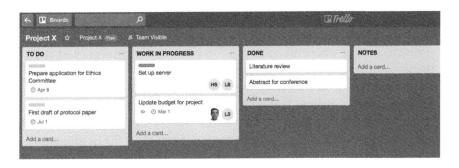

FIGURE 9.2 A typical arrangement of a Trello board, with cards categorised in four lists: To Do, Work in Progress, Done, Notes.

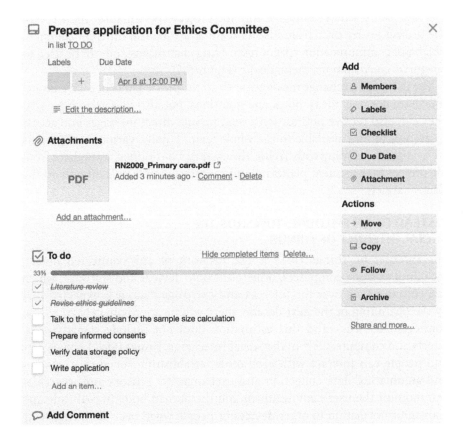

FIGURE 9.3 A card associated to an activity.

- Be assigned to one or more team members who will be responsible for the activity and will receive notifications when there are related updates.
- Provide a space where all team members can post comments and can mention other users, who will receive a notification.
- Include attachments directly from one's computer or from online storage services, such as Dropbox and Drive.
- Have a due date-the members to whom the card is assigned receive notifications, while a calendar provides an overview of the deadlines of the different tasks.
- Feature checklists in which the users can include smaller tasks that need to be completed.
- Be colour-coded with various labels.

Slack

Slack is an online platform which helps with the communication among the team members, makes all exchanged information easily searchable and represents a more effective way for project coordination than email. The project leader can create his/her team and establish different *channels*, which are communication spaces resembling chat rooms and can be used to categorise conversations thematically (Figure 9.4).

The users can exchange messages with all the participants of each channel and share not only ideas, notes and questions, but also files and blog posts. They can also receive notifications, send private direct messages and access an archive of files available to the whole team. Finally, various integrations are available, including with Trello: The users can be notified for updates from the project management platform, and can create new cards directly in the Slack channels.

INSTEAD OF AN EPILOGUE: TOWARDS THE SOCIAL INTERNET OF THINGS

The Internet of Things (IoT) is the network of any connected object, including sensors, computers, other electronic devices and software, which can communicate over the Internet and exchange data. It is expected that by the beginning of the next decade, there will be approximately 20 billion connected devices—and this estimation does not include smartphones, tablets and computers.[33,34] In the Social Internet of Things (SIoT), the objects and people can interact with each other, establishing social relationships and automating data collection and exchange.[35,36] Sensors and wearables can monitor the user's environment and the human body in real time and transmit information to other devices or people when necessary, triggering context-aware and tailored activities (for instance, in ambient assisted living), while aggregated data from multiple sources can produce intelligence for

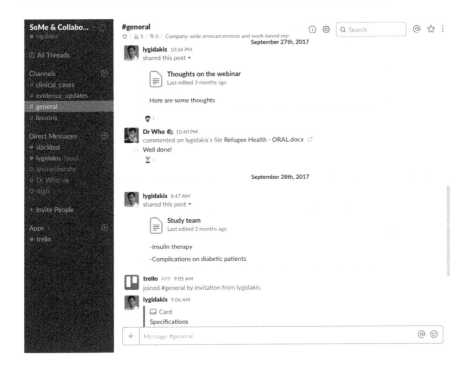

FIGURE 9.4 A team configuration in Slack with various thematic channels.

public-health applications (for instance, determining the quality of the air and alerting asthmatic patients).[37,38] The extension of social networks to smart connected objects will offer new solutions to health care and is a promising research field.

REFERENCES

1. De Bronkart D. From patient centred to people powered: Autonomy on the rise. *BMJ*. 2015;350:h148.
2. Topol E. *The Patient Will See You Now: The Future of Medicine is in Your Hands*. New York, NY: Basic Books; 2015.
3. Stellefson M, Chaney B, Barry AE et al. Web 2.0 Chronic Disease Self-Management for Older Adults: A Systematic Review. Eysenbach G, editor. *J Med Internet Res [Internet]*. 14 February 2013;15(2):e35. Available at: http://www.ncbi.nlm.nih.gov/pmc/articles/PMC3636299/
4. Ryan GS. Online social networks for patient involvement and recruitment in clinical research. *Nurse Res* 2013;21(1):35–9.
5. Fenner Y, Garland SM, Moore EE et al. Web-based recruiting for health research using a social networking site: An exploratory study. *J Med Internet Res* 2012;14(1):e20.
6. Ramo DE, Prochaska JJ. Broad reach and targeted recruitment using Facebook for an online survey of young adult substance use. *J Med Internet Res* 2012;14(1):e28.
7. Hunt JR, White E. Retaining and tracking cohort study members. *Epidemiol Rev [Internet]* 1998;20(1):57–70. Available at: http://www.ncbi.nlm.nih.gov/pubmed/9762509

8. Butler J, Quinn SC, Fryer CS, Garza MA, Kim KH, Thomas SB. Characterizing researchers by strategies used for retaining minority participants: Results of a national survey. *Contemp Clin Trials* 2013;36(1):61–7.

9. Weitzman ER, Adida B, Kelemen S, Mandl KD. Sharing Data for Public Health Research by Members of an International Online Diabetes Social Network. Shea BJ, editor. *PLOS ONE [Internet]* 27 April 2011 [cited 8 January 2018];6(4):e19256. Available at: http://dx.plos.org/10.1371/journal.pone.0019256.

10. Maher CA, Lewis LK, Ferrar K, Marshall S, De Bourdeaudhuij I, Vandelanotte C. Are Health Behavior Change Interventions That Use Online Social Networks Effective? A Systematic Review. Eysenbach G, editor. *J Med Internet Res [Internet]* 14 February 2014;16(2):e40. Available at: http://www.ncbi.nlm.nih.gov/pmc/articles/PMC3936265/

11. Foster D, Linehan C, Kirman B, Lawson S, James G. Motivating Physical Activity at Work: Using Persuasive Social Media for Competitive Step Counting. In: *Proceedings of the 14th International Academic MindTrek Conference: Envisioning Future Media Environments [Internet]*. New York, NY, USA: ACM; 2010. p. 111–6. (MindTrek '10). Available at: http://doi.acm.org/10.1145/1930488.1930510

12. Kreuter M. *Tailoring Health Messages: Customizing Communication with Computer Technology*. LEA's communication series. Mahwah, N.J.: L. Erlbaum; 2000. xiii, 270.

13. Bandura A. Social cognitive theory of mass communication. In: Bryant J, Zillmann D, editors. *Media Effects: Advances in Theory and Research*. London: Mahwah; 2002. p. 94–124.

14. Laranjo L, Lau A, Coiera E. Design and Implementation of Behavioral Informatics Interventions. In: *Cognitive Informatics in Health and Biomedicine*. Springer International Publishing; 2017. p. 13–42.

15. Williams G, Hamm MP, Shulhan J, Vandermeer B, Hartling L. Social media interventions for diet and exercise behaviours: A systematic review and meta-analysis of randomised controlled trials. *BMJ Open* 4:2014.

16. Chou WY, Prestin A, Lyons C, Wen KY. Web 2.0 for health promotion: reviewing the current evidence. *Am J Public Health [Internet]* 2013;103(1):e9–18. Available at: http://www.ncbi.nlm.nih.gov/pubmed/23153164

17. Laranjo L, Arguel A, Neves AL et al. The influence of social networking sites on health behavior change: a systematic review and meta-analysis. *J Am Med Informatics Assoc [Internet]* 2014; Available at: http://www.ncbi.nlm.nih.gov/pubmed/25005606.

18. Cavallo DN, Tate DF, Ries A V, Brown JD, Devellis RF, Ammerman AS. A social media-based physical activity intervention: A randomized controlled trial. *Am J Prev Med* 2012;43(5):527–32.

19. Napolitano MA, Hayes S, Bennett GG, Ives AK, Foster GD. Using facebook and text messaging to deliver a weight loss program to college students. *Obesity* 2013;21(1):25–31.

20. Valle CG, Tate DF, Mayer DK, Allicock M, Cai J. A randomized trial of a Facebook-based physical activity intervention for young adult cancer survivors. *J Cancer Surviv* 2013;7(3):355–68.

21. Brindal E, Freyne J, Saunders I, Berkovsky S, Smith G, Noakes M. Features predicting weight loss in overweight or obese participants in a web-based intervention: Randomized trial. *J Med Internet Res* 2012;14(6):e173.

22. Centola D. The spread of behavior in an online social network experiment. *Science* 2010;329(5996):1194–7.

23. Cobb NK, Graham AL. Health behavior interventions in the age of Facebook. *Am J Prev Med* 2012;43(5):571–2.

24. Weitzman ER, Cole E, Kaci L, Mandl KD. Social but safe? Quality and safety of diabetes-related online social networks. *J Am Med Informatics Assoc* 2011;18(3):292–7.

25. Lau AYS, Sintchenko V, Crimmins J, Magrabi F, Gallego B, Coiera E. Impact of a web-based personally controlled health management system on influenza vaccination and health services utilization rates: A randomized controlled trial. *J Am Med Informatics Assoc* 2012;19(5):719–27.

26. Proudfoot J, Klein B, Barak A et al. Establishing guidelines for executing and reporting internet intervention research. *Cogn Behav Ther* 2011;40(2):82–97.

27. Andrews G, Cuijpers P, Craske MG, McEvoy P, Titov N. Computer therapy for the anxiety and depressive disorders is effective, acceptable and practical health care: A meta-analysis. *PLOS ONE* 2010;5(10):e13196.

28. Coiera E. *Guide to Health Informatics*. 3rd ed. London: CRC Press; 2015. p. 440.

29. Lopez-Pelayo H, Wallace P, Segura L et al. A randomised controlled non-inferiority trial of primary care-based facilitated access to an alcohol reduction website (EFAR Spain): The study protocol. *BMJ Open [Internet]* 2014;4(12):e007130. Available at: http://www.ncbi.nlm.nih.gov/pubmed/25552616

30. Lygidakis C, Wallace P, Tersar C et al. Download Your Doctor: Implementation of a Digitally Mediated Personal Physician Presence to Enhance Patient Engagement With a Health-Promoting Internet Application. *JMIR Res Protoc [Internet]* 4 March 2016 [cited 3 March 2016];5(1):e36. Available at: http://www.researchprotocols.org/2016/1/e36/

31. Pinho-Costa L, Yakubu K, Hoedebecke K et al. Healthcare hashtag index development: Identifying global impact in social media. *J Biomed Inform* 2016;63:390–9.

32. Beguerisse-Díaz M, McLennan AK, Garduño-Hernández G, Barahona M, Ulijaszek SJ. The 'who' and 'what' of #diabetes on Twitter. *Digit Heal [Internet]* 1 January 2017;3:2055207616688841. Available at: https://doi.org/10.1177/2055207616688841

33. van der Meulen R. Gartner Says 8.4 Billion Connected 'Things' Will Be in Use in 2017, Up 31 Percent From 2016 [Internet]. Vol. 2016, Gartner Press Release. 2017. p. 1. Available at: https://www.gartner.com/newsroom/id/3598917

34. Nordrum A. Popular internet of things forecast of 50 billion devices by 2020 is outdated. *IEEE Spectr [Internet]* 2016;0–2. Available at: https://spectrum.ieee.org/tech-talk/telecom/internet/popular-internet-of-things-forecast-of-50-billion-devices-by-2020-is-outdated

35. Thuemmler C, Bai C. *Health 4.0: How Virtualization and Big Data are Revolutionizing Healthcare [Internet]*. 1st ed. Thuemmler C, Bai C, editors. Springer International Publishing; 2017 [cited 20 June 2017]. XII, 254. Available at: http://link.springer.com/10.1007/978-3-319-47617-9

36. Baktha K, Dev M, Gupta H, Agarwal A, Balamurugan B. Social network analysis in healthcare. In: Bhatt C, Dey N, Ashour AS, editors. *Internet of Things and Big Data Technologies for Next Generation Healthcare*. Cham: Springer; 2017.

37. Turcu CE, Turcu CO. Social Internet of Things in Healthcare: From Things to Social Things in Internet of Things. In: Reis CI, Maximiano M, da S, editors. *Internet of Things and Advanced Application in Healthcare [Internet]*. Hershey, PA, USA: IGI Global; 2017. p. 266–95. Available at: http://services.igi-global.com/resolvedoi/resolve.aspx?doi=10.4018/978-1-5225-1820-4.ch010

38. Kranz M, Roalter L, Michahelles F. Things that twitter: Social networks and the internet of things. *What can Internet Things do Citiz Work Eighth Int Conf Pervasive Comput (Pervasive 2010) [Internet]*. 2010;(May 2010):1–10. Available at: https://pdfs.semanticscholar.org/5409/c0eda06876ce479c14fc895bfcdece8872b4.pdf

CHAPTER 10

Quality improvement research in primary care

Andrew W. Knight and Paresh Dawda

WHAT IS QUALITY IMPROVEMENT RESEARCH AND WHY IS IT IMPORTANT IN PRIMARY CARE?

We constantly talk in our staff rooms and on our tea breaks across primary care services about how to improve the way we provide care. Forms are redesigned and processes are tweaked. Do things improve? All improvement requires change but not all changes are an improvement.[1] Did our improvement efforts achieve positive results? Which methods of quality improvement work best? What are the contextual factors which affect success? Rigorous scientific enquiry into these questions is called quality improvement research (QIR). See Box 10.1 for some definitions of QIR and related terms.

BOX 10.1   DEFINITIONS

Quality Improvement: A structured organisational process for involving personnel in planning and executing a continuous flow of improvements to provide quality health care that meets or exceeds expectations.[2]

Quality Improvement Research: Applied research aimed at informing change that improves policy and practice.[3]

Improvement Science: A field of knowledge which applies research methods to help understand what impacts on quality improvement.[4]

Implementation Research: The scientific study of methods to promote the systematic uptake of research findings and other evidence-based practices into routine practice and, hence, to improve the quality and effectiveness of health services.[5]

Quality improvement (QI) appeals to those who work and research in primary care because of its potential to achieve the 'quadruple aim'[6]: improved health outcomes, improved patient experience, reduced costs and increased joy in work. QI can reduce suffering and waste by providing practical solutions to problems that practitioners and patients face every day. Primary care faces many challenges in getting evidence into practice in busy clinical contexts.[7] QI efforts are designed to make best evidence care routine. However, QI efforts are often unsustained, fail, or involve unacceptable and unrewarded extra work for front-line clinical staff.

QIR aims to apply rigorous scientific enquiry to improvement work in order to identify strategies that maximise the chance of good outcomes for patients and health workers. A quality improvement researcher in primary care has two essential roles:

1. Supporting teams to plan well designed quality-improvement interventions
2. Designing rigorous evaluations of quality improvement interventions
   a. So that teams can learn
   b. To add to the body of knowledge about QI in primary care

This chapter provides guidance on these two roles and discusses some issues unique to QIR, including the tension between research and quality improvement, ethics approval and publication challenges.

PLANNING WELL DESIGNED QUALITY IMPROVEMENT PROJECTS

Here we outline some considerations in planning high-quality QI projects. There are numerous resources and courses that provide detail. Some are listed in Box 10.5 at the end of this chapter.

Choose your partners

Consider who to invite to be part of the project. Frontline clinicians understand the problems and can suggest solutions. Leaders provide 'buy-in' required for system and business change. Funders are seeking better outcomes and savings. Consumers experience the health journey and can help target problems and outcomes that they value.[8,9] Improvement agencies and university departments can contribute research expertise. Effective governance is crucial for effective improvement and will vary depending on the size and context of the project.

Problem definition

The first step in designing strong QIR is defining and understanding the problem (see example Box 10.2). Problems may be identified through

- Incident reporting or complaints
- Routine data from your clinical service (variable or low achievement of outcomes)
- Research into evidence/practice gaps
- Brainstorming by consumers or providers

There are a range of tools for problem identification associated with QI.[10] 'Brainstorming' and 'affinity' can help you identify and prioritise issues. 'Pareto' analyses can highlight the small number of problems that have the biggest impact. 'Process mapping' may reveal waste, delay or unnecessary complexity. Links to resources describing these and other QI tools can be found in the resources section in Box 10.5 at the end of this chapter. Problems can be prioritised by size, cost to the system, the availability of known evidence around intervention, funding and likely clinician buy-in.

It is essential to thoroughly understand the problem you have chosen. How big is it? What is its nature? Literature and research (both qualitative and quantitative) can offer deeper understanding, which will greatly increase the likelihood of successful improvement.

Design the intervention

Quality improvement and QIR are more effective if QI interventions themselves are methodologically strong. They will usually employ a strong theoretical

---

**BOX 10.2   EXAMPLE: UNDERSTANDING A PROBLEM
WITH CANCER CARE/GP INTEGRATION**

We conducted a qualitative study interviewing a purposive, diverse sample of 23 GPs about their experience and views of the integration of cancer services in our region. They identified delay in letters about cancer care as an issue. A short fax-back survey attached to discharge letters asked GPs to quantify the delay and set a goal. The steering group agreed that we would aim to decrease letter delay from an average of 27 days to less than seven days.

BOX 10.3   THE THREE MFI QUESTIONS[12]

Q1. What are we trying to achieve? (Aim)
A good improvement aim will be measurable and time-limited.
Q2. How will we know our changes have made a difference? (Measures)
A good improvement measure will be related to the aim and easily collected.
Q3. What changes do we think will make a difference? (Change Ideas)
Good change ideas will be related to the aim and may arise from known evidence and/or team ideas.

approach. There are a number of well recognised theoretical approaches[11] including Statistical Process Control, Six Sigma, Lean, and Plan/Do/Study/Act models such as the Langley and Nolan 'Model for Improvement' (MFI).[12] Quality Improvement Collaboratives[13,14] have been widely used to implement and teach QI in primary care often using the MFI as the core theoretical construct.

Aims, measures and change ideas (see Box 10.3)

Effective improvement projects have clear aims. Useful aims are important enough to be meaningful to clinicians and enthuse funders, and small enough to be achievable. An aim should be specific, measurable, achievable, realistic and timely or 'SMART'.[15]

There is an extensive knowledge base growing around the science of developing useful clinical measures for primary care.[16] Ideal improvement measures relate directly to the aim, have face validity for clinicians and are easily collected (e.g. electronically extractable from clinical records). Some examples of aims and measures from the Australian Primary Care Collaboratives programme can be seen in Table 10.1.

Ideas about effective changes can be collected from consumers, clinicians and literature. Some examples of change ideas from the diabetes work of the Australian Primary Care Collaboratives programme are listed in Table 10.2.[19] Changes are commonly tested using small-scale, rapid-improvement, cycles often referred to as plan/do/study/act cycles (or PDSA cycles).[20] Hundreds of rapid improvement cycles may be carried out in a QI project. By testing small changes and spreading success change can be safely accelerated and spread.

Designing rigorous evaluations of quality improvement interventions

In QI project evaluation the researcher seeks to understand:

1. To what extent an intervention worked and results can be causally attributed to it; and
2. Why or how the intervention worked; that is, what were the explanatory factors associated with the structures and processes of the delivery of the intervention?[21]

Portela et al.[22] and Ovretveit[23] have produced useful resources exploring the different study designs used in QIR. The study of improvement interventions is an emerging field characterised by debate and diversity.[22] A number of frameworks have been developed aimed at summarising and supporting knowledge of effective QIR approaches. The Consolidated Framework for Implementation Research (CFIR)[24] provides a 'menu of constructs' associated with effective implementation. The exploration, preparation implementation,

TABLE 10.1 Examples of improvement project aims and measures from the Australian Primary Care Collaboratives Program[17,18]

Topic	Aim	Sample measures
Coronary Heart Disease	A reduction in the mortality of patients with CHD by 30% in 3 years	% of patients with CHD where LDL cholesterol recorded within the previous 12 months was less than or equal to 2 mmol/L % of patients with CHD whose most recent BP reading taken within the previous 12 months was less than or equal to 130/80 mmHg % of patients with CHD whose smoking status has been recorded
Chronic Obstructive Pulmonary Disease	To reduce by 30% the number of hospital admissions (compared with the previous 12 months)	% of patients with COPD whose smoking status has been recorded % of patients with COPD with a recorded spirometry result % of patients with COPD with a recorded influenza vaccine within the previous 12 months
Diabetes	50% of patients with diabetes within participating practices have an HbA1C of 7% or less	% of patients with diabetes who have had an HbA1C measurement result recorded within the previous 12 months % of patients with diabetes who have had an HbA1C measurement recorded within the previous 12 months categorised as less than or equal to 7%

Source: Knight AW et al. *BMJ Qual Saf* 2012;21(11):948–55; Improvement Measures available for submission to the Improvement Foundation databases. 2016. Available at: https://apcc.org.au/download/if-measure-suite-measure-specifications-v5-8-31-march-2016/?wpdmdl=1210. (Accessed September 2017).

and sustainment (EPIS) framework[25] seeks to provide an evidence-based four-phase model of the implementation process developed from existing literature. The PARiHS (Promoting Action on Research Implementation in Health Services) framework[26] examines the interaction between evidence, context and facilitation (the type of support provided) in successful implementation.

QIR study designs may be divided into two broad categories: Quality improvement projects in which the primary goal is securing change and evaluative studies in which the primary goal is scientific advance.[22] This differentiation can at times be artificial with some studies sharing aims and characteristics of both categories.

Quality improvement projects

Characteristically, these projects are aimed at securing positive change in a particular service rather than research directed towards generating new knowledge. They will usually be designed using principles such as the Model for Improvement that has already been outlined. Statistical Process Control

TABLE 10.2 Some of the diabetes change ideas used in the Australian Primary Care Collaboratives Program[19]

Change principle	Change idea
Establish a system for creating, validating and updating a register of people with diabetes	• Agree on a clear definition of diabetes and the two subdivisions (type 1 and 2) using existing guidelines • Develop a register of people with diabetes • Develop systems to maintain valid registers
Be systematic and proactive in managing the care of people with diabetes	• Establish a multidisciplinary team (micro-team) to manage the care of people with diabetes • Identify a lead health professional to coordinate the care of people with diabetes • Establish practice protocols (or customise existing protocols) for the care of people with diabetes • Embed the use of protocols through the use of computerised templates • Establish proactive call and recall arrangements for people with diabetes • Ensure people with diabetes receive optimal care including the use of drug therapies • Undertake annual cycles of care to claim service incentive payments
Involve patients in delivering and developing their care	• Maximise self-management by people with diabetes • Develop a deliberate strategy for self-management • Integrate the patient's perspective in the design of services • Ensure written communication is appropriate and understood • Pay special attention to the needs of hard-to-reach groups

Source: Knight AW et al. *BMJ Qual Saf* 2012;21(11):956–63.

(SPC)[27] methods which involve repeated measurements over time are often the preferred method of analysis of data in quality improvement projects. Data may be presented graphically in control charts, run charts and frequency plots. SPC is suited to the iteratively evolving nature of improvement work in contrast to methods used for statistical hypothesis testing in more familiar research paradigms.

Evaluative studies
Evaluative studies are characteristically prospectively conceived as research projects which generate new knowledge. They may be commissioned to evaluate improvement projects.

Quasi-experimental and experimental designs
Non-comparative quasi-experimental designs include before/after designs, time series and PDSA testing. These may be used when controlled trials are

not feasible, often for reasons of cost or practicality. Assigning causality is more difficult in the absence of control groups.

Comparative experimental designs (using control groups) include randomised control trials (RCTs) and non-randomised designs such as cross-over comparative and stepped-wedge trials. RCTs provide increased ability for direct inferences regarding causality. They are difficult to implement in complex adaptive systems such as health. Cluster RCT designs, where units or institutions are randomised rather than individuals, may address some issues but require larger sample sizes and may be more expensive. Stepped-wedge designs involve sequential roll out of an intervention so that all clusters receive it by the end of the trial. Reviews find experimental studies in quality improvement frequently suffer from risk of bias.[28] It is common for the intervention to mutate over time while the assumption for RCTs is a stable, well-defined, uniformly delivered intervention. Outcomes may also be strongly influenced by variations in the contexts in which interventions are delivered.

Observational designs
These studies evaluate change without control groups in real world settings using qualitative and/or quantitative data. While attribution of causality in uncontrolled studies is more difficult, these interventions tend to be set in the real world and so may have great applicability to other similar services. They may be used where controlled studies are difficult or unethical. Examples of observational study designs include audit evaluations, cohort evaluations and cross-sectional and case-control studies. Qualitative studies may include single-case evaluations which look at a single clinical service or organisation. Case comparison studies and realist evaluation have been used in observational designs.

Action evaluations
Action evaluation designs allow feedback from the researcher/evaluator to the implementers to permit enhancement of the intervention while it is being implemented. The researcher may present findings to implementers early on and help them redesign the intervention as the project proceeds.

Process evaluations
QIR may use process evaluation to examine components of the intervention and the fidelity and uniformity with which the intervention is applied. Process evaluations can combine longitudinal and cross-sectional approaches and may include surveys and interviews of managers, frontline team members and patients. Direct observation and document review, including medical records, may be used.

Qualitative methods

Qualitative methods can explore what actually happened in a project, helping to understand why and how the activities succeeded or failed. Common methods include interviews, ethnographic observation and documentary analysis[29] described elsewhere in this book. These approaches can explain the contextual factors that contribute to the impact of a quality improvement project and the fidelity with which interventions are implemented.

ISSUES IN QIR

The tension between research and QI

Researchers may challenge the contribution of QI to scientific knowledge of health care. They may be critical of uncontrolled projects, research design rigor and use of unvalidated measures. Those using QI methods may be critical of what are seen as slow timeframes, cautious strategies and unrealistic conclusions drawn from more traditional research designs. RCTs may be seen as artificial, impractical and meaningless in real-life health care in complex adaptive systems. Solberg et al. explored some of these tensions.[30] Their table comparing the differences in measurement for research, quality improvement and accountability is reproduced as Table 10.3.

As QI and QIR continue to develop, this tension is being considered and explored. The risks of precipitate adoption and spread of unproven QI interventions are significant.[31] Methods for increasing the confidence in the effectiveness of QI continue to evolve. The improvement of services in real world health care settings is clearly important for improving value to patients. The drive to increased research rigour to understand what is effective in real-world quality improvement methodologies is an important goal of high-quality QIR.

The importance of context in QIR

QI interventions that work well in one area or organisation often seem to deliver disappointing results when replicated elsewhere. The most common explanation for this variation is context. Contextual factors can be grouped into external factors (such as regulatory requirements), organisational factors (such as size), and teamwork/leadership/safety culture and management tools (such as training and audit). Reviews of studies of the impact of context on QI overwhelmingly focus on the 'meso', or organisational, level.[32] Studies at the micro-level which might be most relevant to primary care teams are few. 'Quality and coherence of policy' and 'supportive organisational culture' are consistently associated with positive findings. Further research is required to understand the impact of context on QI and which interventions might work best in which context.[33]

TABLE 10.3 Characteristics of measurement for improvement, accountability and research

	Improvement	Accountability	Research
Who?			
Audience (Customers)	Medical group Quality improvement team Providers and staff Administrators	Purchaser Payers Patients/members Medical groups	Science community General public Users (clinicians)
Why?			
Purpose	Understanding of a. Process b. Customers Motivation and focus Baseline Evaluation of changes	Comparison Basis for choice Reassurance Spur for change	New knowledge without regard for applicability
What?			
Scope	Specific to an individual medical site and process	Specific to an individual medical group and process	Universal (though often limited generalisability)
Measures	Few Easily collected Approximate	Very few Complex collection Precise and valid	Many Complex collection Very precise and valid
Time period	Short, current	Long, past	Long, past
Confounders	Consider but rarely measure	Describe and try to measure	Measure or control
How?			
Measurers	Internal and at least involved in the selection of measures	External	External and usually prefer to control both process and collection
Sample size	Small	Large	Large
Collection process	Simple and required minimal time cost and expertise Usually repeated	Complex and requires moderated cost and effort	Extremely complex and expensive May be planned for several repeats
Need for confidentiality	Very high (organisation and people)	None for objects of comparison; the goal is exposure	High, especially for the individual subjects

Source: Solberg LI et al. *Jt Comm J Qual Improv* 1997;23(3):135–47.

Ethics in QIR

Research involving humans requires approval by human research ethics committees (HRECs) to protect participants from harm and ensure research activity is likely to produce useful outputs. The ethical rules for QI are currently not clear. Many HRECs recognise that quality improvement

BOX 10.4 TRIGGERS WHICH MAY INDICATE NEED FOR ETHICAL REVIEW (AUSTRALIAN NATIONAL HEALTH AND MEDICAL RESEARCH COUNCIL)[35]

Consider formal ethics application:

- Where the activity potentially infringes the privacy or professional reputation of participants, providers or organisations
- Where there is secondary use of data—using data or analysis from quality assurance (QA) or evaluation activities for another purpose
- When gathering information about the participant beyond that which is collected routinely; information may include biospecimens or additional investigations
- When testing of non-standard (innovative) protocols or equipment
- Where there is comparison of cohorts
- When using randomisation or the use of control groups or placebos
- Where there is targeted analysis of data involving minority/vulnerable groups, whose data is to be separated out of the data collected or analysed as part of the main evaluation activity

projects involve activities that are part of the routine development of services and use routinely collected data. They may make provision for such activities to be carried out and even have associated publications without the requirement of formal ethical approval provided the projects meet strict conditions.

Internationally, the difference between QI which does not require HREC approval and research which does is judged on intent. If the intent is to add new knowledge or test innovations beyond usual care, then the project may be classified as research.[34] The Australian National Health and Medical Research Council has produced a document which addresses ethical approval in quality assurance activities and provides a list of triggers which may indicate the need for formal ethical approval (see Box 10.4).[35] Those carrying out QI projects should seek advice on ethical issues from their relevant HREC and obtain an independent statement, particularly if considering publication. Most rigorous evaluative QIR projects will involve non-routinely collected data obtained from individuals and, so, will require ethical approval.

Publishing QIR

Publishing and disseminating QIR can spread ideas and add to the knowledge of what works in QI. Rubenstein et al.[36] classified QIR literature into six broad groupings of articles:

- Empirical literature on development of QI interventions
- History, documentation or description of QI interventions
- Success, effectiveness or impact of QI interventions
- QI intervention stories, theories and frameworks
- QI intervention literature syntheses and meta-analyses
- Development and testing of QI intervention related tools

Despite increasing recognition of QI and QIR, it can be challenging to find outlets for publishing research. Quantitative analyses such as SPC methodologies may be unfamiliar to peer reviewers schooled in more traditional approaches, leading to rejection even of high-quality, important work. There are journals which focus on quality improvement and implementation research and a link to a list of these is provided in Box 10.5.

Quality improvement projects may be published as 'quality improvement reports' under an established set of publication guidelines known as the Standards for QUality Improvement Reporting Excellence (SQUIRE)

BOX 10.5 RESOURCES

1. *Designing Quality Improvement Projects*:
    a. The Institute for Health care Improvement: http://www.ihi.org/ and http://www.ihi.org/resources/Pages/Tools/Quality-Improvement-Essentials-Toolkit.aspx
    b. Agency for Health care Research and Quality: https://www.ahrq.gov/research/findings/factsheets/quality/qipc/index.html
    c. The Health Foundation: http://www.health.org.uk/
    d. The Improvement Foundation: http://improve.org.au/
    e. The Australian Primary Care Collaboratives: https://apcc.org.au/
2. *Evaluating Quality Improvement Interventions*:
    a. Models for Implementation Research
    b. EPIS framework: http://www.cebc4cw.org/implementing-programs/tools/epis/
    c. Consolidated Framework for Implementation Research: http://www.cfirguide.org/
    d. Recommendations for Quality Assurance Activities: https://www.nhmrc.gov.au/guidelines-publications/e111
    e. Guideline on Ethics in Human Research: https://www.nhmrc.gov.au/guidelines-publications/e72
3. *Publishing*:
    a. SQUIRE statement: http://squire-statement.org/
    b. Journals publishing QI work: https://medicine.yale.edu/chiral/scholarlywork/journals.aspx

statement.[37] The SQUIRE statement is accepted by major journals as a standard for reporting quality-improvement research.

REFERENCES

1. Batalden PB, Davidoff F. What is 'quality improvement' and how can it transform healthcare? *Qual Saf Health Care* 2007;16(1):2–3.
2. Sollecito AS, Johnson, JK. *Continuous Quality Improvement in Health Care*, 4th ed. Burlington, USA: Jones and Bartlett Learning; 2013.
3. Greenhalgh T, Russell J, Swinglehurst D. Narrative methods in quality improvement research. *Qual Saf Health Care* 2005;14(6):443–9.
4. Evidence Scan: Improvement Science. 2011. Available at: http://www.health.org.uk/sites/health/files/ImprovementScience.pdf. (Accessed October 2017).
5. Eccles MP, Mittman, BS. Welcome to implementation science. *Implement Sci* 2006;1(1). https://implementationscience.biomedcentral.com/track/pdf/10.1186/1748-5908-1-1.
6. Bodenheimer T, Sinsky C. From triple to quadruple aim: Care of the patient requires care of the provider. *Ann Fam Med* 2014;12(6):573–6.
7. Lau R, Stevenson F, Ong BN et al. Achieving change in primary care-causes of the evidence to practice gap: Systematic reviews of reviews. *Implement Sc* 2016;11:40.
8. Optimising Consumer Participation in Cancer Services: Model for Consumer Participation in Quality Improvement. 2007. Available at: http://ourhealth.org.au/consumer-rep-support/consumer-and-community-engagement/useful-resources/involving-consumers-research-.Wa5G35MjFmA. (Accessed September 2017).
9. PHCRIS. Introduction to...consumer involvement in research. 2015. Available at: http://www.phcris.org.au/guides/consumer_participation.php. (Accessed September 2017).
10. Quality Improvement Tools: Clinical Excellence Commission; Available at: http://www.cec.health.nsw.gov.au/quality-improvement/improvement-academy/quality-improvement-tools. (Accessed September 2017).
11. Boaden R, Harvey G, Moxham C, Proudlove N. *Quality Improvement: Theory and Practice in Healthcare*. NHS Institute for Innovation and Improvement. 2008. Available at: https://www.rcem.ac.uk/docs/Clinical%20Audit_Improvement/23c.%20Quality%20Improvement%20theory%20and%20practice%20in%20healthcare.pdf. (Accessed September 2017).
12. Langley G, Nolan K. *The Improvement Guide: A Practical Approach to Enhancing Organizational Performance*. San Francisco: Jossey-Bass; 1996.
13. The Breakthrough Series: IHI's Collaborative Model for Achieving Breakthrough Improvement. IHI Innovation Series white paper [Internet]. 2003 Available at: http://www.ihi.org/resources/Pages/IHIWhitePapers/TheBreakthroughSeriesIHIsCollaborativeModelforAchievingBreakthroughImprovement.aspx. (Accessed September 2017).
14. Knight A. The collaborative method. A strategy for improving Australian general practice. *Aust Fam Physician* 2004;33(4):269–74.
15. Dawda DP, Raymond DM. An introduction to quality improvement. *InnovAiT* 2016;9(11):702–6.
16. Campbell SM, Braspenning J, Hutchinson A, Marshall MN. Research methods used in developing and applying quality indicators in primary care. *BMJ* 2003; 326(7393):816–9.
17. Knight AW, Caesar C, Ford D, Coughlin A, Frick C. Improving primary care in Australia through the Australian Primary Care Collaboratives Program: A quality improvement report. *BMJ Qual Saf* 2012;21(11):948–55.

18. Improvement Measures available for submission to the Improvement Foundation databases. 2016. Available at: https://apcc.org.au/download/if-measure-suite-measure-specifications-v5-8-31-march-2016/?wpdmdl=1210. (Accessed September 2017).
19. Knight AW, Ford D, Audehm R, Colagiuri S, Best J. The Australian Primary Care Collaboratives Program: Improving diabetes care. *BMJ Qual Saf* 2012;21(11):956–63.
20. Raymond DM, Dawda DP. Making quality improvement simple: The Model for Improvement. *InnovAiT* 2016;9(12):768–72.
21. Granger BB, Shah BR. Blending quality improvement and research methods for implementation science, part I: Design and data collection. *AACN Adv Crit Care* 2015;26(3):268–74.
22. Portela MC, Pronovost PJ, Woodcock T, Carter P, Dixon-Woods M. How to study improvement interventions: A brief overview of possible study types. *BMJ Qual Saf* 2015;24(5):325–36.
23. Ovretveit J. *Evaluating Improvement and Implementation for Health.* Maidenhead: Open University Press; 2014.
24. Damschroder LJ, Aron DC, Keith RE, Kirsh SR, Alexander JA, Lowery JC. Fostering implementation of health services research findings into practice: A consolidated framework for advancing implementation science. *Implement Sci* 2009;4(1):50.
25. Aarons GA, Hurlburt M, Horwitz SM. Advancing a conceptual model of evidence-based practice implementation in public service sectors. *AdmPolicy Men Health Men Health Serv Res* 2011;38(1):4–23.
26. Hamilton O. PARiHS framework for implementing research into practice McMaster University: National Collaborating Centre for Methods and Tools. 2011. Available at: http://www.nccmt.ca/resources/search/85. (Accessed September 2017).
27. Wheeler DJ. *Understanding Chaos. The Key to Managing Variation.* Knoxville, Tennessee: SPC Press; 2000.
28. Ivers NM, Tricco AC, Taljaard M et al. Quality improvement needed in quality improvement randomised trials: Systematic review of interventions to improve care in diabetes. *BMJ Open* 2013;3(4):e002727. DOI: 10.1136/bmjopen-2013-002727.
29. Pope C, van Royen P, Baker R. Qualitative methods in research on healthcare quality. *Qual Saf Health Care* 2002;11(2):148–52.
30. Solberg LI, Mosser G, McDonald S. The three faces of performance measurement: Improvement, accountability, and research. *Jt Comm J Qual Improv* 1997;23(3):135–47.
31. Auerbach AD, Landefeld CS, Shojania KG. The tension between needing to improve care and knowing how to do it. *N Engl J Med* 2007;357(6):608–13.
32. Kaplan HC, Provost LP, Froehle CM, Margolis PA. The Model for Understanding Success in Quality (MUSIQ): Building a theory of context in healthcare quality improvement. *BMJ Qua Saf* 2012;21(1):13–20.
33. Fulop N, Robert G. *Context for Successful Quality Improvement.* London: The Health Foundation; 2015. Available at http://www.health.org.uk/publication/context-successful-quality-improvement. (Accessed November 2017).
34. Lynn J, Baily MA, Bottrell M et al. The ethics of using quality improvement methods in health care. *Ann Intern Med* 2007;146(9):666–73.
35. NHMRC. Ethical Considerations in Quality Assurance and Evaluation Activities. 2015. Available at https://www.nhmrc.gov.au/_files_nhmrc/publications/attachments/e111_ethical_considerations_in_quality_assurance_140326.pdf. (Accessed November 2017).
36. Rubenstein LV, Hempel S, Farmer MM et al. Finding order in heterogeneity: Types of quality-improvement intervention publications. *Qual Saf Health Care* 2008;17(6):403–8.
37. SQUIRE. Promoting Excellence in Healthcare Improvement Reporting. 2015. Available at: http://www.squire-statement.org/. (Accessed September 2017).

CHAPTER 11

Programme evaluation in primary care

Lauren Siegmann, Robyn Preston and Bunmi Malau-Aduli

WHAT IS EVALUATION?

When understanding evaluation, you will use the research methods, including data collection and analysis, outlined in other chapters. However, the major distinction between research and evaluation hinges on the intention of the activity. Research aims to create generalisable theory or knowledge about the world.[1] Evaluation is concerned with making judgment about the value of something[2] or testing some practical solution to a problem.[3] It is the act of making a judgment about the merit or worth of something that is what makes evaluation a unique discipline and distinct from research.[4]

WHAT CAN BE EVALUATED IN PRIMARY CARE?

Within any primary care organization, there are three domains of decision making and activities: Policy (or governance), management and service provision. These domains are explained more fully by Watson, Broemeling and Wong[5] in their article 'Results-based logic model for Primary Health Care'. A primary care organisation provides services to clients or patients. The demands or needs of patients justify the organisation. In effect, patients are another domain of the organisation which need to be considered in organisational decisions and activities. It is important to note all these domains address different decisions and activities and all contribute to the organisation's effectiveness. Thus, the role of evaluation for any of these domains will differ; yet the input at any domain will contribute to the effective

---

BOX 11.1   EXAMPLES OF WHAT CAN BE EVALUATED IN PRIMARY CARE

- An existing service to determine if improvement could be made
- An existing service in a new format, e.g. location
- A new service
- A new way of working
- A training programme
- A health promotion event (such as a family fun day or mental health week activity)

---

functioning of the organisation. In primary care, there are a range of activities that can be evaluated (Box 11.1).

WHY DO WE NEED EVALUATION?

On a conceptual level, the purpose of an evaluation may be understood differently by the stakeholders involved (see Chapter 6). The interest in, expectation of and funding available for an evaluation tends to differ between contexts. Within any one primary care organisation, evaluation may be seen by some people as a necessary but meaningless activity, while others may believe it is a way to gain insight into what happened and why. Thus, an evaluator must deal with the political realities of the expectations of different groups of stakeholders. For example, programme managers may see evaluation as a means of improving implementation, service providers may perceive it as a means of determining if the programme is meeting need and policy makers may see it as justification of money spent.

Regardless of the evaluator's viewpoint, most evaluations in primary care focus on five broad areas:

1. To determine what changed as a result of the programme being implemented
2. To make a judgment about the extent to which the observed changes are sustainable
3. To work out which parts of the programme are most and least effective in contributing to change
4. To work out if the programme is meeting the needs of the targeted stakeholders and beneficiaries
5. To make an assessment as to the extent that the programme represents value for money

A well-designed evaluation should be able to answer what parts of the programme contributed to the overall success and what parts impeded the achievement of programme or service objectives. Identifying barriers to implementation or reasons for not achieving targets may be as important as measuring success. Unfortunately, identification of failure or lack of success is not as well received as indicators of success. Nevertheless, the information is important to enable primary care staff to fill gaps, review processes and develop new strategies for service delivery.

EVALUATION ACROSS THE PROGRAMME CYCLE

Most, if not all, programmes go through a series of normative stages called the 'Programme cycle', illustrated by Figure 11.1:

1. *Assessment:* To understand need and developing a programme that responds to that need
2. *Implementation:* The programme is enacted or put into place
3. *Reflection:* Stakeholders determine what worked and what did not work
4. *Redevelopment:* Based on the results of reflection, changes are made for the next programme cycle

Primary care services could plan and prepare for one-off evaluations. However, evaluations should also be undertaken continuously for quality improvement. Evaluation in primary care should be an integral part of the programme cycle and not just an activity that is implemented at the end of the programme's life. However, if you receive a grant or funds to provide

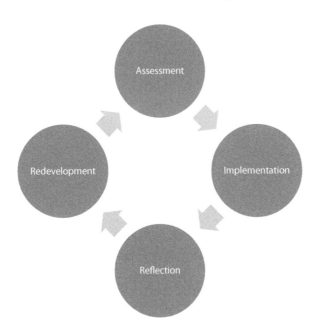

FIGURE 11.1 Basic programme cycle.

BOX 11.2 INTEGRATING EVALUATION INTO DAY-TO-DAY PRACTICE

Using evaluation regularly and becoming familiar with how to plan, perform and implement evaluation findings can help develop an evaluation culture within your practice or organisation. There are many activities that primary care practitioners regularly perform which can be used to develop evaluative practices, including:

- *Daily reflective practice*: To assist with personal reflection of primary health care services or activities, you may ask, 'What happened?' or 'Should it have happened?' or 'How can I avoid that happening in the future?' or 'How can I use that success in other areas?'.
- *Weekly team or mentor meetings*: Using questions such as 'How did that go?', your team can develop strategies to improve services and regularly review them. These sessions can also be used as problem-solving or brainstorming sessions.
- *Monthly reports to team leaders or managers*: Frequently, service providers have to provide monthly meetings; use these as an opportunity to review what you have achieved and what you want to achieve, reviewing the documented processes used in past months to achieve your outcomes. From this, you can determine what did and did not succeed and modify your processes accordingly.
- *Annual review and reporting procedures*: Annual reporting procedures present an excellent opportunity to retrospectively review your progress longitudinally. Over time, you may notice trends which will help you plan for the future.

a specific service or project, the funding body may wish to obtain a report of the outcomes from the project. In this case, you would perform a one-off evaluation to meet their requirements. Remember that the information you collect continuously to improve your practice (see Box 11.2) can be used for the one-off evaluation report for the funding body, which may in turn improve the overall quality of the evaluation.

John Owen, in his book *Program Evaluation, Forms and Approaches* identified five normative approaches to evaluation.[5] Table 11.1 outlines these approaches and demonstrates how they align with the programme cycle.

TOOLS FOR DECIDING WHAT DATA YOU NEED

So far, we have discussed why you might want to do evaluation and the purpose of evaluation and provided some insight into how evaluation can become an everyday activity in a primary care service. During evaluation, you collect and analyse data or evidence so that you can apply judgment about the merit or worth of a programme. Data can be collected and analysed for evaluation using research methods outlined in this book. A common risk in programme

TABLE 11.1 Five normative approaches to evaluation

Types of evaluation	Proactive	Clarificative	Interactive	Monitoring	Impact
Purpose	Identifying the need for the programme and what the programme should look like	Planning the programme and its further evaluation	Implementing change in an empowering and participatory way, while learning from the process of implementation	Measuring the implementation of the programme—is it working?	Measuring the outcomes of the programme
Key approaches	Performing a needs assessment or situational analysis Synthesising the relevant literature in a scoping or systematic review	Developing a logic model for the programme Assessing how to evaluate the programme once implemented	Action research Participatory methods	Assessment of the process of implementation and performance of the programme: key inputs, activities, outputs Systems analysis	Evaluation
Stage of the programme cycle	Assessment	Assessment	Across all stages	Implementation Reflection	Reflection Assessment

Source: Owen JM. *Program Evaluation: Forms and Approaches,* 3rd ed. Crows Nest, N.S.W: Allen & Unwin; 2006. pp 52–3.

evaluation is that practitioners collect reams of data, with much of the data not being relevant or helpful in making judgment about how the programme is going. Without an upfront plan for evaluation, there is a risk that incorrect data may be collected, the evaluation may not evaluate the correct aspects of the service or it may not evaluate the objectives of the service or programme.

If you collect irrelevant information, you will have performed an evaluation which does not meet objectives. You may have a perfectly planned programme which met the initial objectives of the funding organisation, reached the target audience and achieved the impact it proposed, but unless the correct data is collected throughout the programme to reflect this, the evaluation of the effectiveness of the programme will be worthless.

The purpose of the programme determines what is to be evaluated. For this reason, most evaluations have one or more forms of 'conceptual frameworks' that guide evaluation planning, implementation and judgment of the programme. A conceptual framework is an analytical tool that identifies and illustrates the relationship between the relevant factors that may influence a programme and the successful achievement of its goals and objectives.[6]

Programme logic

One of the most popular conceptual frameworks used in evaluation is the programme logic (Table 11.2). The programme logic is a diagram that outlines the causal links between what the programme does and the changes it expects to see. It is a form of clarificative evaluation.[7] You can use your programme logic to:

- Develop a framework to measure the quantity and quality of the planned activities and outputs.
- Identify what kinds of questions you want to ask and who you want to ask (you will know because you will have outlined the types of change you expect to see for different types of stakeholders).
- Identify when you should ask certain questions (you will know because you have outlined when you expect to see changes to occur).
- Communicate the rationale of a programme to stakeholders.

A program logic usually has some or all of the elements shown in Table 11.2.

CONCLUSIONS

The approach to program evaluation outlined in this chapter is illustrated by two practical examples in Boxes 11.3 and 11.4. Additional resources to help you with program evaluation are given in Box 11.5.

TABLE 11.2 Elements of the programme logic

Foundational activities/inputs	What the programme does or provides to create an enabling environment for programme activities to occur
Activities	What the programme does to reach its expected outcomes
Outputs	The tangible products or results that are directly generated by the activities
Immediate outcomes	The change that occurs as a direct result of the output and/or activity being implemented
	Changes at this level usually involve changes to stakeholders' knowledge and attitudes and changes in access to networks and opportunities
Intermediate outcomes	The changes that occur for programme beneficiaries 1–3 years after the activity has been implemented
	Changes at this level usually involve behaviour change of various stakeholders
Programme outcomes	The end goals or objectives of the programme
Social goal	The broader social problem that the programme is seeking to address

BOX 11.3   PRACTICAL PROGRAMME
EVALUATION: EXERCISE ONE

Jane is a health promotion officer with a small mental health charity based in a regional city. She is also a member of the local mental health week committee. The committee obtains funding through a state grant, and this year, allocated funds to five different services:

- A civic reception and awards night for consumer advocates and workers at the Council chambers
- Community fun day at the local park with information stalls (20 different services) and activities for families, including a movie and free rides
- A professional development breakfast for the mental health community and health workers with an internationally renowned speaker
- An open day at 'The Clubhouse', a drop-in centre for people living with mental health issues; and
- A weekend mental health first-aid course for senior high school and university students

The committee is applying for the grant next year to support their own running costs and to allocate funds again to services. There have been grumblings in the community section that the same groups seem to get the funding every year. Jane has been tasked with evaluating the success of the week.

- What is the purpose of this evaluation?
- What tools could Jane use to plan her evaluation?
- What data do they need to collect?
- Who are the stakeholders involved?
- What are some of the issues?

Notes/answers: The issue for Jane is that there is an overall evaluation of the committee/week, as well as individual evaluations for each of the activities. She also has multiple stakeholders. As well as a logical framework for the overall week/committee, Jane should develop simple tools with those who have successfully won the grants. A short, one-page evaluation report should be required with the feedback on expenditure of funds. These could include surveys for those who have attended the fun day, mental health first aid and professional development breakfast. The success of the civic reception could be gauged through media reports and number of attendees. The open day could also be evaluated through surveys or number of attendees, as well as long-term increase in clientele numbers. Jane should also ensure she is using data that services already collects. A report to all of the town's community sector should be developed as well as one for the funding body. This will ensure that the committee is transparent about funding. A short statement on committee membership, who attended meetings and who did what could be ascertained from committee meeting minutes. This would also assist with transparency and may urge those grumbling about funding to help out next year.

BOX 11.4   PRACTICAL PROGRAMME EVALUATION: EXERCISE TWO

Bill is a practice nurse at a metropolitan general practice specialising in services for students at the nearby university. Together with the university's health student group, Bill has received funding from the Student Union for all health students to receive a free flu shot prior to going on placement. The shots will be given by nursing students as part of their placement with the practice. A media article at the start of the programme sparked complaints on social media from education students who said that they should also be eligible for the programme if they are going on placement in schools. The university response was that they would subsidise flu shots for all students on placement, should the programme be successful.

Bill will work with Crystal, a nursing student, to report back to the Student Union on the success of the programme.

- What is the purpose of this evaluation?
- What tools could Bill and Crystal use to plan the evaluation?
- What data do they need to collect?
- Who are the stakeholders involved?
- What are some of the issues?

Notes/answers: Bill and Crystal can use existing tools in the clinic. A simple clinical audit could ascertain if there was an increase in health professional students receiving flu shots compared with the year before. A client survey could also be given to students when they wait in the waiting room after their shot (questions could include would they normally get a flu short, convenience, satisfaction, etc.). An additional indicator of interest to the university could be the number of nursing students who received training in immunisation at the clinic. In the longer term, Bill and Crystal could do a cross-sectional survey after the flu season to see how many of those students did or did not get the flu. The university would also want some indication of the cost of the programme and how increasing the service to other students would increase costs.

BOX 11.5   RESOURCES

The Primary Health Care Research Information Service (PHCRIS): Based at
Flinders University, PHCRIS has a range of free resources for primary
care and primary health care researchers and evaluation. (http://www.
phcris.org.au/guides/evaluation_gettingstarted.php)

The Planning and Evaluation Wizard: The Planning and Evaluation Wizard
(PEW) is designed to allow you simple access to planning and evaluation
tools that are relevant to your Primary Health Care project. It helps
demystify the jargon associated with project planning, evaluation and
report writing, as well as provide practical assistance and examples.
You can progress through the module with your own project. (http://
www.flinders.edu.au/medicine/sites/pew/)

Better Evaluation: Information about more than 300 evaluation options
(methods and processes), organised into 34 different evaluation tasks.
(www.betterevaluation.org)

*Evaluating complex health interventions: A guide to rigorous research
designs*: This resource is particularly useful for those commissioning
evaluations in health and community settings. Designs illustrated
include experimental, quasi-experimental and observational designs—
randomised controlled trial, cluster randomised stepped wedge design,
interrupted time series design, controlled before and after design,
regression discontinuity design and natural experiment. (http://www.
academyhealth.org/evaluationguide)

Evaluation of Straight Talk: Although outside the realm of primary care,
this evaluation won the team (including section author Lauren) the
Australasian Evaluation Society 2016 Indigenous Evaluation Award.
(http://resources.oxfam.org.au/pages/preview.php?ref=1694&
alternative=-1&ext=jpg&k=&search=%22Straight+Talk%22&off
set=0&order_by=relevance&sort=DESC&archive=0&page=16,
https://resources.oxfam.org.au)

Australasian Evaluation Society: Holds workshops and seminars on diverse
evaluation topics, including Monitoring and Evaluation, Introduction to
Programme Evaluation, etc. (www.aes.asn.au)

REFERENCES

1. Stake RE. Generalizability of program evaluation: The needs for limits. *Educ Prod Rep* 1969;2:39–40.
2. Scriven M. *Evaluation Thesaurus*. Thousand Oaks: SAGE Publications; 1991.
3. Guba E. Significant Differences. *Educ Res* 1969;20:4–5.
4. Hawe P, Degeling D, Hall J. *Evaluating Health Promotion: A Health Worker's Guide.* Marrickville, NSW: MacLennan & Petty; 2007.
5. Owen JM. *Program Evaluation: Forms and Approaches*, 3rd ed. Crows Nest, N.S.W: Allen & Unwin; 2006.

6. Miles MB, Huberman AM, Saldaña J. *Qualitative Data Analysis: A Methods Source Book*, 3rd ed. Thousand Oaks: SAGE Publications; 2013.
7. Watson DE, Broemeling, A-M, Wong ST. A Results-Based Logic Model for Primary Healthcare: A Conceptual Foundation for Population-Based Information Systems. *Health Policy* 2009;5(Spec No):33–46.

SECTION III

Preliminary steps to doing primary care research

CHAPTER 12

How to prepare your research proposal

Bob Mash

Proposals may be written for ethics committees in order to receive approval, health services in order to obtain permission or funding bodies in pursuit of a grant. The intended readership will have different concerns, such as the ethical issues raised by the study, the impact on service delivery or the extent to which the proposed study aligns with the objectives of the call for proposals. As the researcher, you will need to ensure you address these concerns and structure the proposal according to their instructions.

Nevertheless, research proposals usually follow a similar structure even though they will describe different methodologies, as shown in Box 12.1. A research proposal is not necessarily a long document, as committees must often assess multiple proposals in a short space of time; nevertheless, it needs to succinctly describe all the important features of the study.

BOX 12.1   STRUCTURE OF A RESEARCH PROPOSAL

1. Title
2. Summary
3. Introduction
4. Aim and objectives
5. Methods
6. Ethical considerations
7. Timeframe
8. Budget and funding
9. References
10. Appendices

The title of the study should accurately reflect the aim and study design. Avoid overly dramatic, colloquial or non-specific titles. Often you will be asked to submit a summary as well as the full proposal. In an ethics committee, for example, the summary may be read by the whole committee, while the full proposal is read by only one or two reviewers. The summary, therefore, is an important element that should be brief, structured and aligned with the full proposal. It may be better to write the summary once the full proposal is complete.

INTRODUCTION

The introduction is an argument for the social and scientific value of your proposed study. The social value speaks to the importance and relevance of your study in terms of society, the burden of disease or the health services. What will this study contribute to solving an important problem, improving the health of the community or the performance of the health services? The scientific value speaks to the knowledge gap that will be addressed by your study. In defining the knowledge gap, you will need to outline what is already known about your specific research topic and, therefore, what is not known. Your research question should then flow logically from the knowledge gap that you have defined.

Your argument for the social and scientific value should be derived from your literature review (see Chapter 14). The literature review, therefore, is purposively used to author your argument. Novice researchers may struggle to use the literature in this way. Try to avoid listing studies that you have read and just describing them sequentially in the introduction. Critical appraisal of the literature is also important in terms of judging the relative credibility of different studies, but your writing should go beyond analysing and comparing studies. Your synthesis, appraisal and interpretation of the literature should support the logical development of your argument.

It may assist your writing to roughly outline your argument as a series of key logical steps and to then expand each key point into a paragraph. The reader should be able to follow the logical connections between paragraphs and the flow of your argument. Typically, the argument will move from the global picture to the regional situation, and finally to local evidence. Use simple language whenever possible and short sentences so that your writing is easy to follow. Focus your literature review on the specific research question and avoid spending too much time on the background. For example, if your study is about factors affecting adherence to tuberculosis (TB) treatment, you do not need to outline all the literature on the pathophysiology of the TB bacillus. Cite the primary sources of evidence to support your key points, and avoid citing secondary sources where the evidence is mentioned tangentially or in passing. Each statement of fact in your argument, however, should be supported by a citation to the evidence.

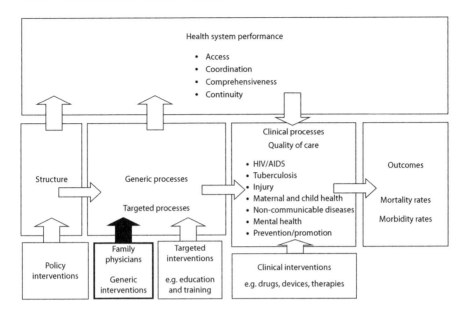

FIGURE 12.1 Example of a conceptual framework.[1,2]

In some proposals, the introduction will also introduce a key theory or conceptual framework for the study. If your study design is relying on existing theory, then this should be outlined in the introduction. For example, a study on behaviour change counselling may rely on an understanding of self-determination theory, which should then be described. Similarly, your study design may have an underlying conceptual framework that has been derived from the literature. For example, a study on the impact of family physicians on the district health system may have a model of the health system as a conceptual framework that guides the design and selection of data collection tools. A conceptual framework is often summarised in a diagram that shows how the key concepts are related (Figure 12.1).

AIM AND OBJECTIVES

Your research question and study aim are usually the same, although one is expressed as a question and the other as a statement. The aim should capture all the key aspects of the study in a sentence. For example, the people or population to be studied, any intervention or exposure, any comparison group, the location or context of the study and the outcome of interest. In experimental or observational studies, the hypothesis being tested may be clearly defined in the aim but, if necessary, can also be stated as a separate hypothesis.

The aim can then be broken down into its subcomponents, each of which will be studied (Box 12.2). These subcomponents are research objectives that

> ### BOX 12.2   EXAMPLE OF AIM AND OBJECTIVES FOR A STUDY[3-6]
>
> The study aims to evaluate the impact of family physicians on clinical processes, system performance and outcomes within the district health system of South Africa. Specific objectives include:
>
> 1. To describe the perceived impact of family physicians in terms of their six roles within the district health system
> 2. To explore the perceptions of district managers regarding the impact of family physicians
> 3. To evaluate the influence of family physicians at primary care facilities and district hospitals
> 4. To evaluate the relationship between an increase in family physician supply in each district on key district health system indicators

need to be answered or addressed by the study and should not be a list of methodological steps. All studies end by reporting on their implications and recommendations, and thus, this does not have to be stated as an objective. The language used in defining the aim and objectives is important as this often implies the type of study design. For example, words such as measure, evaluate or describe may imply a more positivist and quantitative approach (see Chapters 16 to 21), while words such as explore indicate a more interpretative and qualitative approach (see Chapters 22 to 26).

METHODS

Most studies can be outlined using a similar structure for the methods section: The study design, the setting, approach to sample size and sampling, the intervention (if any), data collection and data analysis. Some study designs may require a different structure that relates to their unique methodological steps, for example, quality improvement cycles[7] and participatory action-research cycles.[8]

Study design

The type of study design should be clearly stated in a sentence or two. For example, 'this is a pragmatic clustered randomised controlled trial' or 'this is a descriptive survey'. Most study designs are well known and do not have to be further justified, although the choice of design must be appropriate to address the aim and objectives. Avoid combining descriptors that are vague, confusing or contradictory. For example, studies cannot primarily be both descriptive and experimental as the one describes a single group and the other compares two groups. Avoid describing your study using the dichotomy quantitative or qualitative. Studies that use qualitative techniques should be placed within a particular methodological tradition such as ethnography or phenomenology. Section IV outlines a variety of commonly used study designs.

In some proposals, there are several different types of study. For example, the study outlined in Box 12.2 required a descriptive survey, a phenomenological qualitative study, an observational cross-sectional study and an ecological study of a national database. In this situation, the study design section should list the different studies and how they relate to the objectives and to each other. For example, one study may be needed to inform the design of another or may need to happen in a particular sequence. A diagram is often helpful to clarify the overall design and relationship of different studies. The methods section may then be divided into sections in order to fully describe each study in turn.

Setting

A description of the setting usually involves a description of the primary care services and the community being served. The description should focus on the aspects that are most relevant to the study. For example, in a study that explores the experiences of sexual assault survivors with follow-up care in a health district, the description will focus on the specific services offered to sexual assault survivors, including the health workers involved, and the way care is organised. The setting should also describe the community being studied in terms of its size, culture, language, socioeconomic profile and burden of disease. Specific features that relate to the topic should be described; in this example, male patients are often referred from the local prisons.

In studies using qualitative techniques, it is particularly important to have a 'thick description' of the context and also to describe the researchers and their relationship to the topic and setting. The confirmability of qualitative studies requires attention to the reflexivity of the researcher (see Chapter 23). This could also be presented in a separate subsection of the methods.

Sample size and sampling strategy

Most studies involve the selection of subjects, respondents or participants. The principles on which this is done vary with the methodology but always needs to be explained.

POSITIVIST EXPERIMENTAL AND ANALYTICAL STUDIES

In positivist experimental and analytical studies that collect quantitative data, it is usually necessary to select a sample from a larger study population that is representative of that population so that results from the sample can be generalised to the population. The size of the sample and how it is selected are both critical. The proposal should describe the assumptions made in calculating the sample size, although it does not usually need to give the exact mathematical equation. In a descriptive study, the sample size calculation usually requires you to know the size of the population, the key variable you want to use, the anticipated result, the standard deviation of that variable and the precision with which you want to measure it (the width of the 95% confidence intervals). Some of these items may be difficult to predict, although they can be estimated from previous studies or even a pilot study.

In a study that compares groups, you will also need to decide what variable to use and its standard deviation. In addition, you need to define the acceptable level of error in deciding if the groups are different. Type 1 error (alpha) is typically set at 5% and relates to the chance of saying there is a difference when in fact there is not. Type 2 error (beta) is typically set between 10% and 20% and relates to the chance of saying there is no difference when in fact there is. This also equates to a power of 80%–90%, which is another way of expressing this error. You will also need to decide what difference between the groups would be meaningful to measure (the effect size).

At the end of the day, the final sample size may be a compromise between what is statistically desirable and practically possible, given the available time and resources. One also needs to consider how many additional people to select in order to compensate for non-responders or loss to follow-up. You will often need to consult a statistician to assist you with the sample-size calculation.

Having decided how many people to select, you then need to decide how to select them. The specific inclusion and exclusion criteria to be used need to be defined. Exclusion criteria should be additional to the inclusion criteria and not just the same idea expressed in the opposite direction.

Different approaches are possible and will depend on the context and study design:

- *Simple random sampling*: For example, using computer-generated random numbers to select people from a list.
- *Systematic random sampling*: For example, selecting every 'nth' person from a queue of people. This assumes that the people randomly enter the queue and there is no hidden pattern.
- *Stratified random sampling*: For example, people are selected as above but the number coming from different facilities is stratified according the workload.
- *Cluster random sampling*: For example, people are selected as above in groups or clusters, typically from the same location, and the way in which they share characteristics must be taken into account.
- *Consecutive sampling*: For example, people are selected consecutively as they come as long as they meet the inclusion and exclusion criteria.

Convenience sampling is best avoided if possible as this implies people are selected based on them being conveniently available to the researcher on a particular day or place. The chance for bias in this selection is high. Whichever approach you choose, it must be fully described.

QUALITATIVE STUDIES

In studies that use qualitative techniques, the aim is not to generalise the findings statistically to the study population, but to fully understand and interpret the phenomenon, culture or case that you are interested in. For example, the phenomenon might be how young adults decide whether to use condoms when having sex or how patients experience group diabetes education. People are therefore chosen on the basis that they are fully part of this phenomenon and able to share their perspective. The sample size depends on engaging with sufficient people to fully understand the phenomenon. Usually, the researcher will commit to interviewing a certain number of respondents in the proposal (typically 5–25) and then describe how they will determine saturation of their data. For example, they might state that they will continue interviewing people until the last three interviews fail to identify any new ideas or themes.

The sampling strategies are also different and are usually purposeful in that people are consciously and not randomly selected on the basis of their ability to shed light on the phenomenon of interest:

- *Criterion sampling*: For example, specific criteria are determined for selecting people. Criteria may also be combined in a matrix with the number of people to be selected who meet different criteria.
- *Snowball sampling*: For example, when respondents are difficult to identify, the current respondent may identify other people that they know who meet the necessary criteria.
- *Extreme case sampling*: For example, respondents at the extreme ends of the phenomenon are selected, such as those that attended all sessions of diabetes group education and those that attended none.
- *Purposeful random sampling*: For example, if there is a group of people of equal interest to understanding the phenomenon, they could be chosen randomly. Be sure you understand this is not for statistical purposes.

This section must practically describe how the sampling strategy will be implemented.

Intervention or exposure

If the study involves an intervention, such as in a randomised controlled trial, it should be fully described. You should also describe how you will know that the intervention was actually delivered. Likewise, the exposure in an observational study should be fully defined.

Data collection

Similar principles apply regardless of the methodology. Firstly, you should outline any data collection tools and include the full tool as an appendix (e.g. questionnaire, interview guide). You will need to argue for the validity and reliability of the tool (see Chapter 18) and explain where the tool came from and whether it was developed from scratch or adapted. You may need to explain how you will ensure the content and construct validity of the tool prior to using it. You may also need to explain how you will pilot the tool with your recipients to ensure its face validity and feasibility.

Secondly, you need to practically explain how the data will be collected in terms of who, when, where and how (see Chapter 27). Describe how you will overcome problems such as language barriers or ensuring the capability of research assistants to communicate effectively.

Data analysis

Again, similar principles apply regardless of methodology. Firstly, you should explain how the data will be captured (e.g. in an Excel spreadsheet or in a verbatim transcription) and how it will be checked for errors or omissions. Any additional calculations or categorisations of your data should be explained. Secondly, you should define any software that you plan to use (e.g. Statistical Package for the Social Sciences, Atlas-ti) and any assistance that you expect in the analysis (e.g. statistician, supervisor). Finally, you should explain the tests or steps that you anticipate using in your analysis.

For quantitative data, you will need to outline your descriptive analysis:

- Categorical data is either binary (e.g. yes/no, male/female), nominal (e.g. married, unmarried, widowed, divorced) or ordinal (e.g. strongly agree, agree, unsure, disagree, strongly disagree). Categorical data is presented as frequencies and percentages.
- Numerical data (e.g. age, weight, blood pressure) is presented as a mean and standard deviation if the data are normally distributed (Figure 12.2). If the data is skewed and not normally distributed (Figure 12.3), then it is presented as a median and interquartile range.

The rationale for your selection of inferential statistical tests (e.g. Chi-square test or independent samples t-test) should be explained. Key concepts in deciding on the test are:

- Type of data (numerical, ordinal or nominal).
- Whether or not numerical data is normally distributed.

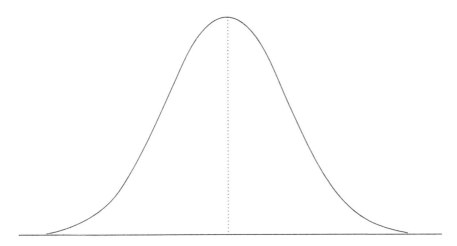

FIGURE 12.2 The normal distribution. The dotted line shows the mean of the data.

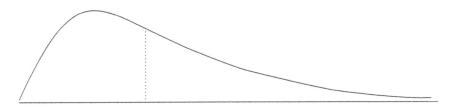

FIGURE 12.3 A skewed distribution. The dotted line shows the median. Compare the shape of the graph with the normal distribution shown in Figure 12.2.

- If there are groups, whether they are paired (the same people) or unpaired (different people).
- If there are comparisons, what is the independent variable (the exposure or risk factor) and the dependent variable (the outcome or response variable)?

For qualitative data analysis, the steps used should be described (e.g. familiarisation, create thematic index, coding, charting, interpretation).

ETHICAL CONSIDERATIONS

The ethical issues that should be considered are described in Chapter 13. Ethics committees are referred to as institutional review boards in some countries. The social, scientific value and methodological rigour of the study have already been described in the proposal, but are also essential prerequisites for the study to be ethical. In this section, you should argue for a favourable risk-benefit ratio, the fair selection of participants, independent review of the proposal, informed consent and how you will respect the rights (particularly in terms of autonomy, confidentiality and privacy) of the study participants or communities.

TIMEFRAME

This section should outline the expected duration and timing for each phase of the proposal. Typically, this would include the time for obtaining approvals, preparation, data collection, intervention, data analysis and report writing. A Gantt chart, as in Figure 12.4, can be used to clarify the timeframe.

BUDGET AND FUNDING

The budget if often better prepared in an Excel spreadsheet with a summary included as a table in the proposal. Text to justify and explain your budget should be included. Key aspects of the budget to consider are:

- *Personnel costs*: Cost of salaries for researchers, research assistants, consultants, administrative support
- *Equipment costs*: Cost of the necessary equipment for the intervention or data collection
- *Supply costs*: Cost of printing, stationary, office supplies
- *Travel and accommodation*: Costs of air and road travel as well as any accommodation and subsistence
- *Financial costs*: Costs of financial management and auditing of accounts
- *Indirect costs*: Costs expected by your institution to cover the support services that your research will use; usually added as a % of the total costs

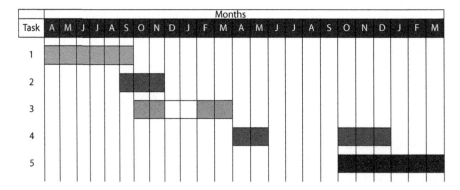

FIGURE 12.4 Example of a Gantt chart for the proposal timeframe. (1) Preparation and training; (2) Recruitment and baseline data collection; (3) Intervention; (4) Outcome data collection; (5) Analysis and report writing.

The funder may stipulate the categories to be used in drawing up the budget and what is eligible. The source(s) of funding for your proposal should be stated or anticipated in this section. Ethics committees and health services may want to know that you have sufficient funds, while funders may want to know what co-funding or in-kind contributions are available.

REFERENCES AND CITATIONS

As with all academic writing, a reference list should be given and cited in the text. Health sciences often use Vancouver style with numerical citations sequentially in the text and a numbered reference list. It is recommended that you use reference manager software to cite and reference consistently. Articles can usually be imported directly from your search (e.g. PubMed, Google Scholar) into the reference manager. References should be complete and correctly formatted.

APPENDICES

A variety of additional documents may be required depending on who you are submitting your proposal to. Usually, your data collection tools should be included as appendices as well as your informed consent forms.

PROPOSALS AND PROTOCOLS

Your research proposal is about what you plan to achieve, the reason you want to do this and how you will do it. It is written for a particular audience such as a funder or an ethics committee and should be concise. You may also choose to write a research protocol. This is a much more detailed document and will outline all the steps required to carry out your study, along with a practical timetable to guide your activities. You should anticipate the potential problems you may encounter and show some forward planning as to how you propose to deal with these issues. It is also possible to publish your protocol in a peer-reviewed journal, for example *JMIR Research Protocols*, which means your methods may be critiqued before you embark on your study.

REFERENCES

1. Lilford RJ, Chilton PJ, Hemming K, Girling AJ, Taylor CA, Barach P. Evaluating policy and service interventions: Framework to guide selection and interpretation of study end points. *BMJ* 2010;341:c4413.
2. Donabedian A. The quality of care: How can it be assessed? *JAMA* 1988;260(12):1743–8.
3. von Pressentin KB, Mash RJ, Baldwin-Ragaven L, Botha RPG, Govender I, Steinberg WJ. The birds-eye perspective: How do district health managers experience the impact of family physicians within the South African district health system? A qualitative study. *South Afr Fam Pract* 2017;4(1):1–8.

4. von Pressentin KB, Mash RJ, Esterhuizen TM. Examining the influence of family physician supply on district health system performance in South Africa: An ecological analysis of key health indicators. *Afr J Prm Health Care Fam Med* 2017;9(1), a1298.

5. von Pressentin KB, Mash RJ, Baldwin-Ragaven L, Botha RP, Govender I, Steinberg WJ, Esterhuizen TM. The Influence of Family Physicians Within the South African District Health System: A Cross-Sectional Study. *Ann Fam Med* 1 January 2018;16(1):28–36.

6. von Pressentin KB, Mash RJ, Baldwin-Ragaven L, Botha RP, Govender I, Steinberg WJ. The perceived impact of family physicians on the district health system in South Africa: A cross-sectional survey. *BMC Fam Pract* 2018;19:24. DOI: 10.1186/s12875-018-0710-0.

7. Van Deventer C, Mash B. African primary care research: Quality improvement cycles. *Afr J Prm Health Care Fam Med* 2014;6(1), Art. #598, 7 pages. http://dx.doi.org/10.4102/phcfm.v6i1.598.

8. Mash B. African primary care research: Participatory action research. *Afr J Prm Health Care Fam Med* 2014;6(1), Art. #585, 5 pages. http://dx.doi.org/10.4102/ phcfm.v6i1.585.

CHAPTER 13

How to ensure your research follows ethical principles

*Christopher Barton,
Sally Hall, Penelope Abbott,
Chun Wah Michael Tam,
Amanda Lyons and Siaw-Teng Liaw*

WHAT ARE ETHICAL PRINCIPLES IN RESEARCH, AND WHERE DID THEY COME FROM? A BRIEF HISTORY OF RESEARCH ETHICS

Contemporary human research ethics is based upon three critical documents: (1) The Nuremberg Code,[1] (2) the Declaration of Helsinki[2] and (3) the Belmont Report.[3] The Nuremberg Code was published in response to the acts of barbarism perpetrated on prisoners in Nazi concentration camps. It emphasises the need for research participants to have the ability to provide voluntary consent and to exercise free power of choice. Despite its historical importance, in the years that followed its release, it was largely ignored.[4]

The World Medical Association adopted the Declaration of Helsinki in 1964 to build upon the Nuremberg Code. The Declaration of Helsinki is an influential code of ethics to guide research involving human participants. Importantly, it is a living document, which is continuously updated to take into consideration changing societal expectations and technological advances affecting the conduct of research with humans. The Declaration of Helsinki is primarily directed towards physicians and has as its starting point the Declaration of Geneva: 'the health of my patient will be my first consideration' and that 'a physician shall act in the patient's best interest when providing medical care'.

The Belmont Report arose in response to the Tuskegee syphilis experiment – a study involving predominately poor African Americans. This experiment tracked the progression of untreated syphilis in participants. However, this continued nearly three decades after a cure had become widely available. The Belmont Report emphasises respect for persons and autonomous decision making, including the need for allowances for vulnerable persons who require more protection.[5] It also provided, for the first time, guidance on the distinction between clinical research and clinical practice[6,7] and the responsibilities of health professionals involved in research.[5]

In the context of these reports, the field of bioethics emerged in the 1970s. Influential authors such as Beauchamp and Childress described common 'principles' for ethically justified human research, including (1) the goal of valuable knowledge, (2) a reasonable prospect that the research will generate the knowledge that is sought, (3) the necessity of using human subjects, (4) a favourable balance of potential benefits over risks to the subjects, (5) fair selection of subjects and (6) measures to protect privacy and confidentiality. Beauchamp and Childress conclude that only if these conditions have been met is it appropriate to invite potential subjects (or their surrogates) to give their informed consent or refusal to participate in research.[8]

In Australia, the National Health and Medical Research Council has developed a National Statement on Ethical Conduct in Human Research (2007, updated 2015) which identifies core values and principles in human research (see Box 13.1). This document is available at www.nhmrc.gov.au/guidelines-publications/e72.

BOX 13.1   ETHICAL PRINCIPLES IN RESEARCH

Research merit and integrity: Research should be justified by its potential benefits and be well-designed and conducted, methodologically appropriate, respectful of participants and conducted by teams with appropriate skills.

Researchers should be committed to integrity in the pursuit of knowledge, honesty in conducting research and disseminating results and to permitting scrutiny of their research practice.

- *Justice*: Research should treat participants fairly in terms of the recruitment process, the burden of participation, the distribution of benefits of participation and access to outcomes and information about results. There should be no exploitation of participants.
- *Beneficence*: The benefits of the research (for participants or the wider community) should justify any risks to participants. Researchers are responsible for the welfare of participants in the research context.
- *Respect*: Researchers should recognise and respect the intrinsic human value of participants including their privacy, confidentiality and cultural sensitivities and their capacity to make independent well-informed decisions.

PHILOSOPHICAL POSITIONS UNDERPINNING RESEARCH ETHICS

Contemporary human research ethics have been shaped by the extraordinary societal change that occurred in the second half of the twentieth century. Principlism, a philosophical approach that uses 'principles' in ethical and moral reasoning, has emerged as the dominant framework.[8] Using a principlism approach (Box 13.1) provides a relatively simple and practical guide for thinking through human-research ethics issues.

Some contemporary ethicists have criticised the primacy given to principlism from a practical perspective, suggesting that it can trend towards operational minimalism[9,10] – for example, when ethical decision making is reduced to checklists focused largely on risk. Others have proposed a communitarian approach as an alternative.[10,11] Communitarianism has a greater focus on the common good and the public interest, for instance, emphasising that research findings should be communicated to and benefit the communities in which the research takes place.[12,13] This approach may have better ethical alignment with the modern emphasis on partnership with communities and their representatives when undertaking research, including in research with indigenous communities,[14,15] and which may be particularly important in the primary health care context. The communitarian approach starts with the questions 'How does this research and treatment benefit the communities of individuals, carers, families, and health and other professionals in the neighbourhood? Is there potential harm to the communities? Do the benefits to the common good outweigh costs of harm? Are there tensions between individual rights to this treatment (autonomy) and the public good and rights of the community (justice, beneficence and non-maleficence)?'[10]

ETHICAL ISSUES SPECIFIC TO THE PRIMARY CARE SETTING

While all researchers share general ethical obligations (Box 13.2), the primary care context is unique. Primary care research includes individual and community-based clinical research, health-services research, public-health research and research that has a focus on education for students and practitioners in primary care.[16]

Different ethical issues arise between primary care researchers conducting research with patients in their own practice and external (e.g. university) researchers recruiting patients from the practice or drawing upon a patient list held by the practice.

Doctor-patient relationships in primary care are typically maintained over long periods of time. The consequences of research projects within a practice raise different ethical issues to primary care research conducted outside the clinical setting. Research within a practice may influence care long after the project is completed[17] and specific ethical issues arise. In particular, the role of clinicians in recruiting patients to research studies can be problematic if there

BOX 13.2 KEY STRATEGIES AND CONSIDERATIONS FOR ETHICAL RESEARCH

Good research practice requires thoughtful consideration and judicious application of ethical principles, which should be embedded in the research design. Ethical guidelines provide advice for the exercise of judgment rather than a set of rules or checklists. In developing research proposals, researchers should consider:

- *Likely risks to participants*: Assessment of risks includes potential for harm, discomfort or inconvenience and the likelihood and potential severity or consequences of these risks. These may be physical, psychological, social, economic or legal.
- *Whether the benefits justify the risks*: Benefits may include direct benefits to participants, families or communities or indirect benefits such as improvements in knowledge and understanding, social outcomes, skills or expertise. Research is ethically justifiable only when its potential benefits justify any risks involved.
- *How risks will be minimised or managed*: In designing research, researchers should minimise risks and have a plan to manage those risks which cannot be avoided.
- *Processes for seeking and obtaining consent*: Consent to participate in research should be voluntary, fully informed and based on a mutual understanding between participants and researchers of the process of the research, the implications and likely benefits of participation for both. This includes transparency when benefits accrue to the researcher. Under some circumstances, it may be legitimate to waive the need for consent, but this should be subject to consideration by an appropriate ethical review body.

  Participants should not suffer disadvantage if they decide not to participate in research and are entitled to withdraw consent after providing it.
- *Capacity*: Participants should have the capacity to provide informed consent. Where consent is provided by someone else, it should be in the best interests of the participant.
- *Coercion*: Participants should not feel coerced or pressured to participate. Reimbursement is appropriate but should be proportionate to participation and not encourage participants to take unacceptable risks.

is undue persuasion or coercion in the context of the power difference in the therapeutic relationship.[17-19] Specific strategies to minimise this risk will be required, such as the use of a third party (e.g. administrative or nursing staff) to explain the research and recruit patients or by ensuring the confidential return of a survey, so that the clinician is unaware of the patient's choice to participate or not.

It is useful for all researchers to keep in mind that patients visit the primary care practitioner with a single outcome in mind – they are sick or require health care. This needs to be recognised by the person doing the recruiting, whether internal or external to the research site. Recruitment strategies which don't involve personal invitations from the primary care practitioner but are framed as invitations to find out more information about a study have been used successfully.[20] It is crucial that invitations to participate in research should emphasise to the patient that their choice to participate, or not, will have no impact on therapeutic relationships or ongoing care provided by the primary care practice.

Maintenance of confidentiality requires special care in primary care research. Identifying and obtaining consent from patients to become research participants may raise questions about confidentiality, as the clinical information used to identify patients who meet study selection criteria was originally collected for a purpose other than research.[17–19] Confidentiality may also be compromised when findings are communicated within primary care teams who are familiar with participants.[17] Even publishing anonymised data may breach confidentiality if the participants can be identified by context. This is a particular issue for qualitative research in primary care[17,19] and research in small, rural communities.

The increasing use of information and communication technologies in health care further creates ethical complexity. There are privacy, confidentiality and ownership issues related to the data contained in primary care information systems, especially where health information derived from patients are used for secondary purposes and potentially shared without the patients' explicit knowledge. This may happen, for example, through clinical audits for quality-improvement initiatives. Although formal ethical review may not be required, such activities must still be conducted ethically and issues such as consent and confidentiality need to be considered.[17,18]

DOES MY RESEARCH REQUIRE ETHICAL REVIEW?

Institutional Review Boards (IRBs) and independent Human Research Ethics Committees (HRECs), 'ethics boards', are charged with protecting the rights and safety of participants involved in human research.[21] Before research can begin, and in many cases before funding will be released, proposals must be submitted to ethics boards for consideration, comment, guidance and approval. Following approval, changes to the protocol (including investigators, participant recruitment material and consent forms) cannot be made without seeking approval for amendment. Research studies in which patients are recruited as participants will nearly always require review by an ethics board, however some research or evaluation and audit activities may not require formal review by a full committee under some circumstances.[18,21,22] Increasingly, scientific journals require evidence of ethics board approval (or an exemption to the need for approval) prior to publishing research so if the intent is to publish findings, even of clinical audit, researchers should seek ethical review or exemption.

Ethics boards form one part of a governance structure for human research. Researchers should make themselves aware of the governance structures and any specific legal requirements for research within their local institution and communities, as these will vary between countries and even within countries depending on local laws and regulations. In reviewing proposals, ethics boards will take into consideration the laws and regulations of the country in which the research is to be performed, as well as applicable international norms and standards. Its deliberations should be independent of the researcher or sponsor but transparent in its functioning and decision making. For example, industry funding of research can create particular ethical considerations relating to transparency and the task of identifying and managing conflicts of interest.[7]

WRITING AN ETHICS APPLICATION

For the new researcher, the initial steps in undertaking a research project and seeking ethical review can seem daunting and have been described as like 'stepping into another country – with a new language and different expectations'.[22] The technical and administrative requirements of ethics boards can seem burdensome. Increasingly, standardised forms have been adopted with the aim of ensuring inclusion of all information required to adequately assess the ethics of a proposal.[21,22] However, these forms typically attempt to cover the gamut of human research from laboratory to clinical to large scale population health research, making them lengthy and complex to navigate.

Researchers need to allow plenty of time to prepare the ethics documentation, including the relevant content at a level of detail that enables the ethics board to conduct the review.[21] A study must be scientifically sound in order to be ethical, which is why ethics boards also comment on the methods. However, while the protocol for a study may have been well developed, perhaps as part of a grant proposal, and have a sound scientific basis, it is often the case that the ethical aspects of the project have not been as fully considered, which may delay approval of the project.[18]

Informed consent from participants is a core focus of ethics committees, who will spend considerable time in their discussions to ensure that research participants' rights are protected, taking into account the unique characteristics of the population at the centre of the research project.[21] In addition to these ethical considerations that apply to all research, additional consideration and protections may be required for vulnerable groups including children and young people, people in dependent or unequal relationships (including those highly dependent on medical care) and people with a cognitive impairment, intellectual disability or mental illness. Further support or protections may also be required for people with poor literacy, limited education or those who may require interpreters.

It is possible that the increasing focus on technical compliance in ethics documentation may obscure rather than facilitate broad ethical thinking in health research. We encourage researchers to frame and embed ethical issues at the beginning of the research process and for novice researchers to seek help and guidance at the outset from experienced primary care researchers or mentors to brainstorm research and ethical questions.[22] The ethical dimensions of research go beyond the mechanical application of guidelines or sets of rules and call for an appreciation of context and individual deliberation regarding the application of ethical values. Box 13.3 outlines the key issues that should be addressed in your research proposal and particularly the section on ethical considerations. Box 13.4 provides links to additional resources on ethics that will be of use to the primary care researcher.

BOX 13.3 ADDRESSING ETHICAL CONSIDERATIONS IN THE RESEARCH PROPOSAL

- *Social and scientific value*:
  - The value of the research should have been argued for in the introduction of the proposal.
- *Scientific validity*:
  - The scientific validity of the methods should have been described in the methods section of the proposal.
- *Fair selection of study population*:
  - Has the study population been fairly chosen?
  - Have any groups been excluded, for non-scientific reasons, that could benefit from the research?
  - Is the study population vulnerable in any way?
- *Favourable risk-benefit ratio*:
  - Have the risks and benefits been assessed as accurately as possible?
  - Is the risk-benefit ratio favourable?
  - What are the local context and risks?
  - How will the biopsychosocial risks to participants, families and communities be minimised?
  - Are there likely to be benefits to the community, especially vulnerable communities?
  - How will you disseminate results and ensure that the benefits of the project can be realised?
- *Independent review*:
  - Will the research be submitted for independent scientific review?
  - What other permissions are needed?

- *Informed consent*:
  - How will you ensure that participants are appropriately informed about what participation involves and obtain consent?
  - Has sufficient information been disclosed in a culturally and linguistically sensitive manner?
  - Do you need to argue for a waiver of informed consent?
  - Does your study involve children, teenagers or other groups who have specific issues with ensuring informed consent?
- *Respect for participants and study communities*:
  - Do the participants know they can withdraw from the study at any time?
  - Have issues of confidentiality and privacy been adequately addressed?
  - How will you ensure confidentiality of participants, including mechanisms for data storage and security?
  - How will you use the information participants provide?[23]

BOX 13.4   USEFUL FREE RESOURCES

- Graf C, Wager E, Bowman A, Fiack S, Scott-Lichter D and Robinson A. Best Practice Guidelines on Publication Ethics: A Publisher's Perspective. *International Journal of Clinical Practice*, 2007;61:1–26.
- A video guide for new GP researchers: https://www.youtube.com/watch?v=p1n2kPvk3iE
- Praxis Online Research Ethics Training: www.praxisaustralia.com.au
- Centre for Clinical and Research Ethics, Washington University in St Louis: http://ethicsresearchcore.org
- Research Ethics Program, UC San Diego: http://research-ethics.net/
- Norwegian University of Science and Technology Ethics Portal: http://www.ntnu.edu/ethics-portal
- NIH Annual Review of Ethics – Case Studies: https://oir.nih.gov/sourcebook/ethical-conduct/responsible-conduct-research-training/annual-review-ethics-case-studies
- Ethics Education Library, Illinois Institute of Technology: http://ethics.iit.edu
- NHS Health Research Authority: http://www.hra.nhs.uk/

REFERENCES

1. The Nuremberg Code. Secondary The Nuremberg Code 1949. https://history.nih.gov/research/downloads/nuremberg.pdf.
2. WMA Declaration of Helsinki – ethical principles for medical research involving human subjects. Secondary WMA Declaration of Helsinki – ethical principles for

medical research involving human subjects 2013. https://www.wma.net/policies-post/wma-declaration-of-helsinki-ethical-principles-for-medical-research-involving-human-subjects/.

3. The Belmont Report. Secondary The Belmont Report 1979. https://www.hhs.gov/ohrp/regulations-and-policy/belmont-report/index.html.

4. Develin S. Introduction to good clinical practice. In: McGraw M, George A, Shearn S et al. editors. *Principles of Good Clinical Practice*. London: Pharmaceutical Press; 2010.

5. Miracle V. The Belmont Report: The triple crown of research ethics. *Dimens Crit Care Nurs* 2016;35(4):223–28.

6. Beauchamp T, Saghai Y. The historical foundations of the research-practice distinction in bioethics. *Theor Med Bioeth* 2012;33:45–56.

7. Friesen P, Kearns L, Redman B et al. Rethinking the Belmont Report? *Am J Bioeth* 2017;17(7):15–21.

8. Beauchamp T, Childress J. *Principles of Biomedical Ethics*, 7th ed. New York: Oxford University Press; 2013.

9. Callahan D. Minimalist ethics. *Hastings Cent Rep* 1981;11(5):19–25.

10. Liaw S-T, Tam C. Ethical research or research ethics? *Aust Fam Physician* 2015;44(7):522–23.

11. Callahan D. *The Roots of Bioethics: Health Progress, Technology, Death*. New York: Oxford University Press; 2012.

12. Barton C, Tam C, Abbott P et al. Can research that is not intended or unlikely to be published be considered ethical? *Aust Fam Physician* 2017;46(6):442–44.

13. Rajan K. The experimental machinery of global clinical trials: Case studies from India. In: Ong A, Chen N, editors. *Asian Biotech: Ethics and Communities of Fate: e-Duke Books*, Durham, NC, USA: Duke University Press; 2010.

14. Dunbar T, Scrimgeour M. Ethics in Indigenous Research – Connecting with Community. *J Bioeth Inq* 2006;3(3):179–85.

15. Ross L, Loup A, Nelson R et al. Human subjects protections in community-engaged research: A research ethics framework. *J Empir Res Hum Res Ethics* 2010;5(1):5–17.

16. Beasley J, Bazemore A, Mash B. The nature of primary care research In: Goodyear-Smith F, Mash B, editors. *International Perspectives on Primary Care Research*. Boca Raton, Fl.: CRC Press/Taylor & Francis; 2016.

17. Rogers W, Schwartz L. Supporting ethical practice in primary care research: Strategies for action. *Br J Gen Pract* 2002;52:1007–11.

18. Barton C, Tam C, Abbott P et al. Ethical considerations in recruiting primary care patients to research studies. *Aust Fam Physician* 2016;45(3):144–48.

19. Jones R, Murphy EAC. Primary care research ethics. *Br J Gen Pract* 1995;45:623–26.

20. Reed R, Barton C, Isherwood L, et al. Recruitment for a clinical trial of chronic disease self-management for older adults with multimorbidity: a successful approach within general practice. *BMC Fam Pract* 2013;14(125).

21. Jacobs R. Institutional review boards and independent ethics committee's In: McGraw MJ, George A, Shearn S et al. editors. *Principles of Good Clinical Practice*. London: Pharmaceutical Press; 2010.

22. Liaw S-T, Tam C. Research ethics and approval process: A guide for new GP researchers. *Aust Fam Physician* 2015;44(6):419–22.

23. Emanuel EJ, Wendler D, Killen J et al. What makes clinical research in developing countries ethical? The benchmarks of ethical research. *J Infect Dis* 2004;189(5):930–7.

CHAPTER 14

How to search and critically appraise the literature

Celeste Naude and Taryn Young

INTRODUCTION

New research is usually not done in a vacuum, and most research builds on what has come before. Even 'ground-breaking' research usually relies on previous work in that field or in a related one. There are not many major unrelated research 'breakthroughs'. By doing research, we seek to increase our knowledge of the world around us through systematic processes of experimentation and observation, and each piece of good quality research contributes to increasing our knowledge in a specific field in an incremental way.

The principle that research is cumulative makes it very important to have a thorough understanding of previous research in your area of interest when you start a new study. This requires you to find and read this previous research by searching the scientific literature. But, very importantly, not all published and unpublished research is of equal value and sufficient quality, as it may not have been conducted using satisfactory methodological rigour. For this reason, we need to appraise the validity of all the research we find and read. This concept was well captured by Professor Trisha Greenhalgh when she said, 'If one is deciding whether a paper is worth reading, you should do so on the design of the methods section and not on the interest value of the hypothesis, the nature or potential impact of the results or the speculation in the discussion'.[1]

In this chapter, we focus firstly on searching the literature and secondly on critically appraising the research you find. Useful tips and resources are detailed in the boxes.

STEPS IN SEARCHING THE LITERATURE

Searching the literature successfully to find the evidence you are looking for involves various stages. You may need to do multiple searches in various databases to find and read a broad range of literature on important aspects of your area of interest. The relevant evidence from the different searches can then be integrated to inform your precise research question and to make an argument for the social and scientific value of your study. You can use the five steps outlined in this chapter to do a targeted search. An illustrated example is provided in Figure 14.1.

Step 1: Formulate your search question

Formulating a clear, answerable question can get your searching off to a good start. Using a mnemonic, like PICO or PECO, to formulate your question helps to identify and organise the key aspects of a complex research question, where P = Patient or Population, I = Intervention or Indicator, E = Exposure, C = Comparison or Control or Context and O = Outcome.

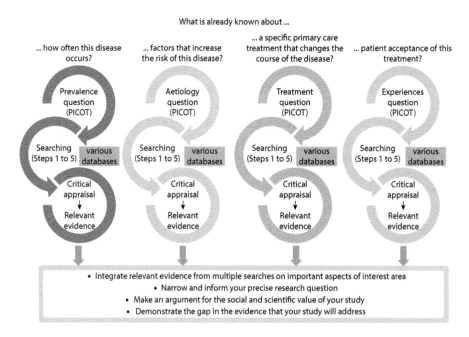

FIGURE 14.1 Illustrated example of doing multiple literature searches to gain a thorough understanding on what is already known about important aspects of your area of interest, using five steps.

Ask the following questions to help you formulate your question:

P: *What is the patient group or population of interest?*
I: *What is the intervention or issue of interest?*
or
E: *What is the exposure of interest?*
C: *What is the comparison intervention of interest? What is the context?*
O: *What is the primary outcome of interest?*

The mnemonic PICO can be extended to PICOT or PECOT, if your question has a time component (see Box 14.1 for examples):

T: *What is the relevant time period?*

BOX 14.1   EXAMPLES OF FORMULATING CLEAR, ANSWERABLE QUESTIONS USING PICOT/PECOT

Does aspirin improve survival after myocardial infarction?	In patients with first episode, acute myocardial infarction (P), does daily, low-dose, oral aspirin (I) lead to higher survival rates (O) compared to placebo (C)?
Does counselling help improve breastfeeding?	In pregnant women (P), what is the effect of breastfeeding counselling (I) compared to no counselling (C) on the number of babies being exclusively breastfed (O) for the first 6 months of their lives (T)?
Does measles, mumps, rubella vaccination lead to autism?	Are infants (P) that received the MMR vaccine (E) more at risk to be diagnosed with autism (O) in the first 5 years of life (T) than babies that did not receive the MMR vaccine (C)?

You also need to identify what type of question your search question is (see Box 14.2). Different types or categories of questions depend on the nature or focus of your question. Diagnosis or diagnostic test questions are used to determine which test is more accurate in diagnosing a condition. Prevalence or incidence questions are used to study the burden of a disease. Risk factor questions are used to determine the greatest risk factors or causes of a condition. Questions about harm help to understand the safety of a treatment. Prognosis or prediction questions are used to determine the clinical course over time and likely complications of a condition. There are intervention or prevention questions that are used to determine which treatment or preventive intervention leads to the best outcome. Cost-effectiveness questions weigh the costs and benefits of interventions for conditions. Experiences and meaning questions help us to understand the significance of an experience for an individual, group or community.[2]

BOX 14.2   EXAMPLES OF THE TYPICAL NATURE OR FOCUS OF DIFFERENT CATEGORIES OR TYPES OF QUESTIONS

Category	Typical nature or focus of questions
Diagnosis and screening	How accurate is this test?
Frequency/prevalence/incidence	How often does this disease occur?
Risk/aetiology/cause	What factors increase the risk of this disease?
Harm	Is this intervention safe?
Prognosis	What are the consequences of this disease?
Treatment/intervention	Does treatment change the course of this disease?
Prevention/intervention	Does early intervention keep this disease from occurring, or does it slow its development?
Cost-effectiveness	Are the benefits of the treatment worth the costs incurred?
Experiences and meaning	Why do patients behave in a certain way and how do they experience the disease, test or treatment?

Step 2: Identify the study design that will best answer your type of question

Study design refers to the structured approach followed by researchers to answer a particular research question. The study design is important because it determines how we sample the population of interest, how we collect and measure data and how we analyse data. While no research study design is considered more valuable than another, some study designs are more appropriate for different types of questions (see Box 14.3). This is because

BOX 14.3   QUESTION TYPES AND THE BEST STUDY DESIGN TO ANSWER THEM

Question type	Best study design to answer
Therapy or prevention	Randomised controlled trial
Risk factor and aetiology	Cohort or case-control study
Diagnosis and screening	Cross-sectional and randomised controlled trial, respectively
Prognosis and incidence	Cohort study
Prevalence	Cross-sectional study
Meaning and experiences	Qualitative study

As we know from the hierarchy of evidence, for each type of question, a systematic review of all available relevant studies is better than an individual study.

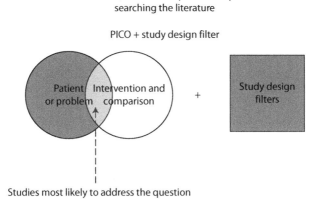

FIGURE 14.2 The link between a clear, answerable question and searching the literature.

these study designs are likely to provide the least biased answer to the specific type of question.

Knowing the most appropriate study design for your question can help you narrow your searches by study design to find studies that are most relevant to your focused question.

The mnemonic PICOT can be extended to PICOTS or PECOTS, where S = study design, to remind you that different types of study designs are best used to answer different types of questions.

Figure 14.2 depicts how Steps 1, 2 and 3 can help with searching the literature and finding the evidence you are looking for.

Step 3: Select appropriate database(s) to search

There are numerous electronic research databases available to search, such as Medline and Embase. Most of these database are accessed using a dedicated search engine, for example, PubMed is a free search engine accessing primarily the Medline database of references and abstracts on life sciences and biomedical topics. Ovid is a platform that hosts more than 100 core and niche databases in health and other sciences.

For all types of primary studies, Medline (PubMed) is a good place to start searching. If you are looking for trials, then a collection of more than 1 million randomised and other controlled clinical trials can be found in the Cochrane Library. If your interest has a national, regional or other geographic focus, you may need to search databases or journals that are specific to a region, as many regional journals may not be included in bibliographic databases such as Medline. For example, the World Health Organization (WHO), in collaboration with the Association for Health Information and Libraries in Africa (AHILA),

---

BOX 14.4   DATABASES FOR SYSTEMATIC REVIEWS

Start by searching the Cochrane Database of Systematic Reviews in the Cochrane Library.	http://www.cochranelibrary.com/
Epistemonikos is a collaborative, multilingual database of health evidence. It is the largest source of systematic reviews relevant for health-decision making.	https://www.epistemonikos.org/
Database of Abstracts of Reviews of Effects is a database containing abstracts of systematic reviews that have been quality-assessed. Each abstract includes a summary of the review together with a critical commentary about the overall quality.	http://www.cochranelibrary.com/
Trip database is another resource that can be searched for primary studies and systematic reviews.	https://www.tripdatabase.com/

---

has produced an international index to African health literature and information sources, called African Index Medicus (AIM), to improve access to health information published in or related to Africa (more information at http://indexmedicus.afro.who.int/). African Journals OnLine (AJOL) is another regional resource, hosting a large online library of peer-reviewed, African-published scholarly journals (more information at https://www.ajol.info/). LILACS is a comprehensive index of scientific and technical literature of Latin America and the Caribbean (more information at http://lilacs.bvsalud.org/en/). In most databases, you can choose to restrict your search by language or not. Databases that focus on collections of systematic reviews are shown in Box 14.4.

Step 4: Putting together a search strategy

Your question will inform which search terms to use. The search is usually started with two of the four PICO or PECO components, usually P and I. Depending on the question and retrieval, the search can be further focused by adding the rest of the components of the question. The more components you add to your search, the more you will limit your search, that is, the fewer total search results you will retrieve.

It is recommended that you start by searching for the specific study design that best answers your question, unless you search in a database or library where the articles have been pre-sorted according to certain study designs.

There are two general approaches one can use for searching an index or database, namely (1) keywords (or textwords) and (2) controlled vocabulary terms. The type of search terms you use will mainly depend on the database you are using. It is always good to know whether the databases you choose use keyword searching, a controlled vocabulary or both.

For your search, you need to identify relevant keywords, synonyms and controlled vocabulary terms for components of your question, including the study design. And you combine your search terms with Boolean operators.

Keyword searching

Keyword searching is also known as natural language, free text or textword searching. Unless limited to certain fields, such as 'Title' or 'Title/Abstract', the entire text is searched (all fields). Keyword searching does not consider variant spellings of a word (e.g. the US pediatrics vs. the British paediatrics), and does not search for synonyms of a keyword, for example, a search done on hypertension will not retrieve articles that use the term high blood pressure. Using synonyms for keywords can help overcome this, such as, infant, neonate, baby, babies, newborn. Searches can also be limited to certain fields such as 'Title/Abstract' to narrow search results.

How to perform an effective keyword search

- *Truncation:* This is an effective means of finding plurals, variants of terms or terms with various endings. Truncation allows you to add a symbol to your search term so that all variants of the word appear, and is usually added to the end of the root of a word to instruct the database to search for all forms of a word. For example, the word health* retrieves articles with the words: health, healthy, healthier and healthful. With some databases, you can also use truncation in the middle of a term: wom*n will retrieve women or woman. The rules and symbols (*, #, $) for truncation searching vary from database to database. Truncation will broaden your search.
- *Wildcard (?):* This is similar to truncation, but is really useful when there are multiple ways to deal with the middle of a word. Wildcard will assist with finding the same word with alternative spellings. The word behavio?r will look for behavior and behaviour. The '?' tells the database that you want a given character in a word to be any letter. With some databases you can use the wildcard symbol '#'; this tells the database that you want an additional character inside the word, for example, an#emia would find results containing either anaemia or anemia.
- Use inverted commas if searching for a specific phrase, such as 'evidence-based health care' or 'primary health care'.

Controlled vocabulary terms

Controlled vocabularies use a specific term for a number of synonyms. Once you find the correct term, you do not need to use synonyms in order to perform your search. A controlled vocabulary employs a thesaurus that prescribes which term should be used for a concept. For example, Medline (PubMed) employs the MeSH (Medical Subject Headings) thesaurus. The MeSH term for lung cancer is lung neoplasms. An article written about lung cancer will be indexed under the term lung neoplasms even if the phrase lung neoplasms does not appear in the article. A factsheet on MeSH is available at https://www. nlm.nih.gov/pubs/factsheets/mesh.html and tutorials on MeSH are available at https://learn.nlm.nih.gov/rest/training-packets/T0042010P.html.

A controlled vocabulary allows you more control in choosing search terms. Techniques that you can use when searching with a controlled vocabulary include hierarchical structure, broader, narrower and related terms, major or starred terms and working backwards.

Boolean operators

The Boolean operators (AND, NOT and OR) are then used to join keywords, synonyms and controlled vocabulary terms to create search strings. Joining terms with AND finds articles with both terms, joining terms with NOT finds articles with the first term and without the term that follows the operator NOT; and joining terms with OR finds articles with either term.[3] The Boolean operator OR is usually used to link together similar concepts, enclosing these in parenthesis, and then AND is used to link these search strings together (see Box 14.5).

BOX 14.5   BOOLEAN OPERATORS

(infant* OR neonate* OR baby OR babies OR newborn* OR 'Infant, Newborn'[MeSH])
AND
(dummy OR dummies OR soother* OR pacifier* OR comforter*)
AND
(breastfeeding OR 'breast feeding' OR 'breastfeed' OR 'breast feed' OR 'Breast Feeding'[MeSH])
AND
('randomized controlled trial' OR 'randomised controlled trial' OR 'controlled trial' OR 'clinical trial' OR 'randomized trial' OR 'randomised trial' OR 'Randomized Controlled Trial' [Publication Type])

Search terminology

- *Search terms*: The keywords, phrases you are going to have in your search.
- *Search string*: Example (infant* OR neonate* OR baby OR babies OR newborn*). Usually, you will have one search string per PICO(TS) component that you search for, but not always; for example, an

Intervention search string could be made up of 2 search strings, as follows: ('vitamin C' OR 'ascorbic acid') AND (supplement OR pill OR tablet).

- *Search strategy*: All search strings joined together with Boolean operators.

Step 5: Perform the search and select studies

Once you have put together your search strategy and selected your databases, perform your search. Further resources on how to perform the search are listed in Box 14.6.

Depending on the yield of your search, you can also limit your search further (if relevant) using filters, for example, by language, publication type or date. In most databases, you can also sort your search results by date of publication or by relevance. You will also be able to view the title and abstract in most databases.

Once you have selected the studies most relevant to your question and research topic, the next very important step is to obtain the full texts of these articles and to read and critically appraise them, as explained in the next section. This will stand you in good stead for gaining a thorough understanding of previous research around your question.

BOX 14.6   RECOMMENDED SEARCHING RESOURCES

Textbook on searching skills: de Bruin C and Pearce-Smith N. *Searching Skills Toolkit: Finding the Evidence.* Wiley-Blackwell and BMJ Books; 2012.

YouTube video on searching: Search Smarter, Search Faster. https://www.youtube.com/watch?v=Oa66AxTbjxA

PubMed tutorial (covering 'building the search', managing results', 'saving the search', 'getting the articles' and 'review exercises'): http://www.nlm.nih.gov/bsd/disted/pubmedtutorial/

PubMed help: https://www.ncbi.nlm.nih.gov/books/NBK3827/#pubmedhelp

---

CRITICAL APPRAISAL

Good quality research is important because it builds the evidence base that informs our health care practices and policies. Additionally, identifying and reading good-quality research helps you to improve your knowledge about previous important and relevant work as you prepare to do a new study. The extent to which any study can draw valid conclusions depends on whether the study used rigorous methods. Just because an article has been published in a journal does not mean it is sound and rigorous.

Some common problems with studies include unclear objectives, poor research design, methodological weaknesses, inadequate data reporting, selective use and reporting of data, unsupported conclusions and conflicts of interest, which may bias behaviour and decision making during research.

Critical appraisal is an appraisal of a study based on careful analytical evaluation, where the research is appraised to assess its validity (closeness to the truth) and its usefulness (applicability). Use the following four questions to guide your critical appraisal:

1. Does this study address a clearly focused question?
2. Did the study use valid methods to address this question?
3. What are the results of this?
4. Are these valid, important results applicable to my patient or population?[3]

'Study validity' is 'the degree to which the inference drawn from a study, is warranted when account is taken of the study methods, the representativeness of the study sample and the nature of the population from which it is drawn'.[4] There are two types of validity: internal and external validity.

Internal validity is determined by the degree to which bias has been reduced by the rigour of the methods used. Threats to internal validity include random error, systematic error (bias) and confounding. Bias is any systematic error in the design, conduct or analysis of the study that results in a mistaken estimate of the exposure's effect on the risk of disease. Bias can cause you to get the wrong answer or an invalid answer about a relationship between exposure and outcome. There are two main types of bias: (1) selection bias – refers to flaws in the selection of study subjects and (2) information bias – refers to flaws in procedures for gathering information from study subjects. Confounding refers to a 'mixing of effects' in which the association between an exposure and outcome is distorted because of the involvement of a third variable that is associated with both exposure and outcome.

External validity (generalisability) is the extent to which the results obtained from the study sample are applicable to the target population. Generalisability depends on the extent to which participants, context, interventions etc. in a study are representative of the people to whom the findings are to be applied.

Critical appraisal can be applied to both quantitative and qualitative research using the same four questions, but slightly different concepts. What differs is the nature and type of processes that ontologically and methodologically distinguish quantitative and qualitative research from

BOX 14.7   TOOLS THAT CAN BE USED TO GUIDE CRITICAL APPRAISAL

Centre for Evidence-Based Medicine Critical Appraisal Worksheets	Provide step-by-step questions for articles about diagnosis, harm, prognosis, systematic reviews (of therapy) and therapy http://www.cebm.net/critical-appraisal/
Critical Appraisal Skills Programme (CASP) Checklists	Provide set of 8 critical appraisal tools designed to be used when reading research. These include tools to critically appraise systematic reviews, randomised controlled trials, cohort studies, case control studies, economic evaluations, diagnostic studies, qualitative studies and clinical prediction rules http://www.casp-uk.net/casp-tools-checklists
Other resources for critical appraisal of qualitative studies	Lincoln YS, Lynham SA, Guba EG. Vol. 4. *Paradigmatic controversies, contradictions, and emerging confluences, revisited. The Sage Handbook of Qualitative Research*; pp. 97–128. Sage Publications; 2011. Meyrick J. What is good qualitative research? A first step towards a comprehensive approach to judging rigour/quality. *J Health Psychol* 2006;11:799–808.

each other. Quantitative research is primarily concerned with numerical data and their statistical interpretations under a reductionist, logical and objective paradigm. Qualitative research uses non-numerical information and its interpretation, which are intricately linked to human senses and subjectivity, to improve knowledge about psychosocial aspects of health care. There are various tools available to guide critical appraisals of quantitative and qualitative research (see Box 14.7). Remember that systematic reviews use a structured approach to take stock of existing studies, and reading an up-to-date systematic review provides a useful starting point for getting to know the existing body of research.

CONCLUSION

Research is incremental and builds on what has been done before. Therefore, finding and reading previous research is a very important part of gaining a thorough understanding of previous work in your area of research when you start a new study. However, reading the previous research is not enough. We must also critically appraise the validity of all the research we find and read so that our knowledge and new research is informed by good quality and relevant previous work.

REFERENCES

1. Greenhalgh T. How to read a paper. Getting your bearings (deciding what the paper is about). *BMJ* 1997;315(7102):243–6.
2. Echevarria IM, Walker S. To make your case, start with a PICOT question. *Nursing* 2014;44(2):18–9.
3. Centre for Evidence-based Health Care Nuffield Department of Primary Care Oxford University. EBM tools. Secondary EBM tools. http://www.cebm.net/category/ebm-resources/tools/.
4. Last JM. *A Dictionary of Epidemiology*, 4th ed. New York: Oxford Universities Press; 2001.

SECTION IV

Methods and techniques for doing primary care research

CHAPTER 15

Taking stock of existing research: Approach to conducting a systematic review

Taryn Young and Celeste Naude

INTRODUCTION

With the growth in research outputs, it is important to take stock of existing research to inform both practice and new research. As put by Egger, '... Two processes are at work side by side, the reception of new material and the digestion and assimilation of the old; and as both are essential...'.[1] Research is not done in a vacuum and most research builds on what has come before.

The current emphasis on reducing research waste requires a thorough assessment or review of existing research as a key first step before embarking on any new research. This is also called research synthesis and there are many different types of reviews ranging from scoping reviews to systematic reviews to overviews of reviews.[2] In this chapter, we focus on scoping and systematic reviews. Useful tips and resources are detailed in the boxes.

Scoping reviews can be defined as a form of knowledge synthesis that addresses an exploratory or emerging research question aimed at mapping key concepts, types of evidence and gaps in research related to a defined area or field, by systematically searching, selecting and synthesising existing knowledge. Scoping reviews address a broad question about what has been done in a well-defined field and can inform the need for a new systematic review. For additional resources on methods for, and examples of, scoping reviews see Box 15.1.

A scoping review should have a protocol detailing the criteria that will be used to include and exclude studies to identify what data are relevant, how searching for studies will be done, and how the data will be extracted and mapped. It is important to report all details of the methods undertaken in a scoping review, and a reporting guideline for scoping reviews (PRISMA-ScR) is currently being developed as part of the Enhancing the QUAlity and Transparency Of health Research (EQUATOR) Network. For more information, visit http://www.prisma-statement.org/Extensions/InDevelopment.aspx.

A systematic review is 'a review in which bias has been reduced by the systematic identification, appraisal, synthesis, and, if relevant, statistical aggregation of all relevant studies on a specific topic according to a predetermined and explicit method'.[3] It can consider various types of questions (Table 15.1). The key aspects which differentiate systematic reviews from other reviews are that they include:

BOX 15.1   ADDITIONAL RESOURCES

There are five basic steps for preparing a scoping review:

1. Identify the broad research question(s).
2. Identify the relevant studies.
3. Select studies.
4. Extract the data.
5. Collate, summarise and report the data.

Open access papers on methods for scoping reviews

- Levac D, Colquhoun H, O'Brien KK. Scoping studies: Advancing the methodology. *Implementation Science*: IS 2010, 5:69.
- Peters MD, Godfrey CM, Khalil H, McInerney P, Parker D, Soares CB. Guidance for conducting systematic scoping reviews. *International Journal of Evidence-Based Health care* 2015, 13(3):141–146.

Examples of scoping reviews available in open access journals

- van Dongen JJ, van Bokhoven MA, Daniëls R, van der Weijden T, Emonts WW et al. Developing interprofessional care plans in chronic care: A scoping review. *BMC Fam Pract* 2016 Sep 21;17(1):137.
- Khanassov V, Pluye P, Descoteaux S, Haggerty JL, Russell G et al. Organizational interventions improving access to community-based primary health care for vulnerable populations: A scoping review. *Int J Equity Health* 2016 Oct 10;15(1):168.

TABLE 15.1 Examples of systematic reviews in open access journals

Type of question	Systematic review example
Prevalence	Usenbo A et al. Prevalence of Arthritis in Africa: A Systematic Review and Meta-Analysis. PLOS ONE 2015; 10(8):e0133858. http://journals.plos.org/plosone/article?id=10.1371/journal.pone.0133858
Diagnostic test accuracy	Creavin ST et al. Mini-Mental State Examination (MMSE) for the detection of dementia in clinically unevaluated people aged 65 and over in community and primary care populations. Cochrane Database of Systematic Reviews 2016, *Issue* 1. *Art. No.: CD011145.* http://onlinelibrary.wiley.com/doi/10.1002/14651858.CD011145.pub2/full
Treatment	Gera T et al. Integrated management of childhood illness (IMCI) strategy for children under five. Cochrane Database of Systematic Reviews 2016, *Issue* 6. *Art. No.: CD010123.* http://onlinelibrary.wiley.com/doi/10.1002/14651858.CD010123.pub2/full
Qualitative	Glenton C et al. Barriers and facilitators to the implementation of lay health worker programmes to improve access to maternal and child health: Qualitative evidence synthesis. Cochrane Database of Systematic Reviews 2013, *Issue* 10. *Art. No.: CD010414.* http://onlinelibrary.wiley.com/doi/10.1002/14651858.CD010414.pub2/full
Health systems	Flodgren G, Rachas A, Farmer AJ, Inzitari M, Shepperd S. Interactive telemedicine: Effects on professional practice and health care outcomes. Cochrane Database of Systematic Reviews 2015, *Issue* 9. *Art. No.: CD002098.* http://onlinelibrary.wiley.com/doi/10.1002/14651858.CD002098.pub2/full

- A clear and specific question;
- Explicit pre-defined eligibility criteria for considering studies for inclusion;
- Comprehensive searches in electronic databases and other sources to identify all potential studies;
- Duplicate independent selection of studies and data extraction; and
- Critical appraisal of the quality (risk of bias) of included studies, which is used together with the results to formulate conclusions.

STEPS IN CONDUCTING A SYSTEMATIC REVIEW

Conducting a systematic review involves various stages, such as clarifying the rationale and checking if there are already any existing systematic reviews on the topic, developing and refining a clear question, developing a clear protocol, registering the title and key features of the protocol and conducting and reporting the findings of the systematic review (Figure 15.1).

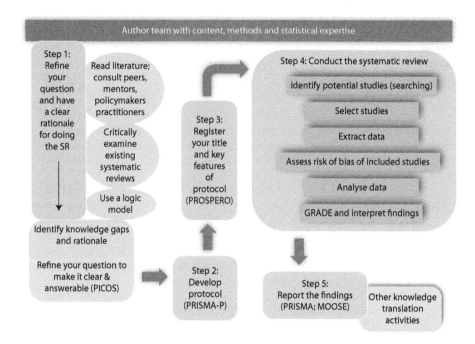

FIGURE 15.1 Steps in conducting a systematic review.

Step 1: Refine your question and be clear on the rationale for doing the systematic review

Conducting a systematic review is a transparent, comprehensive, reproducible and ordered way of assessing the total body of research (all relevant studies) on a well-defined topic in order to (1) inform policy and practice and (2) inform new research. The foundation for a systematic review is a clear, answerable question.

The process of defining and refining your research question is often iterative and can take time, as you need to consider various aspects, such as what is the problem? Why is this the problem? What do you know about potential solutions to the problem? How do these solutions potentially work? What are the gaps in knowledge? Often this is done by reading current literature and consulting others, such as talking to peers and mentors, to policymakers and to practitioners. This will help refine the question to make it clear and answerable. The question should detail the participants (P), the issue or intervention (I), the context or comparison (C), the outcomes of interest (O) and the study design(s) (S).

Often there may be a tension between a broader versus a narrow question, for example, 'assessing the effects of strategies to improve vaccination coverage' (broader) versus 'parent and learner education for improving the uptake of HPV vaccines in female learners older than 9 years' (narrower). Determining the final scope of the question will depend on a number of things, such as relevance of the question, the knowledge gap, the alignment with theoretical models, generalisability and resource availability.

To support the background and rationale for complex systematic reviews, logic models are often used to make sense of the complexity. It is a useful method to understand and display the various facets of an intervention, how they link and interact and other important contextual elements.[4] Logic models can be very useful to help refine your question.

It is also important at this stage to assess existing reviews on the topic to determine what is known already, to assess how well previous reviews were conducted and to make sure there is a clear gap in the evidence base, thus providing a rationale for your new review. See Box 15.2 for information on where to search for ongoing and existing systematic reviews. Tools are available to assess the methods used to conduct systematic reviews such as AMSTAR (https://amstar.ca/)[5] and ROBIS (http://www.bristol.ac.uk/population-health-sciences/projects/robis/).[6]

Step 2: Develop the protocol for the systematic review

Like all other research, you need a clear protocol for conducting a systematic review. Conducting a systematic review involves various judgments, and to minimise bias being introduced, a clear *a priori* protocol should detail the rationale, question and methods to be followed. Box 15.3 provide some further practical considerations to sort out at protocol development stage.

BOX 15.2   WHERE TO SEARCH FOR ONGOING AND EXISTING SYSTEMATIC REVIEWS

Epistemonikos: A collaborative, multilingual database of health evidence. It is the largest source of systematic reviews relevant for health-decision making (https://www.epistemonikos.org/).

Cochrane Database of Systematic Reviews: A database in http://www.cochranelibrary.com/ which includes all Cochrane Reviews (and protocols) prepared by Cochrane Review Groups.

Database of Abstracts of Reviews of Effects: A database in http://www.cochranelibrary.com/ which contains abstracts of systematic reviews that have been quality-assessed. Each abstract includes a summary of the review together with a critical commentary about the overall quality.

PubMed: Comprises more than 21 million citations for biomedical literature from Medline, life science journals and online books (www.pubmed.com).

PROSPERO: A database of ongoing systematic reviews (https://www.crd.york.ac.uk/PROSPERO/).

BOX 15.3   ON A PRACTICAL NOTE

Software: There are various software packages available for systematic
reviews, including:
- RevMan is the software used for preparing and maintaining
  reviews. RevMan facilitates preparation of protocols and full
  reviews, including text, characteristics of studies, comparison
  tables and study data. It can perform meta-analysis of the data
  entered and present the results graphically (available for free at
  http://community.cochrane.org/tools/review-production-tools/
  revman-5/revman-5-download).
- Eppi-Reviewer is an online software tool for evidence synthesis
  that is web-based and can manage and analyse data. It has been
  developed for all types of systematic review such as meta-analysis,
  framework synthesis and thematic synthesis (http://eppi.ioe.ac.uk/
  cms/Default.aspx?tabid=3396).
- DistillerSR is a web-based reference screening, data extraction
  and reporting solution for systematic reviews (https://www.
  evidencepartners.com/products/distillersr-systematic-review
  -software/).
- Systematic Review Data Repository (SRDR) is a tool for the
  extraction and management of data for systematic review or meta-
  analysis. It is also an open and searchable archive of systematic
  reviews and their data (https://srdr.ahrq.gov/).

Referencing: If you are not using a software package, such as RevMan, you
will need good referencing software such as https://www.mendeley.
com/ or http://endnote.com/.

Author team: You need more than one person to conduct a review. In
convening the team, consider who has content, methodological and
statistical expertise. A first-time author may want to involve a senior
author/mentor to provide guidance. Clarify roles and ensure the team
is familiar with the review project plan.

Typical sections in a protocol include:

- Background and rationale
- Objectives
- Methods
  - Criteria for considering studies for the review
  - Approach for identifying studies for the review
  - Selection of studies
  - Data extraction and management
  - Risk of bias assessment of included studies
  - Data analysis and synthesis

- Contribution of authors
- Conflicts of interest

See Box 15.4 for a useful guide and checklist for protocols of systematic reviews.

Step 3: Register your title and key features of your protocol

Once you have defined your question and developed your question, the next step is title registration. PROSPERO, the website - https://www.crd.york.ac.uk/PROSPERO/, is 'an international database of prospectively registered systematic reviews in health and social care, welfare, public health, education, crime, justice, and international development, where there is a health related outcome'. 'PROSPERO aims to provide a comprehensive listing of systematic reviews registered at inception to help avoid duplication and reduce opportunity for reporting bias by enabling comparison completed review with what was planned in the protocol'. If you are conducting a Cochrane review, your title is automatically registered.

The following information needs to be captured when registering your review on PROSPERO: question detailing PICO elements, types of studies to be included, information on the proposed search approach to identify studies, process for selection of studies, data extraction and risk of bias assessment, contact details and proposed timeline.

BOX 15.4   USEFUL GUIDE AND CHECKLIST FOR PROTOCOLS FOR SYSTEMATIC REVIEWS

Preferred Reporting Items for Systematic review and Meta-Analysis—Protocols (PRISMA-P), http://prisma-statement.org/Extensions/Protocols.aspx, was published in 2015 aiming to facilitate the development and reporting of systematic review protocols. It includes a checklist with recommended items to address in a systematic review protocol.

Step 4: Conduct the systematic review

Identify potential studies

A combination of structured searches in electronic databases and other sources are typical for systematic reviews, as well as a detailed report of the searches used. You want to be as comprehensive as possible to identify published, unpublished and ongoing studies linked to your question. To search electronic databases such as PubMed (Medline) and EMBASE you will need the assistance of an information specialist to develop a robust search strategy. For details of a useful tutorial on searching see Box 15.5. Searches of these databases are supplemented by checking conferences, contacting experts in the field, checking reference lists of included studies and by searching for ongoing studies in trial registries.

**BOX 15.5   WANT TO KNOW MORE ABOUT
SEARCHING ELECTRONIC DATABASES?**

PubMed tutorial (covering 'building the search', 'managing results', 'saving the search', 'getting the articles' and 'review exercises'): http://www.nlm.nih.gov/bsd/disted/pubmedtutorial/

Select studies

Search results are then reviewed using the pre-specified eligibility criteria. Two authors will independently screen the search results (titles and abstracts) and compare their selection of studies. They then obtain full text articles of all shortlisted, potentially eligible titles and abstracts, and by reading the full texts, make the final decision on whether the study meets the inclusion criteria or not. Data from this stage is then typically summarised in a flow diagram detailing the selection of studies, as well as a table of included studies, table of excluded studies, table of ongoing studies (where relevant) and the table of studies awaiting assessment (if there was missing data and a judgment could not be made).

Extract data

For all studies included in the systematic review, the author team will extract key data using a piloted data extraction form to guide the process. Information to extract aligns with the review question. This typically includes descriptive information about the study participants, the interventions/issue, the comparisons/context, which outcomes were assessed and how, as well as data on outcome assessment, funding, ethics, etc. Data extractions are usually conducted independently by two authors and then compared.

Assess risk of bias of included studies

Key to systematic reviews is the independent, duplicate appraisal and assessment of the risk of bias of all included studies. The extent to which a systematic review can draw valid conclusions depends on whether the data and results from the included studies are valid. Risk of bias assessments are usually done using existing tools developed for this purpose, with well-defined domains that are specific to the study design (Box 15.6).

BOX 15.6 SOME RISK OF BIAS ASSESSMENT TOOLS FOR DIFFERENT STUDY DESIGNS

Experimental studies: Cochrane risk of bias tool for randomised controlled trials; The Critical Appraisal Skills Programme (CASP) checklist for randomised controlled trials; The Risk Of Bias In Non-randomized Studies of Interventions (ROBINS-I) assessment tool; Methodological index for non-randomized studies (MINORS)

Observational studies: Risk of Bias Assessment tool for Non-randomized Studies (RoBANS); Newcastle-Ottawa Scale for cohort studies; CASP Checklist for cohort studies; CASP Checklist for case-control studies; Newcastle-Ottawa Scale for case-control studies; ARHQ Methodology Checklist for Cross-Sectional/Prevalence Study; Quality Assessment of Diagnostic Accuracy Studies (QUADAS) tool; CASP Checklist for Diagnostic test study.

Analyse data

Firstly, it is important to decide which comparisons will be made and which outcome data will be required for these comparisons. Depending on the type of data, there are various methods that can be used to summarise and synthesise the outcomes assessed in the included studies. In systematic reviews with more than one study, which are considered to be combinable, one can conduct a meta-analysis (a statistical aggregation of the quantitative outcome data). This synthesis can be conducted in software such as RevMan. Not all systematic reviews include a meta-analysis as this is dependent on the type of data, differences between included studies or poor reporting of data in primary studies.

Key to considering a meta-analysis is the assessment of differences between studies, also referred to as clinical, methodological and statistical heterogeneity. When you perform a meta-analysis, you have to measure and report the heterogeneity. You can identify statistical heterogeneity by means of visual inspection of forest plots (the graphical representation of a meta-analysis) and the Chi-squared test, and you can quantify heterogeneity using the I-squared statistic. In your review protocol, you should indicate which strategies will be used for addressing heterogeneity. Combining results from heterogeneous studies is often meaningless and can result in invalid conclusions, so the decisions about combining studies are very important. The Cochrane handbook (http://training.cochrane.org/handbook) has detailed guidance on meta-analysis. If meta-analysis is not possible, results should not be reported per study, but rather synthesised narratively per outcome, taking into account the risk of bias of the included studies that report on that outcome.

GRADE and interpret the findings

The Grades of Recommendation, Assessment, Development and Evaluation Working Group (GRADE Working Group) has developed a system for grading the certainty of evidence. This factors in risk of bias, precision, inconsistency (heterogeneity), indirectness and publication bias. It is done for each outcome and defines the 'quality of a body of evidence as the extent to which one can be confident that an estimate of effect or association is close to the quantity of specific interest' (http://handbook.cochrane.org/chapter_12/12_2 _assessing_the_quality_of_a_body_of_evidence.htm).

Following the GRADE assessment of the research evidence on your specific question, you can then, based on your findings, put forward implications for practice and/or implications for further research. More information on GRADE is available at http://www.gradeworkinggroup.org/.

Step 5: Report the findings of the systematic review

For publication, it is important to adhere to reporting guidelines to ensure transparent reporting of your review (Box 15.7). Beyond publication, other knowledge translation activities to disseminate and communicate the findings of your systematic review can take many different forms depending on your message and your audience. It is useful to spend time with your author team to consider this and decide what you will use. This can include presentations at conferences or research meetings, plain language summaries for practitioners, evidence summaries for busy decision-makers or a policy brief for policymakers.

BOX 15.7   REPORTING GUIDELINES

Preferred Reporting Items for Systematic Reviews and Meta-Analyses (PRISMA) http://www.prisma-statement.org/ outlines a minimum set of items for reporting in systematic reviews and meta-analyses and provides a good guide to authors writing up their intervention systematic review.

Methodological Expectations of Cochrane Intervention Reviews (MECIR) are methodological standards to which all Cochrane Protocols, Reviews and Updates are expected to adhere. They are divided into sections for the conduct of and reporting the reviews of interventions.

MOOSE (https://www.equator-network.org/reporting-guidelines/meta-analysis-of-observational-studies-in-epidemiology-a-proposal-for-reporting-meta-analysis-of-observational-studies-in-epidemiology-moose-group/) provides a guide for systematic reviews on observational studies.

CONCLUSION

Systematic reviews are comprehensive, transparent and reproducible assessments of the existing body of research on a specific topic. They inform both new research and evidence-informed policy and practice decisions. Importantly, key steps must be in place to minimise bias when conducting a systematic review.

REFERENCES

1. Egger M, Davey Smith G, Altman D. Systematic Reviews in Health Care: meta-analysis in context, 2nd Edition. London: BMJ Books, 2001.
2. Grant MJ, Booth A. A typology of reviews: An analysis of 14 review types and associated methodologies. *Health Info Libr J* 2009;26(2):91–108.
3. Moher D, Cook DJ, Eastwood S et al. Improving the quality of reports of meta-analyses of randomised controlled trials: The QUOROM statement. Quality of reporting of meta-analyses. *Lancet* 1999;354(9193):1896–900.
4. Rohwer A, Pfadenhauer L, Burns J et al. Series: Clinical Epidemiology in South Africa. Paper 3: Logic models help make sense of complexity in systematic reviews and health technology assessments. *J Clin Epidemiol* 2017;83:37–47.
5. Shea BJ, Reeves BC, Wells G et al. AMSTAR 2: A critical appraisal tool for systematic reviews that include randomised or non-randomised studies of healthcare interventions, or both. *BMJ* 2017;358;j4008.
6. Whiting P, Savovic J, Higgins JP et al. ROBIS: A new tool to assess risk of bias in systematic reviews was developed. *J Clin Epidemiol* 2016;69:225–34.

CHAPTER 16

Statistics in primary care research

Richard Stevens

WHY DO STATISTICS?

'If your experiment needs a statistician, you ought to do a better experiment'

– apocryphal, attributed to Ernest Rutherford

If you can conduct a large experiment with precise measurement, ruling out all unwanted sources of variation, you do not need a statistician: results will speak for themselves. For experiments in the real world of primary care, however, statistics is necessary to account for all the variability that arises when studying human beings. After obtaining a study result (e.g. a numerical difference, on average, between two groups), statistical methods exist to answer questions:

- How confident can I be in this result, given the size of my study?
- Should I believe this result, or could it be attributable to chance alone?

WHEN TO DO STATISTICS

A common mistake is to wait until data has been collected, and then consult a statistician about the analysis. One of the founders of biostatistics, R. A. Fisher, is said to have told the First Indian Statistical Congress in 1938 that 'to consult the statistician after an experiment is finished is merely to ask him to conduct a post mortem examination. He can perhaps say what the experiment died of'. Since Fisher's day, there is more gender diversity in the statistical profession, but the sentiment remains true. For any quantitative study, a consultation with the statistician will be less depressing for all concerned if it happens early in the process.

As discussed later in this chapter, a statistician's advice can tell you if your planned study is unnecessarily large, or too small to hope to succeed. In the latter case, the statistician can also, very often, suggest simple changes to rescue the proposed study. Increasing sample size is not the only way to increase statistical power. The chance that a study succeeds can also be greatly increased by design changes (e.g. using a paired or crossover design) or even by changes as simple as recording a continuous outcome instead of a dichotomous outcome. Involving a statistician in the planning stages will be rewarded with better, more efficient and more successful quantitative studies.

KEY STATISTICAL CONCEPTS
Confidence intervals and standard errors

Variability between people, and within people from day to day, has this consequence: every time we calculate the result from a study, we are conscious that if we did the study again, we would not get exactly the same result. A statistic called the 'standard error' answers the question, 'roughly how different might the answers be if several researchers all tried to do exactly the same study?' Whether we are studying prevalence, or averages, or average differences or almost any numerical result, we can ask our statistical software for a 'standard error' estimate. A large standard error estimate tells us to treat the study with caution; a small standard error encourages us to have faith that if the study were repeated, a similar result would occur.

Standard errors are used to calculate what we call 95% confidence intervals. For example, if the prevalence of autism in your study is 2%, but the 95% confidence interval is between 1% and 5%, you would interpret it this way: 'in our study the prevalence was 2%, but in general, we are 95% sure that the true prevalence is between 1% and 5%'.

p-values and statistical significance

Variability also has the consequence that any difference observed between groups (e.g. between treated and control groups in a trial) may be due to chance alone (rather than a real effect of treatment, for example). As you look at your results, ask yourself this question: 'if there was no real effect, what are the chances that my study would give a difference as large as this or larger?' The *p*-value answers this question. The primary care researcher can safely ignore any debate among theoreticians about the definition and use of the *p*-value,[1] and instead, think of it as a marker for the play of chance. If the *p*-value is large, we can't rule out the play of chance; if the *p*-value is small, we can. By convention, if the *p*-value produced by appropriate statistical software is below 5% (0.05), then medical journals allow you to report that your study found a difference between groups.

A comparison with a small *p*-value is called 'statistically significant' or 'significant' for short, but beware: statistical significance is not clinical significance. In a large study, a trivially small difference between groups may still achieve *statistical* significance. In a small study, a result without statistical significance may nevertheless be large enough to suggest possible *clinical* significance.

Statistical power

Some studies are so small that they are unlikely to succeed even if they are based on a sound hypothesis. For example, suppose a drug, or a vitamin, reduces the lifetime risk of cancer by one-half in adults who take it daily. A study of just a few patients over 6 months would be too small to demonstrate an effect convincingly. Even though the drug has a clinically significant effect, the study result would probably not be statistically significant. Such studies are called 'underpowered'.

Formally, statistical power is the chance that a study succeeds (in demonstrating a difference) assuming that the expected difference exists. To avoid research waste, researchers typically aim for a study that has power of 80%, 90% or even 95%. Higher power is clearly desirable but study size, and hence cost, escalate rapidly as higher powers are sought. Power at the lower end of the range (say, 80%) is more common in fields where recruitment is difficult, interventions are invasive or costs are high per patient. The highest powers (above 95%) are usually only sought in studies whose procedures are non-invasive and cheap per patient, such as postal or electronic surveys.

The concept of power is crucial when planning a study. After concluding a study, the concept of power becomes less important: the study either was significant or it was not. However, it may still be used descriptively: a study whose result suggests clinical significance, without reaching statistical significance, can usefully be described as 'underpowered' to imply that a future, larger study could be worth pursuing.

Relative risk and odds ratio

A simple definition of risk is the number of people who (will) get a disease, divided by the total number of people. A risk of 1 (which is the same as 100%) represents a certainty and 0 (or 0%) an impossibility. In research, generally risk lies between these two extremes. The relative risk is the risk in one group divided by the risk in another. (It may also be called risk ratio; the terms are synonymous and both are abbreviated RR) For example, if the first group is a treated group of patients, and the second group is an untreated group of patients, then the RR measures how much higher, or lower, the risk is in the treated group. An RR greater than 1 denotes increased risk (e.g. RR = 2 denotes a doubling of risk with treatment) and an RR less than 1 denotes decreased risk (e.g. RR = 0.5 denotes a halving risk with treatment).

For some study designs and some analyses, it is easier (or even necessary) to report changes in risk as odds ratios (ORs) instead of RRs. When the outcome is rare, odds ratios are approximately equal to risk ratios and may be interpreted as such. For example, Dikshit reported an odds ratio of 2.0 for oral leukoplakia in women with versus without diabetes; since oral leukoplakia is not common, it would be reasonable to think of this as a doubling of risk.[2] However, when outcomes are not rare, interpreting ORs as RRs will exaggerate the size of the effect. For a full discussion see A'Court.[3]

Another trap in interpretation is to conflate large RRs with large changes in absolute risk. An RR of 2.0 or 0.5 can sound impressive ('doubles risk' or 'halves risk'), but the benefit to patients depends also on the absolute level of risk. For illustration, if a preventive treatment could halve my lifetime risk of insulinoma, I would not be interested: my lifetime risk of insulinoma would change from very, very small to very, very small. A treatment that could halve my lifetime risk of any cancer, on the other hand, would be much more valuable, even though both have the same RR (0.5). The usefulness of RR and OR for scientific analysis does not make them ideal for patient communication, for which a separate literature exists on statistics such as absolute risk difference, number needed to treat and number needed to harm (https://www.cebm.net/2014/03/number-needed-to-treat-nnt/).

HOW TO DO STATISTICS IN PRIMARY CARE RESEARCH

It is no longer necessary to be a mathematician to carry out statistical analyses, since good statistical software can be installed on ordinary desktop computers and used to implement statistical procedures. Nevertheless, specialist knowledge is required to decide which statistical procedures are appropriate and to understand the limitations of the results. Designing and analysing a quantitative study without any specialist statistical advice should be a last resort, because it can so easily lead to unpublishable research: see the excellent satirical article 'How to ensure your paper is rejected by the statistical reviewer'.[4]

For simple studies, a researcher without statistical training but with adequate software could carry out analyses themselves after obtaining statistical advice. Studies comparing two groups, with a well-defined outcome measured at a particular time point, will often fall into this category. Statistical advice is typically available in-house for researchers in university departments, but researchers in clinical practice may have to look elsewhere. For more complex studies, it will increasingly be desirable to involve a statistician in the research team. Issues that raise the statistical complexity include, but are not limited to, multiple outcomes per participants, more than two groups to compare in a study, necessity to adjust for missing data and non-independence of participants (e.g. in a cluster-randomised trial).

Commonly used software for medical statistics includes the Statistical Package for the Social Sciences (SPSS), which is popular for its menu-driven interface and modest price. Statistical Analysis Software (SAS), which is the industry standard in pharmaceutical statistics and statistical software produced by StataCorp, used in many university medical research departments, are more powerful and correspondingly more expensive. The open-source software R is free, but requires a high degree of computer literacy, and ideally some programming skills. Spreadsheet programmes such as Microsoft Excel are superficially appealing for the simplest analyses, but rapidly become unwieldy. Although it is easy to obtain simple statistics such as an average or proportion, obtaining a complete and coherent set of results may well require more mathematical and computing skills in a spreadsheet than in dedicated statistical software such as SPSS. A small literature exists in the statistical journals documenting the hazards of analysis by Microsoft Excel.[5,6]

CONCLUSION

Disraeli famously wrote that 'there are three kinds of lies: lies, damned lies, and statistics' (attributed to Disraeli). Bad statistics are deceptive: the role of a good statistical analysis is to force the statistics to tell nothing but the truth. An early consultation with a statistician will be rewarded with a better study, better science and a better chance of a publication, which can contribute to a better evidence base for treating patients.

REFERENCES

1. Perezgonzalez JD. Fisher, Neyman-Pearson or NHST? A tutorial for teaching data testing. *Front Psychol* 2015;6:223.
2. Dikshit RP, Ramadas K, Hashibe M, Thomas G, Somanathan T, Sankaranarayanan R. Association between diabetes mellitus and pre-malignant oral diseases: A cross sectional study in Kerala, India. *Int J Cancer* 2006;118(2):453–7.
3. A'Court C, Stevens R, Heneghan C. Against all odds? Improving the understanding of risk reporting. *Br J Gen Pract* 2012;62(596):e220–3.
4. Stratton IM, Neil A. How to ensure your paper is rejected by the statistical reviewer. *Diabet Med* 2005;22(4):371–3.
5. McCullough D, Heiserb A. On the accuracy of statistical procedures in Microsoft Excel 2007. *Comput Stat Data Anal* 2008;52(10):4570–8.
6. Knüsel L. On the accuracy of statistical distributions in Microsoft Excel 2003. *Comput Stat Data Anal* 2005;48(3):445–9.

CHAPTER 17

How to conduct a survey in primary care

Lauren Ball and Katelyn Barnes

Many health professionals are familiar with surveys as a way to gather information from the perspective of people, usually patients. Health professionals generally view surveys as a 'safe' introduction to conducting research, as well as an 'easy' project to undertake in practice. However, there are many factors to consider to ensure that the data generated truly reflect the information needing to be collected. These factors include the structure of the survey, wording of the questions, response options and interaction with participants. This chapter provides an overview of these important aspects of conducting a survey in the primary care setting.

WHAT IS A SURVEY?

'Survey' is a broad term that refers to collecting quantitative data from a representative sample of people and then analysing the results statistically. Questionnaires are the instruments or lists of questions used in a survey, often with predefined answers, that seek standardised information from the respondents. The benefits of using surveys are that they are usually quick, inexpensive and convenient for both researchers and respondents.

A high-quality survey requires a clear study aim and research question. The aim and research question should help to clarify the type of survey required, the types of questions that may be involved, the statistics needed to analyse the results and the sample needed to accurately capture information. A clear aim and research question may also help to highlight whether or not there are questionnaires already existing that could be used or adapted or if a new questionnaire needs to be developed.

TYPES OF SURVEYS

Surveys are commonly descriptive and collect data to measure a phenomenon (such as events, behaviours or attitudes) in a specific population. For example, the 'BEACH Program' (Bettering the Evaluation and Care of Health) describes general practice activity in Australia.[1] Each year for 18 years, until 2017, a standardised questionnaire was completed by a randomised sample of 1,000 GPs on 100 patient encounters.

Descriptive surveys can also be used to determine associations or trends between variables. Using the example of the BEACH Program, patient encounters are examined in more detail by looking at the demographic characteristics of the GPs that completed the questionnaire, as well as their patients.[1] This can provide information such as whether or not the gender of age of the GP or patient influences the content of encounter.

Surveys can be 'cross-sectional' or 'longitudinal'. A cross-sectional survey is administered once and collects information as a 'snapshot in time'. A benefit of cross-sectional surveys is that they only require one contact with the sample. However, cross-sectional surveys do not consider any changes over time. In contrast, longitudinal surveys are administered more than once and can therefore measure changes over time. A 'retrospective longitudinal' survey asks respondents about previous events and relies on the memory of respondents. For example, a national survey was conducted in Australia in 2011 investigating GPs' previous experiences with aggressive patients.[2] It may also use existing datasets such as medical records collected for another purpose. A 'prospective longitudinal' survey asks respondents about current and future events, needing multiple contacts with the sample over time. For example, an ongoing prospective cohort study in New Zealand is investigating Maori individuals' cardiovascular disease outcomes through multiple surveys on the sample over time.[3] Prospective studies require the collection of new data.

TYPES OF QUESTIONS

The format in which an item is presented and the way in which it is posed can elicit different answers to the same question. Careful consideration should be given to each question to ensure it will provide a valid and reliable response that accurately reflects the research aim. Table 17.1 outlines some common question and answer formats and the type of data that is produced, as well as key benefits and limitations to consider.

Keeping each question as simple as possible helps to elicit more consistent responses. Instructions or additional information on how to interpret and answer the question may also help to ensure the data being collected is a true reflection of the respondents' views. This is particularly helpful for question formats such as ranking or multiple choice.

TABLE 17.1 Different types of survey question and answer formats

Format	Answer format	Example question	Example answer options	Data output	Type of data and analysis	Benefit	Limitation
Dichotomous	Select one of two available pre-defined answers	Do you wash your hands after each procedure in a patient encounter?	Yes No	Nominal: Binary output under single variable	Descriptive: Frequency of each answer option	Quick to answer, low burden on respondent	Predefined answers may not reflect the diversity of respondents' opinions
Numeric	Enter any number	How many times in the last month have you washed your hands after a procedure in a patient encounter?	1 5 50 100	Scale: Numerical response	Descriptive: Mean and standard deviation Median and interquartile range	Allows a respondent to nominate an answer rather than selecting from predefined answers, which facilitates more power in the analysis	Opportunity for error when entering a response. More difficult to compare between participants without grouping answers.
Multiple choice (single answer option)	A predefined list of answers with the ability to only select one option	Which of the following best describes your hand washing practices during patient encounters?	Never wash hands Sometimes wash hands Always wash hands	Nominal: Binary responses to each answer option	Descriptive: Frequency of each answer option	Predefined answers make descriptive analysis straightforward	Predefined answers may not be reflective of the respondents' actual thoughts

(Continued)

TABLE 17.1 (*Continued*) Different types of survey question and answer formats

Format	Answer format	Example question	Example answer options	Data output	Type of data and analysis	Benefit	Limitation
Multiple choice (multiple answer options)	A predefined list of answers, with the ability to select as many options as applicable.	Which of the following describes your hand washing practices during patient encounters?	I use alcohol-based solutions I use water I use soap I dry my hands I continue my discussion with the patient	Nominal: Binary responses to each answer option	Descriptive: Frequency of each answer option	Predefined answers make descriptive analysis straightforward	Predefined answers may not be reflective of the respondents' actual thoughts
Ranking	Prioritisation of a list of predefined answer options.	Please rank in order of importance which procedures you would consider washing your hands after	Verbal discussion Examination of skin Examination of eyes or ears Internal examination	Nominal: Each answer option will present as a variable with the ranking for 1st, 2nd, 3rd, 4th listed	Descriptive: Frequency of each answer option and reverse scored so top ranking answer has the highest score, then summed for overall ranking	Allows a single preferred option to be easily identified	Predefined answers may not be reflective of the respondents' actual thoughts

(Continued)

TABLE 17.1 (*Continued*) Different types of survey question and answer formats

Format	Answer format	Example question	Example answer options	Data output	Type of data and analysis	Benefit	Limitation
Likert-scale	Select a number or position along a scale with typically five options to choose from	On a scale of 1–5, how would you rate your hand washing practices during patient encounters?	1. (very poor) 2. (poor) 3. (unsure) 4. (good) 5. (excellent)	Ordinal: Selected number response under one variable	Descriptive: Frequency of each answer option	Provides a quantitative response to a subjective topic	The difference between two points (e.g. 1–2, 2–3) may be subjective and therefore may not be equal, which prevents use of means and standard deviation
Open ended	Long or short response, no pre-defined answer	Please describe your hand washing practices during patient encounters	Text response	String: Text response	Can be converted into categories to produce quantitative data	Minimises assumptions by researchers as allows respondents to describe an answer	Data in a questionnaire often not rich enough for full qualitative data analysis

Pilot testing is important when developing questionnaires. Pilot testing involves asking a small sample from the research population to review the questions and answer options and to give feedback on their interpretation and understanding. This process helps to ensure the questions and answer options are interpreted as intended by the researchers. Changes to the wording of questions and answer options should be made in accordance with consistent feedback from the pilot test. Pilot testing can also help to establish the feasibility of the questionnaire, in terms of completion time and proportion of incomplete responses. Questionnaires that take a long time to complete, or result in a lot of uncompleted answers, may need to be revised. Pilot testing should occur until it is expected that new feedback will not markedly improve the interpretation and completion rate of the questionnaire among the sample.

VALIDITY AND RELIABILITY

The 'validity' of a questionnaire relates to the ability of the questions to measure what they are supposed to measure. The 'reliability' of a questionnaire relates to the ability to provide consistent results, given the same context. Validity and reliability are important considerations when developing questionnaires to ensure that the results obtained are meaningful. There are many different types of validity and reliability, some of which require statistical analysis and interpretation. Table 17.2 outlines the types of validity and reliability to which questionnaires may be subject.

PRE-DEVELOPED QUESTIONNAIRES

Some researchers choose to use existing questionnaires to gather data to answer their research question. Although this approach can save time, existing questionnaires will vary in the level of validation testing that has been applied. A literature search should be undertaken to ensure any available tools are identified and considered for use or adaptation. Using questionnaires that have not been validated, or questionnaires validated in a different setting (such as a hospital) or population group, may increase error in the results and interpretation of data. Selecting an established and appropriately validated questionnaire can save time and effort in creating and validating a new questionnaire and can help to increase the rigour of research. Furthermore, using an established questionnaire can assist in the comparison of findings with other research that has applied the same questions. If questions need to be modified or added to the survey, further pilot testing may be required to ensure validity and reliability has been retained. For example, the Royal Australian College of General Practitioners lists validated patient-feedback questionnaires that can be used or adapted in practices.[4]

TABLE 17.2 Types of validity and reliability for surveys

Type	Description	Reason
	Validity	
Content	The extent to which questions are related to the topic being investigated and identifies the relevance of each indicator and criterion	Ensures the content of the survey is relevant to the research aim
Face	The extent to which respondents find the questions to be clear and logical and to measure what the survey is meant to investigate	Ensures that the respondents will understand the questions
Construct	The extent to which different sections of the survey to which the items are as closely associated as expected, according to theory	Increases the likelihood that the questions provide an in depth and comprehensive exploration of the topic
Criterion	The correlation between the survey and a 'gold standard' measure of the same topic. Predictive, concurrent and convergent are types of criterion validity	Provides empirical support for the use of the tool. However, an existing tool is needed that measures the same topic.
	Reliability	
Test-retest	Similarity of answers to the same questions at different time points	Ensures consistent responses to questions over time; caution needed to ensure that questions selected for test-retest reliability are not ones that could change over time due to external influence
Inter-rater	Similarity of answers to the same question obtained by two different researchers (e.g. measuring a patient's height)	Ensures that the question is delivered the same way by different researchers
Internal consistency	Similarity of answers to different questions about the same concept. Applicable to Likert-Scale or multi-choice questions	Useful when there are multiple aspects of the same concept explored in the same questionnaire

RECRUITING PARTICIPANTS

Adequate numbers of participants must be used to draw appropriate conclusions from a questionnaire. An adequate sample size will vary based on the research question and main outcome measures. Descriptive questionnaires will require an adequate sample size to represent the population being researched. If comparisons are being made between groups of respondents (such as exploring the influence of demographic characteristics), an adequate sample size to detect a meaningful difference or change in the main outcome measure is needed. Sample-size calculations are used to identify an adequate number of participants. Previous research can also inform researchers about the response rate they can expect and, consequently, the number of potential participants they will need to approach to ensure they obtain an adequate sample size. More information on sample size calculations can be found in Chapter 16.

Recruitment of participants to complete and return the survey can occur in several ways. A pre-defined list of contacts may be available to telephone, email or post questionnaires to specific groups or individuals. Alternatively, targeted or open invitations can be sent via email, post, newsletters, social media or by approaching potential participants in person. Pre-defined lists (such as email or postal lists) provide a clear number of potential participants contacted that will help to ensure adequate sampling and allow the response rate to be calculated. However, more open methods of invitation can increase the reach of the survey and therefore potentially increase the number of responses. To further enhance response rate, researchers may decide to offer non-coercive incentives (e.g. the chance to win a prize). The most effective recruitment methods will depend on the population required for the study, the sample size needed to provide adequate statistical power and by the method of questionnaire administration.

ADMINISTERING QUESTIONNAIRES

Surveys can be administered in a variety of ways. The most common methods of administration include internet-based, paper-based and verbal. Each method can influence recruitment, reach and researcher effort.

Online surveys can be created, distributed and administered using internet-based survey tools such as SurveyMonkey and LimeSurvey. Some internet-based survey tools are free to use, though they may have restricted features without a paid subscription. A URL must be provided to participants via advertisement or email invitation to allow participants to complete the survey. Most internet-based survey tools allow quick data export into analysis programs such as SPSS, STATA, Microsoft Excel and R. The use of online surveys significantly reduces the amount of hours devoted to data collection and inputting data into analysis software. A limitation of online surveys is that not all respondents may have access to a computer or the internet. Furthermore, practitioners in general practice may be less likely to respond to online questionnaires compared with other modes. As such, it is important to consider the characteristics of the target population when administering an internet-based questionnaire.

Paper-based surveys can be distributed and administered to respondents in a format where they can write their responses. Paper-based surveys can be appropriate when using mail-outs for recruitment and for inviting specific people or groups to participate. Paper-based surveys in primary care typically elicit good response rates for mail-out surveys (with a return, paid envelope), compared to an email invitation for an online survey. Once data has been collected through paper-based surveys, a researcher is required to enter the responses into data-analysis software. Inputting data can be time-intensive and can increase the likelihood of error in transcribing responses. Furthermore, printing and mailing surveys (with return, paid envelopes) can be costly.

Verbally administered surveys require a researcher to talk to each respondent to ask each question. Respondents' verbal answers can then be recorded on the paper-based questionnaire or preferably can be captured directly using an electronic device (e.g. mobile phone, tablet or laptop computer) into a database on the hard drive, internet or data-analysis software. Verbal administration of surveys may allow further instructions to be provided to respondents and allows for the survey to be administered in a conversation-like manner. Verbally administered surveys may also allow researchers to capture more open-ended detail from respondents as they talk about their answers. Verbal administration is also valuable when there is a language barrier and questions or answers must be translated by the researcher or for respondents who have low literacy skills. Researcher time may be more intensive for verbally administered surveys, though verbal administration may reduce the burden experienced by respondents. If more than one researcher verbally administers the survey, training is needed to ensure questions and extra instructions are delivered in the same way to increase inter-rater reliability.

REFERENCES

1. Australian Institute of Health and Welfare. General practice activity in Australia 2009-10. Australian Government, Canberra, ACT. Available at: https://www.aihw.gov.au/reports/primary-health-care/general-practice-activity-in-australia-2009-10/contents/table-of-contents
2. Forrest LE, Herath PM, McRae IS, Parker RM. A national survey of general practitioners' experiences of patient-initiated aggression in Australia. *Med J Aust* 2011 Jun 6;194(11):605–8.
3. Cameron VA, Faatoese AF, Gillies MW et al. A cohort study comparing cardiovascular risk factors in rural Māori, urban Māori and non-Māori communities in New Zealand. *BMJ Open* 2012 Jan 1;2(3):e000799.
4. Royal Australian College of General Practitioners. Validated patient feedback questionnaires. In: *Resources for the Standards for General Practices*, 4th ed. 2013, East Melbourne, Australia. Available at: https://www.racgp.org.au/your-practice/standards/resources/patient-feedback/validated-questionnaire/

CHAPTER 18

Validation studies: Validating new tools and adapting old ones to new contexts

Sherina Mohd Sidik

INTRODUCTION

Validation studies determine the accuracy, dependability and consistency of a tool in measuring what it is supposed to measure. A tool is valid if it measures what it is purported to measure. For example, validation of a tool which detects depression in the community should determine the accuracy of the tool to detect depression in the specified population and prove that it is measuring what it is supposed to measure and is consistent throughout its usage.

The different types of validity are outlined in Chapter 17 on how to conduct a survey. Briefly, 'face validity' is confirmation from a group of experts or other stakeholders as to whether this tool appears to be a reasonable measure of the concept as they understand it. 'Content validity' checks whether all the items in the tool that should be included are included and identifies the relevance of each indicator and criterion. This can be attained through asking experts whether or not the tool appears to contain all the important concepts, behaviours and elements of the concept; it can be more formally assessed by observing patients to see behaviours (interview them or review records) or base the tool on previously reported measures. 'Construct validity' is the extent to which the items in the tool are as closely associated as expected, according to theory. 'Criterion-related validity' determines the ability of each criterion of the tool to measure accurately a specific concept or condition. To assess this ability, the criterion is compared with a 'gold', or reference, standard. This is the strongest form of validity.

MEASURES OF TEST ACCURACY

The accuracy of a test is the degree of closeness of the measurement to the true value of what is being measured. It can be measured against a reference standard that confirms a person has a condition. Properties of a diagnostic or screening test include sensitivity, specificity, predictive values and likelihood ratios (see also Chapter 19). In Table 18.1, true and false positive, false and true negative are represented by A, B, C and D, respectively (the total population is A + B + C + D.

'Sensitivity' is the ability of the test to detect the condition or disease (true positive rate) and is the number of people with the disease who have a positive test divided by the number with the disease (i.e. if all those with the disease were detected, the sensitivity would be 100%). A test with high sensitivity will have few false negatives. 'Specificity' is the ability of the test to correctly identify people who do not have the condition or disease (true negative rate). This is the number of people without the disease who have a negative test divided by the number of people without the disease (i.e. if all the people without the disease were identified as testing negative, the specificity would be 100%). A test that has high specificity will have few false positives. The 'likelihood ratio' (LR) incorporates both the sensitivity and specificity of the test and provides a direct estimate of how much a test result will change the odds of having a disease. The likelihood ratio for a positive result (LR+) tells you how much the odds of the disease increase when a test is positive, whereas the likelihood ratio for a negative result (LR−) shows how much the odds of the disease decrease when a test is negative.

The 'false positive rate' measures those testing positive who have no disease, calculated by the number of people with a positive test with no disease divided by the number of all people without disease: B/(B + D). Similarly, the 'false negative rate' is the rate of those with the disease who test negative, calculated by the number of people with a negative test who have the disease divided by

TABLE 18.1 Measures of validity

	Has condition A + C	Does not have condition B + D	
Positive test A + B	A True positive	B False positive (type I error)	Positive predictive value A/(A + B)
Negative test C + D	C False negative (type II error)	D True negative	Negative predictive value D/(C + D)
	Sensitivity A/(A + C)	Specificity D/(B + D)	

the number of all people with disease: C/(A + C). There is also the 'positive predictive value' of a test: How well does it predict that someone has a disease? This is calculated by the number of people with a positive test who have the disease divided by the number of all the people with a positive test. The 'negative predictive value', therefore, will be the number of people with a negative test who do not have the disease divided by all the people with a negative test.

The probability that a person has the target condition before a diagnostic test result is known (pre-test probability) is also important. If the condition being screened for is of very low probability, then there will be many false positives. This can be ameliorated by only screening a selected (higher-risk) population.

There are three different scenarios when conducting a validation study:

1. Construct a questionnaire from scratch, and validate it against a gold standard.
2. Adapt a questionnaire that was validated elsewhere to be used in a new context (e.g. different country, different population).
3. Translate the questionnaire into another language for cross-cultural adaption.

Chapter 17 covers how to develop a questionnaire or survey and how to adapt it to a new setting. However, many researchers in low- and middle-income

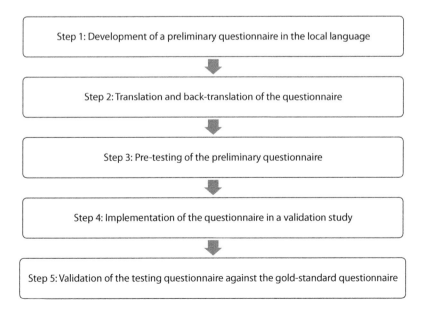

Step 1: Development of a preliminary questionnaire in the local language

Step 2: Translation and back-translation of the questionnaire

Step 3: Pre-testing of the preliminary questionnaire

Step 4: Implementation of the questionnaire in a validation study

Step 5: Validation of the testing questionnaire against the gold-standard questionnaire

FIGURE 18.1 Cross-cultural adaption of a questionnaire.

countries will want to adapt validated questionnaires from English-speaking countries and will need to translate these into local languages and validate them in new settings. There are several guidelines for cross-cultural adaptation of self-report measures. This process may take anywhere from six months to three years, depending on the stages of validation involved. The flowchart in Figure 18.1 shows the steps which need to be taken in validating a new questionnaire in primary care research in a non-English speaking country.[1]

Step 1: Development of a preliminary questionnaire

The questionnaire to be translated and adapted should be identified through a literature review, including a check that a questionnaire has not already been developed or adapted for the target population or country.

Step 2: Translation and back-translation of the questionnaire

The questions can first be prepared in English and then translated into the local language using the back-translation method. There are five stages which are needed to fulfil two steps: (1) first step, the original items of all the measures are translated into the local language and (2) second step, the local language version is then translated back into English. In the second step, any items that appear discrepant to the meaning of the original items are translated again. The final version is the one agreed upon by the translators involved (see Figure 18.2).

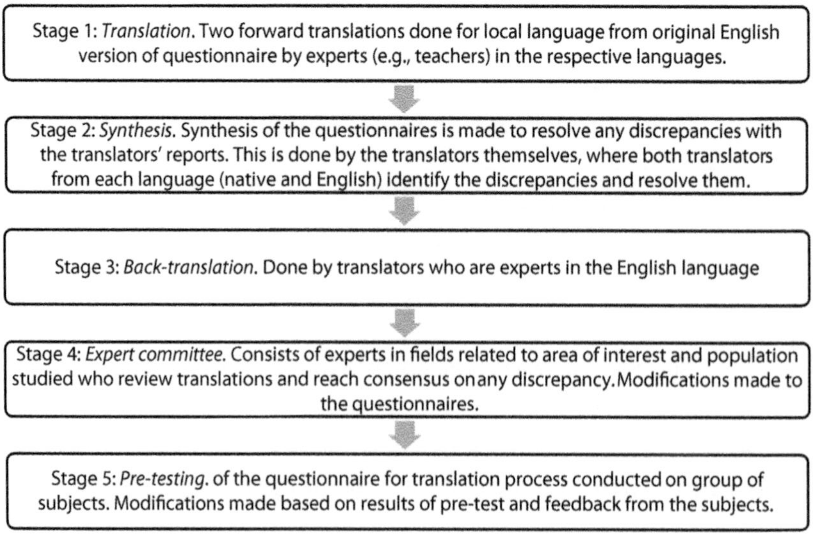

Stage 1: *Translation*. Two forward translations done for local language from original English version of questionnaire by experts (e.g., teachers) in the respective languages.

Stage 2: *Synthesis*. Synthesis of the questionnaires is made to resolve any discrepancies with the translators' reports. This is done by the translators themselves, where both translators from each language (native and English) identify the discrepancies and resolve them.

Stage 3: *Back-translation*. Done by translators who are experts in the English language

Stage 4: *Expert committee*. Consists of experts in fields related to area of interest and population studied who review translations and reach consensus on any discrepancy. Modifications made to the questionnaires.

Stage 5: *Pre-testing*. of the questionnaire for translation process conducted on group of subjects. Modifications made based on results of pre-test and feedback from the subjects.

FIGURE 18.2 Five stages in the translation process of the questionnaire.

Step 3: Pre-testing of the preliminary questionnaire

To assess whether the questionnaire is acceptable to the participants, the preliminary questionnaire is pre-tested (piloted) on subjects who are not included in the study. These subjects should be representative of the study population.

The pre-test is carried out to ensure that:

- The right questions are being asked (has face validity)
- All important and relevant areas are covered (has content validity)
- The questions are properly worded and flow in a logical manner
- The questions are understandable and acceptable to the participants

Feedback and ideas from the subjects are collected, and where necessary, further formal discussions can be conducted with the expert team to finalise the questionnaire.

Following the pre-testing of the questionnaire, internal consistency reliability for the newly developed questionnaire can be done using Cronbach's alpha. For criterion validity, suitable questionnaires should be chosen where either scores of a testing questionnaire are correlated to another questionnaire which measures the same domains (convergent validity), or the results obtained from the testing questionnaire are compared to a well-established questionnaire or interview considered as a gold standard (concurrent validity).

VALIDATION OF THE TESTING QUESTIONNAIRE AGAINST THE GOLD-STANDARD QUESTIONNAIRE

To find a gold-standard questionnaire may require an extensive literature search for an appropriate reference standard. Based on the literature review and formal discussions with the expert team, the best reference standard (gold standard) to validate the testing questionnaire is chosen.

Validation of the testing questionnaire can be done through various study designs. One of the recommended study designs is a double-blinded randomised controlled trial, where both the researchers and participants do not know the questionnaires which are being tested or used as the gold standard.

IMPORTANCE OF VALIDATING NEW QUESTIONNAIRES IN PRIMARY CARE RESEARCH AND ADAPTING OLD ONES TO NEW CONTEXTS

Most validation studies in primary health care currently involve questionnaires assessing behaviours, knowledge, attitude and practices of patients with regards to common health problems in primary care. These include mental health, depression, anxiety, somatisation, pain, hypertension, diabetes, heart disease, asthma, chronic obstructive pulmonary disease, self-care, health risk and health screening, among others. This situation is similar in developed countries, including the US and in Europe, as well as in developing countries, such as Malaysia.

The importance of validating new questionnaires in primary care research is to have new measures that accurately determine the presence and severity of existing and emerging diseases in primary care. This will not only be helpful in determining the focus of care management in primary health care but also improve the quality of treatment which is being provided in primary care clinics.

However, there is also a need to adapt old questionnaires to new contexts in primary care research, especially well-established and validated questionnaires which have been proven to be simple and effective in determining common health care problems. Adapting these questionnaires to new and current contexts is more cost-effective and time-effective than developing and validating new questionnaires.

REFERENCE

1. Beaton DE, Bombardier C, Guillemin F et al. Guidelines for the process of cross-cultural adaptation of self-report measures. *Spine* 2000;25(24):3186–91.

CHAPTER 19

Clinical and other diagnostic tests: Understanding their predictive value

Sarah Price, Robert Price and Willie Hamilton

INTRODUCTION

Testing is fundamental to both clinical practice and research. In primary care, it is a core part of patient management, often being used to select patients for further investigation. National UK guidelines often include recommendations on test indications and subsequent action; for example, National Institute for Health and Care Excellence (NICE) guidelines on suspected cancer: recognition and referral.[1]

Researchers use diagnostic test results to implement a study design, to define inclusion criteria, cases or outcomes, or to classify participants into subgroups for analyses. This chapter starts by reviewing test characterisation and interpretation. It illustrates how decision trees can help you to avoid common pitfalls in test result interpretation.[2] It moves on to describe aspects of testing in primary care research.

TEST CHARACTERISATION AND INTERPRETATION

The simplest form of testing produces a binary result: positive or negative for a target condition.[3,4] Here, target condition includes condition, disease, stage of disease or response to treatment. A simple example is the urine test for pregnancy, which is one of the most commonly carried out point-of-care diagnostic tests in primary care.[5]

Test characterisation

Test characteristics, including *sensitivity* and *specificity*, are determined in validation studies (see Chapter 18). Sensitivity and specificity are both probabilities that are calculated by comparing the test performance with that of a gold standard (or, more commonly, a reference standard) (Table 19.1).

Sensitivity is the probability ('*p*') that the test will give a positive result ('Test +ve'), given that ('|' —note, this is *not* a division slash) the patient has the disease ('Disease +ve'). Mathematically, this conditional probability is written as

$$\text{Sensitivity} = p(\text{Test +ve} \mid \text{Disease +ve})$$

Using a test with a high sensitivity reduces the chances of missing cases of the target condition.

Specificity is the probability ('*p*') that the test will give a negative test result ('Test −ve'), given that the patient is truly healthy ('Disease −ve'). As a conditional probability, it is written as

$$\text{Specificity} = p(\text{Test −ve} \mid \text{Disease −ve})$$

Using a test with a high specificity reduces the chances of incorrectly identifying healthy subjects as having the target condition.

TABLE 19.1 A 2 × 2 contingency table showing how sensitivity and specificity are conditional on knowing the true patient status, whereas positive (PPV) and negative (NPV) predictive values are conditional on knowing the test result

		True patient status for target condition			
		Positive	**Negative**	**Total**	
Test result for target condition	Positive	True positive	False positive	All positive test results	PPV = True positives/All positive test results
	Negative	False negative	True negative	All negative test results	NPV = True negatives/All negative test results
Total		All patients with target condition	All healthy patients		
		Sensitivity = True positives/All patients with target condition	Specificity = True negatives/All healthy patients		

Sensitivity and specificity can be usefully combined into a single index of test accuracy called the positive likelihood ratio (**LR+**):

$$\textbf{LR+} = \text{Sensitivity}/(1 - \text{Specificity})$$

The greater the value of LR+ above 1, the greater the likelihood of disease. A test which yields a lot of information has a high LR+.

Test interpretation

In clinical practice, we really want to know how likely it is that the person has the disease (i.e. Disease +ve), given that they have tested positive (Test +ve). This is commonly called the positive predictive value (PPV) of the result. Alternatively, we may wish to know how likely it is the person is healthy (Disease −ve), given that they have tested negative (Test −ve). This is called the negative predictive value (NPV). PPV and NPV are also probabilities but, in contrast to sensitivity and specificity, they are conditional on *knowing the test result.*

As conditional probabilities, PPV and NPV are written as

$$\text{PPV} = p(\text{Disease +ve} \mid \text{Test +ve})$$
$$\text{NPV} = p(\text{Disease −ve} \mid \text{Test −ve})$$

Notice that, compared with sensitivity (i.e. p[Test +ve|Disease +ve]) and specificity (i.e. p[Test −ve|Disease −ve]), the test and disease terms have swapped places. Note also that the symbol '|' means 'given that' and is not a sign for division.

Calculating PPV and NPV

Unless a test has 100% specificity and 100% sensitivity, it will make errors. So, a positive test result may occur in people who truly have the target condition (true positives) and in those who do not (false positives). Likewise, negative test results occur in people who are truly healthy (true negatives) and in those who have the target condition (false negatives) (Table 19.1).

The contingency table shows how to calculate PPV and NPV (Table 19.1):

$$\text{PPV} = \text{True Positive}/(\text{True Positive} + \text{False Positive})$$
$$\text{NPV} = \text{True Negative}/(\text{True Negative} + \text{False Negative})$$

Crucially, PPV and NPV are not fixed properties of the test; rather, they vary with prevalence of the target condition being sought. The prevalence of the target condition in the studied population should always be reported alongside values of PPV and NPV and, arguably, should be included in the recommendations for reporting diagnostic studies (Box 19.1).[3,4]

Using decision trees forces you to consider the impact of the disease prevalence on PPV and NPV, and has been shown to reduce errors.[2] Testing for human immunodeficiency virus (HIV) illustrates how much PPV varies with prevalence.[6]

Effect of prevalence on PPV
The low-risk population of blood donors in high-income countries has an HIV infection rate of 0.003% (95% confidence interval 0.001%–0.04%), that is, 30 in a million.[7] Testing 1,000,000 American blood donors with a conventional HIV test will produce 1,030 positive results. Of these, only 30 people will actually have HIV—the other 1,000 will have received a false-positive result. Thus, the chance of *actual* HIV infection in a blood-donor whose initial HIV test is positive (the PPV) is 3% (Figure 19.1).

Repeating the test in a high-risk population of males attending a sexually transmitted diseases clinic, where the prevalence of HIV disease is 4%, the PPV for a positive test is 98% (Figure 19.2).

This demonstrates the importance of knowing the prior probability of disease before choosing to carry out a test. It also portrays the difficulties associated with screening of low-prevalence populations. Unless a test has a specificity of 100%, it will always give some false-positive results, the impact

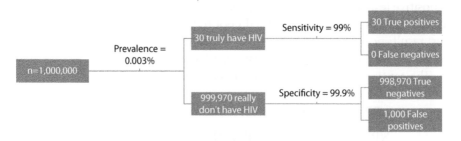

FIGURE 19.1 Decision tree to estimate PPV of a positive HIV test in a low-prevalence population. Strictly, there should be one-third of a person with a false-negative test result, which we have rounded down to zero.

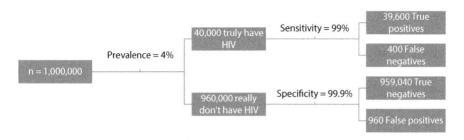

FIGURE 19.2 Decision tree to estimate the PPV of a positive HIV test in a high-prevalence population.

of which will rise as the prevalence falls. False-positives generally require additional testing before being shown to be false and cause considerable worry to the patient, as well as bringing costs.

Bayes' theorem

Clinicians may find Bayes' theorem a useful way to interpret a positive test result as it is explicit in its inclusion of disease prevalence through the prior odds:

$$\text{Post-test odds} = \text{Prior odds} \times \text{Positive likelihood ratio}$$

Odds (a relative measure of risk) are commonly used to express Bayes' theorem. Odds are familiar to gamblers, but less so to others. Odds are simply the chance of something happening (such as a disease being present) divided by the chance of something not happening (disease being absent).

It is straightforward to then convert the post-test odds into PPV (an absolute measure of risk) using this formula:

$$\text{PPV} = \text{Post-test odds}/(1 + \text{Post-test odds})$$

THE CONSISTENCY OF TEST PERFORMANCE CHARACTERISTICS

Researchers often overlook the fact that test characteristics are not completely fixed. This 'spectrum effect' arises from a number of sources, as discussed in the next section.[8,9]

Definition of the target condition

The first source relates to the definition of the target condition, which is particularly germane to primary care, where it may not be a single disease. In clinical practice, finding the right diagnosis is more important than finding a specific single disease. For example, if faecal calprotectin identifies both colon cancer and inflammatory bowel disease (it may, though it's not certain at present), it could be appropriate to measure its performance characteristics with the outcome being *either* cancer *or* inflammatory bowel disease. Even more practically, it would be important to know whether calprotectin is able to identify patients who would benefit from a colonoscopy (identifying either cancer or inflammatory bowel disease, both useful to discover). Therefore, one of the first requirements for researchers conducting studies that characterise tests is to agree on a clear definition of the target condition.[3,4]

The effect of no, or a poor, gold standard

The ideal way of estimating test accuracy is to compare its performance with that of an 'error-free' gold standard. Only then can all the errors be attributed with certainty to the test. However, gold standards are rarely available in practice; usually, reference standards are used instead.[10]

All reference standards are imperfect and can misclassify patients to varying degrees, particularly in primary care. For example, there is no gold standard for a diagnosis of depression. Even if a research team studying a new test for depression had all subjects seen by a psychiatrist, psychiatrists are not infallible. The problem is amplified in observational studies, which analyse information recorded as part of everyday clinical care rather than specifically to meet the study design. Take the example of case definition in a case-control study reporting the PPV of symptoms and test results for lung cancer.[11] The reference standard required histological evidence or written consultant opinion that the patient had lung cancer. However, it likely missed patients with advanced disease in whom biopsy was too risky or clinically inappropriate, as well as those patients who were diagnosed post-mortem.

Reference standards should include a combination of different tests, the joint results of which are used to determine a patient's 'true' status. This minimises misclassification by the reference standard, averting (or nearly so) biased estimates of sensitivity and specificity (Table 19.1).[10]

Misclassification related to the test
Using a reference standard that misses patients with disease has two consequences for validation studies. It will

1. Underestimate the total number of diseased patients, which overestimates sensitivity
2. Overestimate the total number of healthy patients, which underestimates specificity

The opposite effect is seen when reference standards misclassify healthy patients as having the disease. This might occur when the reference standard includes symptoms or markers that are not unique to the disease being sought, but also feature in other diseases.[9] These effects can be mitigated by pre-defining strict exclusion criteria for diagnoses that share the symptom or marker contributing to the reference standard.

Misclassification related to disease severity in the population being studied

Misclassification will also occur because diseases are rarely binary states, but exist at varying degrees of severity. Patients with severe disease are easy to identify and have a relatively low probability of misclassification. In contrast, patients whose disease severity is close to the cut-off point between 'presence' and 'absence' have a relatively high probability of being misclassified. Misclassification tends to be more common in primary care settings, where the disease severity is typically less than in secondary care. A good case in point is lung tumours, which are generally larger in secondary than in primary care (as you enter secondary care later in the disease pathway). So a chest radiograph taken in primary care is less likely to identify a 5-mm-diameter tumour than it is a 2-cm-diameter tumour in the chest clinic. The primary care chest radiograph may be truly normal, or the radiologist may not spot a tiny lesion: They – like psychiatrists—are not infallible.

Researchers should conduct fresh validation studies when planning to implement existing tests in a new setting, as diagnostic tests developed in a secondary care population generally have a lower sensitivity and higher specificity when they are applied to a primary care population.[9] Unfortunately, this rarely happens. Spectacular results are published from an enriched population in secondary or tertiary care, and the test is lauded as being appropriate for primary care.

The effect of variation in test procedure or interpretation

Variation in the interpretation and conduct of tests also contributes to the spectrum effect through misclassification. A simple example is testing the performance of chest radiographs for lung cancer. How do you classify the minor patch of shadowing that in itself doesn't signify cancer, but for which a 6-week repeat radiograph is suggested? Alternatively, the spectrum effect may be rooted in measurement errors arising from badly calibrated machines or simple mistakes in procedure. For example, while urine microscopy detects non-visible haematuria very accurately and with a very low false-positive rate, this is only when it is performed by trained technicians or nephrologists under strictly defined conditions that are not feasible in a primary care setting.[12,13] Researchers can minimise clinical errors arising through the incorrect application or interpretation of tests by

1. Conducting studies under standardised conditions that are achievable in the setting in which they will be applied. For primary care diagnostic studies, that essentially means conducting them in primary care.
2. Agreeing beforehand how to interpret test results.
3. Publishing the above information alongside the test results.

RESEARCH ASPECTS

An important purpose of primary care research is to provide evidence to inform national guidelines on patient pathways.[1] This is particularly relevant for primary care diagnostic research, as many primary care tests are not definitive, but are used to select a population as higher risk of disease for definitive (usually secondary care) testing. Thus prostate-specific antigen, when raised, identifies a group of men at high risk of harbouring a prostate cancer. Only once definitive testing is done can the prostate cancer be diagnosed or ruled out. This ignores the awkward fact that 'definitive testing' may be imperfect too. Needle biopsies may miss the prostate cancer, giving a false-negative.

Health care systems have a duty to strike the right balance between the risk of missing disease and the risk of causing harm through unnecessary investigation. This is all the more difficult in the primary care setting, in which there is a population with early-stage disease that has a low prevalence.

Opting for sensitivity or specificity

When the consequences of a missed or late diagnosis are significant and the risks associated with investigation are low, it may be preferable to optimise testing so that it reduces the chances of missing people with the disease. Here, researchers should focus on identifying a panel of candidate tests that have a high sensitivity that work independently. Parallel testing regimens (i.e. applying tests all at the same time) further optimise sensitivity.

When the consequences of a missed or late diagnosis are less important and the risks associated with investigation are relatively high, it may be preferable to choose tests with a high specificity. This will reduce the chances of exposing healthy patients to unnecessary risk. Again, researchers are encouraged to identify a battery of independent tests, but this time to explore serial rather than parallel testing. Serial testing tends to increase specificity, because not all the tests are applied to everyone deemed to be at risk of the disease.[14]

Selecting the right balance between sensitivity and specificity, deciding on the risk threshold for investigation and choosing the optimal strategy for multiple testing are all complex processes.

Primary care research has a vital role in informing these choices, through well-designed studies in areas such as health economics and modelling, patient preferences and ethics. Such research will examine 'test strategies' rather than individual tests. For example, in our population, does test A work? Or test A performed simultaneously with test B? Or test A then test B? Or what about test C? ('Work' is a qualitative word, as it means different things to different people. Some contexts will be sensitivity driven, or specificity driven, or driven by health economics. Or a mixture of these. Or a compromise, as different stakeholders will have different views. For example, patients choose extremely high sensitivity when a cancer test is offered (they do not want a cancer to be missed). Yet clinicians performing the test would settle for a lower sensitivity, in part to reduce the false-positive rate, and in part to keep their workload manageable. Policymakers, and those paying for the test may well have a different view again).

Health economics and modelling studies

From the point of view of the health care system, health economics and modelling studies are needed to quantify the consequences of the proposed policy for further investigation. For example, studies advocating the liberalisation of testing should be accompanied by health economics analyses modelling the costs of investigating greater numbers of patients. Crucially, these must include the costs associated with investigations of patients who transpire not to have the target condition. For example, a new triage test to select patients for colonoscopy for possible inflammatory bowel disease may well find more cases—and earlier—but the benefits be swamped by the sheer numbers of negative colonoscopies.

Potential topics to cover include

- The savings associated with earlier diagnosis.
- The costs associated with harms arising from follow-up investigations.
- The opportunity costs; that is, the loss of other alternatives when one option is chosen. This is a particular concern in health care systems with constrained resources.

Studies of patients' and practitioners' views of testing

It is well recognised that people are driven more strongly to avoid a loss than to achieve a gain.[15] This suggests that, collectively, patients would prefer highly sensitive tests and referral thresholds set at a low PPV. This has been demonstrated in a vignette study when the appetite for cancer testing was very high even when the chance of cancer was small, with the exception of black patients who were much less keen on testing.[16] Furthermore, whether a patient consents to a procedure/test also depends on the framing of the probabilities of good or bad outcomes; for example, a 2% chance of injury with the test versus a

98% chance of success. Test acceptability is an important factor here, suggesting the need for (probably qualitative) studies addressing questions such as

- Is the test found to be invasive/unpleasant and, if so, does that reduce patient consent for testing?
- Is the test safe to be carried out in the proposed setting?
- Does acceptability vary among different patient groups?
- What is the association between acceptability of the test and risk of the target condition being sought?

Ethics of testing

Ethics studies may also be required, examining test results that

- Have implications for family members (e.g. *BRCA2* testing in breast cancer)
- Identify disease that has a poor prognosis and few treatment options
- Have implications for eligibility for health or life insurance
- Will not necessarily change patient management

There is a strong overlap here with patient-preference studies. In addition, ethics studies may also have a useful role in resolving conflicts between the results of health economics and patient preference studies.

Arguably, there is also a place for ethics studies examining the thorny issue of how much the taxpayer is willing to spend to achieve patient-reported preferences for investigation. Such studies could also investigate whether the proposed testing strategy results in a net benefit to the health of the whole population or a net harm. This is a difficult topic to get across in patient-preference studies.

Safety netting

Safety netting means different things to different people. In the context of research into diagnostics, we use it to mean one (or both) of two concepts:

1. A procedure whereby patients who are not initially selected for testing are reviewed to reconsider whether testing is appropriate at a later point, or
2. Review of those who test negative, but who have continuing symptoms.

Where it has been decided to maximise specificity, this second group may be large. Well-designed safety-netting studies can inform the management of patients with a negative test result but whose symptoms persist. Such studies could examine aspects of false reassurance:

- Will a negative result falsely reassure the patient and/or practitioner?
- If so, what safety-netting steps should be put in place to avoid diagnostic delay in patients whose symptoms persist?

Problems of low incidence or low prevalence: Large study size

As alluded to many times above, clinical testing in primary care is complicated because it seeks to quantify the likelihood of disease which is of low prevalence and may be in its early stages. This has implications for the size of study needed to yield sufficient power. Cohort studies in such a situation may be prohibitively large. While case-control studies are generally placed relatively low in the hierarchy of study design,[14] they can be a practical solution to the problem of researching rare diseases. This is particularly true when they are conducted using prospectively collected data, as provided by electronic medical record databases, such as the Clinical Practice Research Datalink in the UK.

Serendipitous findings

Furthermore, researchers have to consider how to handle 'serendipitous findings.' In the SIGGAR trial of computed tomography (CT) colonography versus colonoscopy for suspected colon cancer, CT identified a small number of non-colonic diseases which probably were the cause of the symptoms.[17] Strictly, this was conducted in the referred population, though it could just as well have been performed in primary care. A pure primary care example would be chest X-ray for cancer identifying mesothelioma (cancer, but was that the study outcome?) or pneumonia (again clinically ever so helpful). Clinically that's very useful—but how will you deal with it in the study?

METHODOLOGY OF PREDICTIVE MODELLING

Many methods are available to researchers interested in developing clinical prediction models that report the probability that a particular disease is present. Detailed discussion of the models, which include logistic regression, generalised linear models, decision tree learning, and Bayesian methods, is well beyond the scope of this book. Whatever the method chosen, researchers are advised to adhere to guidelines on the transparent reporting of multivariable prediction models for individual prognosis or diagnosis (TRIPOD).[18]

REFERENCES

1. National Institute for Health and Care Excellence. Suspected cancer: Recognition and referral [NG12]: NICE, 2015.
2. Gigerenzer G. Making sense of health statistics. *Bull World Health Organ* 2009;87(8):567–67.
3. Bossuyt PM, Reitsma JB, Bruns DE et al. STARD 2015: An updated list of essential items for reporting diagnostic accuracy studies. *Radiology* 2015;277(3):826–32.
4. Cohen JF, Korevaar DA, Gatsonis CA et al. STARD for abstracts: Essential items for reporting diagnostic accuracy studies in journal or conference abstracts. *BMJ* 2017; 358:j3751.

5. Howick J, Cals JWL, Jones C et al. Current and future use of point-of-care tests in primary care: An international survey in Australia, Belgium, The Netherlands, the UK and the USA. *BMJ Open* 2014;4(8):e005611.
6. World Health Organization. *HIV Assays: Operational Characteristics. Report 14. Simple/Rapid Tests.* Geneva: World Health Organization; 2004.
7. World Health Organization. Blood safety and availability, 2017.
8. Leeflang MM, Rutjes AW, Reitsma JB et al. Variation of a test's sensitivity and specificity with disease prevalence. *CMAJ: Canadian Medical Association Journal = Journal de l'Association Medicale Canadienne* 2013;185(11):E537–44.
9. Usher-Smith JA, Sharp SJ, Griffin SJ. The spectrum effect in tests for risk prediction, screening, and diagnosis. *BMJ* 2016;353:i3139.
10. Rutjes AW, Reitsma JB, Coomarasamy A et al. Evaluation of diagnostic tests when there is no gold standard. A review of methods. *Health Technol Assess* 2007;11(50):iii, ix-51.
11. Hamilton W, Peters T, Round A et al. What are the clinical features of lung cancer before the diagnosis is made? A population based case-control study. *Thorax* 2005;60(12):1059–65.
12. Kelly JD, Fawcett DP, Goldberg LC. Assessment and management of non-visible haematuria in primary care. *BMJ* 2009;338:a3021.
13. Rodgers MA, Hempel S, Aho T et al. Diagnostic tests used in the investigation of adult haematuria: A systematic review. *BJU Int* 2006;98(6):1154–60.
14. Fletcher RW, Feltcher SW. *Clinical Epidemiology: The Essentials.* Baltimore: Lippincott, Williams and Wilkins; 2014.
15. Kahneman D. *Thinking, Fast and Slow.* London: Penguin; 2011.
16. Banks J, Hollinghurst S, Bigwood L et al. Preferences for cancer investigation: A vignette-based study of primary-care attendees. *Lancet Oncol* 2014;15(2):232–40.
17. Atkin W, Dadswell E, Wooldrage K et al. Computed tomographic colonography versus colonoscopy for investigation of patients with symptoms suggestive of colorectal cancer (SIGGAR): A multicentre randomised trial. *Lancet (London, England)* 2013;381(9873):1194–202.
18. Collins GS, Reitsma JB, Altman DG et al. Transparent reporting of a multivariable prediction model for individual prognosis or diagnosis (TRIPOD): The TRIPOD statement. *Br J Cancer* 2015;112(2):251–9.

CHAPTER 20

How to conduct observational studies

Tibor Schuster

OBSERVATIONAL STUDIES

Observational studies are an increasingly popular type of investigation to gather data, information and evidence on a particular research question in almost all quantitative domains of primary care research. Areas of application include studies on programme and policy evaluation, field studies and surveys obtaining representative or purposive sample data from target populations. Due to the rapid advancements in information technology, recent observational studies are employing more and more administrative databases and electronic medical or health record data (see also Chapter 8 on the use of big data). Observational studies, as the name suggests, involve acquiring information (data) based on observation without intervening, and are therefore also referred to as non-interventional studies. In other words, observational studies allow investigation of various aspects of a research question under real-life conditions, without any external modification of the processes or procedures that relate to the population under study.

The fundamental concepts and methods relevant to observational studies have evolved from the broader discipline of epidemiology. A major limitation of observational studies is the inevitable risk of confounding bias when estimating effects of exposures. An association or correlation does not necessarily mean causation. However, observational studies may still have great value in situations where rigorously controlled experimental designs such as randomised controlled trials are infeasible, impractical or unethical.

Despite the commonalities of epidemiological research and observational studies in primary care research, the latter may benefit from a better conceptual understanding of mechanisms for why observation units (e.g. patients, health care providers) were, or were not, exposed to the intervention under study. For instance, in an observational study evaluating the effect of a readily available screening method, a doctor's reasoning on when to perform (and not to perform) screening is crucial to identifying relevant confounding factors. In situations where the exposure mechanisms are well understood, 'propensity score' methods are particularly appealing to reduce potential confounding bias. The propensity score is the probability of being exposed to an intervention or treatment, given 'covariates'. Covariates are variables that are possibly predictive of the outcome under study. One can either use stratification, weighting or matching based on the propensity score to account for confounding factors. This is in contrast to the conventional multivariable regression approach where confounding variables are included as adjustment variables in a regression model for the outcome. If the outcome is rare, propensity score methods are typically preferred. If the exposure is rare, classic regression modelling may be more suitable than propensity score methods. Regardless of the chosen analytical approach, *a priori* identification of potential confounding variables is required. Data-driven confounder selection based on significance tests is an outdated and misguided practice.

Observational studies typically aim on estimating the population-level (average) effect of the exposure in the target population. Confidence intervals and, increasingly used Bayesian credible intervals, provide a measure of uncertainty for such estimated mean effects. Prediction intervals, on the other hand, depict a range of exposure effects that are expected to apply to most individuals in the target population. While average effects offer important population-level evidence for policy makers, case-based decisions need to take into account the expected effect of heterogeneity across individuals. For instance, doctors and patients who wish to understand the risks and benefits of medications will be more interested in the expected range of effects in the population, rather than the average effect in the population.

The study design and the way data on exposures, outcomes and covariates are collected and analysed play a fundamental role in determining that an effect estimate is unbiased, and that the associated confidence, credible and prediction intervals are valid. Depending on the context and the available data, some study designs are preferable over others. In many situations, the optimal design choice is not immediately obvious, and advantages and disadvantages of the various options need to be carefully balanced against each other. The ultimate choice of the design will determine the feasibility, time and costs of the research and will inevitably affect the quality and acceptability of the findings.

TABLE 20.1 Overview of design properties of the three observational study types

Study design properties	Observational study design		
	Cross-sectional	Case-control	Cohort
Possibility to study multiple outcomes	☑	☒	☑
Possibility to study multiple exposures	☑	☑	☒
Estimation of outcome prevalence	☑	☒	☑
Estimation of exposure prevalence	☑	☑	☑
Estimation of odds ratios	☐	☑	☑
Estimation of risk differences and risk ratios	☐	☒	☑
Estimation of incidence rates and hazard ratios	☒	☒	☑
Time and cost efficiency	☑	☐	☒
Level of evidence (scientific acceptability)	☒	☐	☑

The symbols represent different levels of feasibility or value: ☑ very feasible/high level; ☐ feasible under assumptions/medium level; ☒ not or hardly feasible/low level.

Before planning and conducting an observational study, make yourself familiar with the STROBE (STrengthening the Reporting of OBservational studies in Epidemiology) statement and its extensions (https://www.strobe-statement.org/). While developed for epidemiology, these guidelines apply equally to observational studies in primary care. The statement provides checklists for various study types, and outlines fundamental requirements on reporting standards and data transparency, as well as on the importance of registration and publication of study protocols.

The following sections cover the three most common observational study designs: Cross-sectional, case-control and cohort studies. For each design, the typical research setting and purpose, common strengths and weaknesses, potential challenges in the planning and conduct of each study type that might need to be addressed and caveats regarding analysis and reporting of study findings are outlined.

The design properties of these three observational study designs are shown in Table 20.1.

CROSS-SECTIONAL STUDIES

Cross-sectional studies are the simplest observational study design. They typically provide data on the entire population under study at one moment in time – effectively a 'snapshot'. The purpose of cross-sectional studies is often to gather information on relevant unknown characteristics of a target population and to determine the distribution, i.e. the prevalence, of exposure and outcome variables. This information may then be used to identify subpopulations with atypical frequencies of critical outcomes, which may reflect unmet current or future health needs in these individuals. Cross-sectional studies may also serve as baseline data for assessing exposure-outcome associations to gain preliminary evidence about the causes of outcomes of interest.

Compared with other study designs, cross-sectional studies are the most time- and cost-efficient, because information is gathered only at a single time point (or a short time period). Data sources may include registries, clinical or administrative databases, surveys, and any type of individual record data in paper or electronic format. However, due to the lack of individual longitudinal data information, cross-sectional studies have limited value in assessing possible aetiological associations between certain exposures or interventions and outcomes. It can be difficult to determine the temporal order of events from cross-sectional data alone, i.e. whether the exposure or outcome of interest occurred first. For instance, in a cross-sectional study assessing the association of weight and doctors' prescription of antidepressants, it would be difficult to infer if weight was the determining factor in a doctor's treatment decision or, if actually the prescription (and therefore likely exposure to the treatment) had affected the weight of the patient.

Another downside of cross-sectional data can be the lack of opportunity to assess the consistency over time of data patterns or associations found in the study sample. For instance, a cross-sectional survey among doctors to determine their current involvement in health promotion (e.g. advertising flu vaccinations) may strongly vary by time or season and can be a poor indicator of doctors' general engagement in health promotion in this population. Lastly, when comparing subpopulations (e.g. exposed versus unexposed individuals) in a cross-sectional study, group differences in outcomes may reflect factors determining their selection into the groups rather than effects of the actual exposure. Careful adjustment for likely confounder variables in the statistical analysis is essential, as the study design does not address this selection bias. There is a risk of adjusting for variables that are not confounders, but actually consequences of the exposure (so called exposure-outcome mediators). A covariate that is influenced by two or more other variables is called a collider, and adjustment for such factors might introduce a 'collider-stratification bias' which may increase the overall inaccuracy of the effect estimate. It is also noted that, while cross-sectional studies allow for estimation of prevalence, they do not enable the estimation of incidence rates (the number of new cases in the population at risk in a given time period).

CASE-CONTROL STUDIES

Case-control is a type of observational study in which the study sample includes a predetermined number of subjects that have experienced a specific critical event (cases) and, often matched on an individual base to each case, subjects that have not experienced the same critical event (controls). For both cases and controls, exposure history is determined using interviews, questionnaires or other available data sources. The information about an individual's exposure history is therefore retrospective in nature. A special type is the nested case-control study. In this design, both cases and controls are sampled from the same cohort which minimises selection bias in conventional case-control study designs.

Case-control studies are conducted to investigate the potential association of one or several past exposure(s) with the study-specific condition (critical event) that is used to define cases. The primary purpose is to see whether the odds for the occurrence of an event is different (higher or lower) among the exposed compared to the unexposed.

The great advantage of case-control studies is their application in scenarios where rare or long-term events are of primary interest. The retrospective study design allows recruitment of cases from health service centres, disease registries or patient networks, avoiding large time- and cost-intensive cohort studies where the uncertain number of prospectively occurring events is a major limiting factor. Because controls are, in the broadest sense, not required to meet very particular inclusion criteria (except for being event-free), the feasibility of a case-control study mostly depends on a sufficient and accessible source for recruitment of cases. Another advantage of case-control studies is the possibility to study multiple potential causes for the same event of interest. For instance, in a case-control study investigating factors possibly leading to early onset of type-2 diabetes mellitus, exposure variables may simultaneously include past lifestyle factors, family history of diabetes and genetic information.

A major limitation of the case-control design is that cases are typically over-represented in the study sample. For this reason, the only valid effect measure that can be computed from the study data is the odds ratio. If the prevalence of the event in the target population is not rare (>10%), the odds ratio overestimates the actual risk ratio (RR) for RR > 1 and underestimates the RR for RR < 1. For rare events, the odds ratio and risk ratio take very similar values.

It is also possible to estimate the prevalence of exposures among cases and controls, however, the determination of the actual event risks for exposed and unexposed requires further assumptions. This is the reason why it is not immediately possible to estimate risk ratios from case-control study data.

The choice of appropriate controls is crucial for dealing with confounding factors. Unsuitable sampling of controls may compromise the study validity. Control individuals should be as similar as possible to cases, except for their event status. However, the sampling scheme must not depend on the exposure(s) under investigation. It is advised to sample controls from the same general population to which the cases belong. For instance, a case-control study on family planning (where a case is defined as having at least one child before the age of 20) may inquire about knowledge of contraceptive methods among young women. Cases could be recruited from local centres providing services for pregnant women. If some cases travel to the clinics from rural areas, the sampling scheme for controls needs to take this into consideration, otherwise the socio-demographic characteristics of controls and cases may differ.

The retrospective nature of case-control studies makes them prone to recall bias, i.e. misclassification of the exposure status due to false statements by respondents. The risk for recall bias is lower if the exposure history is retrieved from reliable data sources. In nested case-control studies that employ clinical or administrative databases, misclassification error may also apply when identifying cases and controls, due to inaccurate or missing data on diagnosis, for example. Lastly, case-control studies only allow one to study exposure-outcome relationships based on one specific event (outcome) definition. It is therefore necessary to carefully choose the outcome of interest. Clinical relevance, reliability of the outcome assessment, and prevalence in the population are key points to consider.

COHORT STUDIES

The key defining concept in this study design is that a group of individuals (the cohort) share partially similar baseline characteristics and are prospectively followed over time. In the course of follow-up, measurements of time-varying features, including exposure variables, covariates and outcome measurements, are recorded.

In general, one can distinguish between prospective and retrospective cohort studies. Prospective cohort studies are characterised by a current definition of the cohort, plus a specified set of variables to be measured in future follow-up assessments (i.e. prospectively). Retrospective cohort studies retrieve data on covariate, exposure and outcome trajectories that were collected before the study protocol was established. That means data used for a retrospective cohort study were initially not collected for the purpose of answering the study's research question(s).

Among all types of observational studies, cohort studies are the most sophisticated design to provide real-world evidence for the efficacy, effectiveness or safety of interventions or exposures. Because of the timely order of variable assessments in cohort studies, it is feasible to adequately model the direction of relationships between variables as causes must precede effects.

The advantage of prospective cohort studies is that, at the planning stage, considerations regarding important covariates and relevant time-varying confounding variables can be taken into account. Variables that may affect the level of exposure to an intervention (including variables affecting adherence) are crucial to adjust for when analysing the study data. Only a prospective cohort design can ensure that all relevant confounder variables are measured at appropriate intervals. One further advantage is the opportunity to study the aetiologies of multiple outcomes that possibly relate to characteristics of the cohort, i.e. exposed and unexposed individuals.

A caveat to prospective cohort studies is the relatively long waiting period from the initiation of the study until usable data become available. For instance, in a prospective cohort study comparing the effects of different beta-blockers prescribed by family physicians, it may take more than one year to collect sufficient data that will allow for an assessment of even short-term effects. The reason for this is that the entire study period is composed of recruitment time (i.e. identifying and consenting eligible doctors and patients), as well as follow up time.

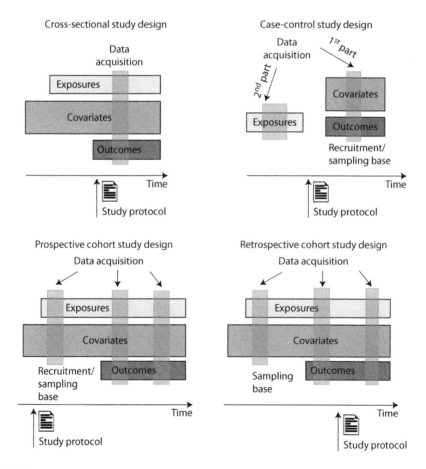

FIGURE 20.1 Overview of timeline in protocol establishment, recruitment/sampling and data acquisition for the various observational study designs.

Retrospective cohort studies, sometimes also called historic cohort studies, use existing data sources to define cohorts based on inclusion and exclusion criteria that were measured in the past. The related databases, however, contain follow-up information of individuals that may reach up into the present. The disadvantage of historic cohort studies is that there is often only limited opportunity to gather additional data that were not recorded but are deemed relevant to answering the research question. For instance, it may be impossible to measure relevant confounding variables that may distort the study findings.

Figure 20.1 summarises the timeline for writing the research protocol, sampling and data collection the three different study designs discussed in this chapter.

CHAPTER 21

Randomised trials in primary care

Gillian Bartlett-Esquilant, Miriam Dickinson and Tibor Schuster

BACKGROUND

The randomised control trial (RCT) design arguably is one of the most important methodological developments in medical research. Researchers in Europe and the US developed in the 1940s what is now considered the method that produces one of the highest levels of evidence, with further refinements occurring that make this a relevant and useful tool for primary care research. The RCT evaluates treatments or interventions in an experimental setting that is under control of the investigator. Evaluation is achieved by comparing pre-specified trial outcomes between at least two treatment or intervention arms. A key element in the method is that participants in the trial are 'randomised', or divided into the study groups by chance to receive either the intervention being tested or to be a 'control', that is, a participant who receives a comparison intervention or a 'placebo'.[1] The random allocation of participants to different interventions minimises allocation bias and, theoretically, should balance between groups both known and unknown factors that might be related to the health outcome.[2]

EQUIPOISE, PARTICIPANTS AND RANDOMISATION

Although RCTs are considered to provide very strong evidence in terms of deciding whether a treatment or intervention works, there are several key considerations that must be contemplated before deciding to use this study design in primary care research. These include determining if equipoise exists, establishing the inclusion and exclusion criteria, deciding on the randomisation strategy and assessing whether and what type of blinding (also called masking) can be done. The first issue, the principle of equipoise, is key to ethically justifying randomisation of one group of participants to a control arm.[3] In general, the investigator should establish that equipoise exists or, in other words, that there is genuine uncertainty with experts in the field whether or not the treatment or intervention will be beneficial.[3] If that condition is satisfied, the investigator then determines the inclusion (characteristics participants must have to be recruited for the study) and exclusion criteria (characteristics that would make potential participants ineligible).[4] Note that the inclusion criteria usually define the target study population in which the investigator would expect to see a benefit such as age, sex or morbidity. Exclusion criteria are meant to be applied to potential participants who have met all the inclusion criteria and further restricts the participants to ensure patient safety and that the primary outcomes of the study are reached. An example of a common exclusion criterion is inability to provide informed consent. Regardless of the inclusion and exclusion criteria, they must be clearly stated and justified. At this stage, the investigator will be able to assess the feasibility of the RCT in terms of number of potential participants who meet these criteria. Participants are only randomised after they have been assessed for eligibility.

There are many ways to allocate participants through randomisation, but the process should maximise statistical power and minimise selection bias and confounding (sometimes referred to as allocation bias).[5] The different methods to randomise participants vary from simple, which is the equivalent of a coin toss, to the complex methods such as co-variate adaptive randomisation.[6] The selection of a randomisation method will depend on the study objectives and participants. There are many published resources to help investigators select and complete the randomisation process,[7] including online tools (www.randomization.com). Again, whatever choice is made must be clearly described and justified. Along with the randomisation process, the study investigator should endeavour to maintain allocation concealment. Allocation concealment is critical to minimising bias in RCTs and comprises the procedures taken to ensure that the patient and the investigator are not made aware of which group they are being randomised to before they enter the study.[8] The allocation concealment method needs to be detailed in the study protocol and any publications reporting the trial results.

BLINDING (MASKING)

Allocation concealment refers to procedures that occur to conceal the results of the randomisation, so that the research team members responsible for recruitment remain impartial in terms of which participants end up in the different treatment or intervention groups. Another important and related procedure is blinding or masking in the trial.[9] While allocation concealment should occur in every RCT, blinding is not always possible or appropriate. Blinding refers to methods that are used to prevent study participants, study investigators and/or the research team members who collect and analyse the study data from being aware of which group each participant belongs to. Who is blinded to what needs to be reported while avoiding ambiguous terms such as 'single-blinded'.[2] The impact of blinding is more crucial when the outcomes are subjective versus objective, and even in trials where blinding of the participants and study investigators is not possible, as is often the case for interventions favoured in primary care, it is still possible to blind those who measure or collect outcomes.

STUDY TYPE

After all of these issues have been assessed and decided to determine the feasibility of conducting an RCT, with detailed reporting in a trial protocol,[10] the investigator also needs to determine the type of trial they are conducting and the study design that will be used.[11,12] In general, there are two different types of RCTs. The first are those trials that focus on efficacy (i.e. does it work?), that by design are highly controlled with extensive inclusion and exclusion criteria to minimise any potential biases or confounding. The second are the trials more commonly found in primary care and are referred to as pragmatic trials that test effectiveness (i.e. does it work in everyday practice?) where the participants are not as highly selected, and the exclusion and inclusion criteria tend to be less stringent.[13] The evidence from pragmatic RCTs often informs decisions about practice, which is why they are favoured in primary care research.

STUDY DESIGN

Included in the two types of RCTs are many different study designs. The most common RCTs are parallel group, crossover, factorial and cluster.[14] Parallel groups trials are the most common design, with participants randomised either to the new treatment or intervention or to the control group (which might be the standard treatment). All participants receive the intervention or control at the same time and stay in their group for the entire trial. In crossover trials, participants are randomised to different sequences of treatments or interventions, but all patients eventually get all treatments or interventions in random order so that the participant ends up being their own control.[15] This trial design assumes that the effect of the intervention is not permanent. Factorial trials assign participants to more than one treatment-comparison group that are randomised at the same time, creating several possible

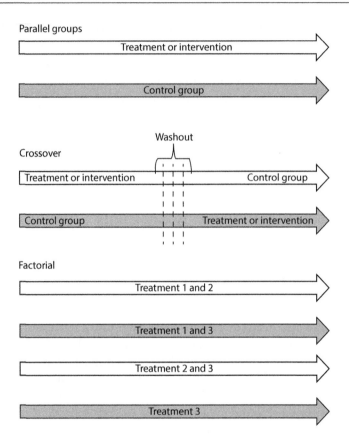

FIGURE 21.1 Basic trial designs.

intervention or treatment combinations (regimens). The cluster design refers to when groups are randomised instead of individual participants, and each of the previously listed designs can be used within cluster randomised trials. The details of the different trial designs are illustrated in Figure 21.1.[16]

CLUSTER RANDOMISED TRIALS

Cluster randomised trials are particularly useful for primary care research where interventions are more likely to be under evaluation, rather than medications or individualised treatments.[17] For this trial design, complete social units or groups, i.e. the clusters, are randomised to receive the intervention.[18] For example, the unit of randomisation might be by clinic, or by practitioner, rather than by the patient who is receiving either the intervention or the control. This is done to prevent contamination that might occur when an educational intervention is applied within a family medicine clinic. For example, as providers often discuss treatment options or practice decisions, it would be impossible to blind the other providers in the clinic to the intervention and not have each other's behaviours affected. There may be other reasons why individual randomisation is not possible for logistical, financial or ethical reasons. As a result, the cluster trial design is commonly used for the evaluation of service delivery or policy intervention at the level of the cluster.

STEPPED WEDGE DESIGN

For the remaining portion of the chapter we will focus on a trial design that is relatively new and particularly relevant and useful in primary care. A relatively new trial design within the cluster randomised trials is the stepped wedge, which is also referred to as the waiting list or phased implementation design.[19,20] This design determines for all groups to successively switch from control to intervention conditions,[21] implying an exclusively unidirectional crossover as illustrated in Figure 21.2.[22] At the beginning of the trial, all clusters are randomised to an *order* as to when to switch and are assigned to a step based on that order. A random number generator can be used to assign the order and there can be multiple clusters per step (e.g. groups of practices). In the first time block, all clusters are in the control phase but all clusters ultimately receive the intervention. Randomised intervention initiation order determines *when* (not if) a cluster receives the intervention, so that by the last time block all clusters are in the intervention phase.

This design addresses several of the limitations of the more common RCTs that are often problematic for primary care. In parallel groups design, the intervention must be implemented in half the clusters simultaneously,

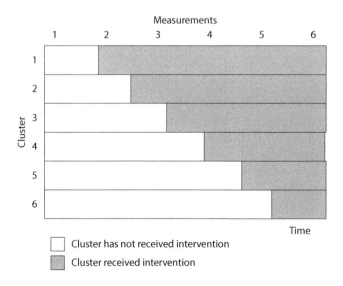

FIGURE 21.2 Stepped wedge RCT design.

which is not always possible for interventions requiring intensive training, if resources are limited or if there are geographical constraints, i.e. the clusters are located over a large area such as several clinics located in different regions of a country. In these situations, there would be a need for phased or sequential implementation of the intervention, which the stepped wedge allows for. The conventional crossover design assumes that carryover effects are absent, which would be an erroneous assumption for interventions that are in the form of training as is the case for most practice-based improvements. With a stepped-wedge design, carry-over effects are limited because crossover is only permitted from control to intervention conditions. The design is therefore particularly suitable for studying interventions with non-removable effects such as educational programmes or the implementation of new policies, in comparison to standard practice. Furthermore, when there are only a few clusters available, the stepped wedge may be a better option than a parallel group cluster randomised trial due to the greater power of the new design.[20] Randomisation is basically ineffective if the number of clusters is small.

A final important point is that the stepped wedge design addresses several ethical considerations that occur frequently in primary care interventions. It allows an investigator to assess an intervention that is believed likely to do more good than harm, and therefore, where equipoise is minimal. This would be the case for the evaluation of therapies or interventions when withholding the intervention from some participants (i.e. controls) is not acceptable, when evaluating the effectiveness (not efficacy) in real-world settings at the population level, when interventions have been shown to be effective in more controlled research settings and are ready for a large scale pragmatic trial or when there is a lack of definitive evidence of effectiveness but belief that intervention will do more good than harm. The design therefore removes the consideration of equipoise and minimises the impact of lack of blinding.

STEPPED WEDGE DESIGN ASPECTS

There are several design features that an investigator needs to consider with the stepped wedge, including the number of clusters, the number of individuals per cluster, the number and length of steps between receiving the intervention and the number of clusters randomised at each step. These design considerations will impact the duration and cost of the trial. The decisions about the design are generally influenced by logistical and statistical considerations. The logical issues are the number of suitable or available clusters, the number of participants considered to be eligible to participate in the study within each cluster and the maximum number of clusters that can simultaneously 'receive' intervention. The statistical issues are mainly the magnitude of expected intervention and time effects and the expected intra-cluster correlation (ICC), which is determined by the within and between cluster variance of the outcome.

WORKING WITH DESIGN EFFECTS

Once the logistically-driven considerations are taken into account, different aspects of the design can be modified to maximise the trial's resources and statistical power. The first step is to conduct a sample size calculation for a standard parallel randomised control trial.[23] To do this, the investigator must have established the primary trial outcome and the outcome characteristics (i.e. categorical versus continuous), the effect size and the common standard deviation of the outcome. To determine the sample size for the stepped wedge, the RCT sample size is multiplied by a design effect that corrects for clustering and the stepped randomisation. A calculation for design effect is illustrated in Figure 21.3 to demonstrate key design factors that can influence the feasibility and planning of the trial.[24] For the sake of simplicity, this model assumes the same number of clusters switch at each step, where a step represents a new group of clusters receiving the intervention, and that the number of measurements is constant. Note that according to Figure 21.3, the design effect decreases as number of measurements after each step (t) increases. This is due to the longitudinal repeated measures aspect of the design. The design effect also decreases as number of measurements at baseline (b) increases and as the number of steps (k) increases. Reasonable estimates of ICC must be chosen from context and/or previous comparable studies. As the ICC increases, the design effect slightly increases, thereafter $\rho = 0.05$ starts to decrease. Although there is some debate, a larger ICC usually increases sample size. The investigator should keep in mind that the efficiency in going from two to three steps is much larger than six to 12 steps. Additionally, the

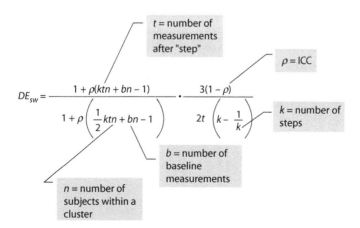

FIGURE 21.3 Calculating design effect.

efficiency gained by increasing number of steps is modest compared with efficiency gained from adding clusters or measurements to the design. Also, it may not be possible to obtain sufficient power only by increasing cluster size. These calculations assume there are random cluster effects, fixed time effects and no cluster by time interactions.

There are some final modelling considerations with the stepped wedge design. Recruitment of participants should be conducted before allocation of intervention (unexposed or exposed period), *or* participants should be recruited completely blind to their exposure status. This would need to be the case when the clusters have members entering and leaving over time. For both participant entry and measurement, calendar time is a crucial and potentially confounding factor. The assessment of effect of time (seasonality and time since implementation) on intervention effectiveness is possible. This is key, as time has an impact in two ways for the stepped wedge design. First, there are learner effects where either the trainer or implementers get 'better' over time at delivering the intervention. This can be adjusted by modelling of calendar time. The other effect is commonly referred to as a 'rising tide' where an intervention that at first seems to be effective might no longer be effective when calendar time is adjusted. This happens when there is a general move to improve patient outcomes and is a reason to consider shorter times between steps. To verify source of bias, look at 'within-wedge' analysis as a secondary or sensitivity analysis. Two effect estimates (stepped wedge and within-wedge) can be compared in a ratio of rates.

While being a particularly well-adapted design for primary care research, there are some disadvantages to the stepped wedge that an investigator needs to consider. The stepped wedge requires sophisticated statistical methods, as any analysis needs to consider (nested) cluster effects (e.g. hospital, ward, clinic, individual measurements over time). Generally, it is more difficult to run than the traditional parallel group RCT in that there is a heavier data collection burden with outcomes measured for every cluster at every time point. Informed consent of individuals in the cluster, if needed, can be complicated. The trial duration can be long if there is a complex implementation or prolonged time needed to influence outcomes. This design is impractical if comparing multiple interventions. Despite these issues, this trial design remains very popular in primary care research.

CONCLUSION

When considering conducting an RCT, use the Consolidated Standards of Reporting Trials (CONSORT) statement (www.consort-statement.org) as a guide. Time and cost considerations of an RCT need to be balanced against its ability to reduce bias and spurious causality. The evidence from RCTs is often synthesised in systematic reviews that are the bedrock of many evidence-based medicine recommendations. Other study designs can provide equivalent evidence,[25] but the RCT has the major advantage of straightforward investigation of cause–effect relationships with minimal bias and confounding factors.[26] When the trial design has high internal and external validity, the evidence can be very compelling. As well as CONSORT, there are many other excellent resources to help investigators design a sound trial, including the PRECIS-2 tool (www.precis-2.org). Remember that you should enter your study on a clinical trial registry and obtain a unique trial registration number before you start your research. Many journals will now only accept a trial for publication if it has been registered.

REFERENCES

1. Randomized Control Trial (RCT). PubMed Health. https://www.ncbi.nlm.nih.gov/pubmedhealth/PMHT0025811/.
2. Moher D, Hopewell S, Schulz KF et al. CONSORT 2010 explanation and elaboration: Updated guidelines for reporting parallel group randomised trials. *BMJ* 2010;340:c869.
3. Freedman B. Equipoise and the ethics of clinical research. *N Engl J Med* 1987;317(3):141–5.
4. Van Spall HGC, Toren A, Kiss A, Fowler RA. Eligibility criteria of randomized controlled trials published in high-impact general medical journals: A systematic sampling review. *JAMA* 2007;297(11):1233–40.
5. Lachin JM. Statistical properties of randomization in clinical trials. *Control Clin Trials* 1988;9(4):289–311.
6. Lin Y, Zhu M, Su Z. The pursuit of balance: An overview of covariate-adaptive randomization techniques in clinical trials. *Contemp Clin Trials* 2015;45:21–5.
7. Kim J, Shin W. How to do random allocation (randomization). *Clin Orthop Surg* 2014;6(1):103–9.
8. Schulz KF, Grimes DA. Allocation concealment in randomised trials: Defending against deciphering. *Lancet* 2002;359(9306):614–8.
9. Wood L, Egger M, Gluud LL et al. Empirical evidence of bias in treatment effect estimates in controlled trials with different interventions and outcomes: Meta-epidemiological study. *BMJ* 2008;336(7644):601–5.
10. CONSORT Group. CONSORT 2010. consort-statement.org. Consort-statement.org.
11. Loudon K, Treweek S, Sullivan F, Donnan P, Thorpe KE, Zwarenstein M. The PRECIS-2 tool: Designing trials that are fit for purpose. *BMJ* 2015;350:h2147.
12. PRECIS-2. precis-.org. http://www.consort-statement.org/.
13. Zwarenstein M, Treweek S, Gagnier JJ et al. Improving the reporting of pragmatic trials: An extension of the CONSORT statement. *BMJ* 2008;337:a2390.
14. Hopewell S, Dutton S, Yu L-M, Chan A-W, Altman DG. The quality of reports of randomised trials in 2000 and 2006: Comparative study of articles indexed in PubMed. *BMJ* 2010;340:c723.
15. Wang D, Lorch U, Bakhai A. Crossover trials. In: Wang D, Bakhai A, editors. *Clinical Trials: A Practical Guide to Design, Analysis and Reporting.* London: Remedica; 2006. p. 91–9.
16. e-Source. Clinical Trials. esourceresearch.org. http://www.esourceresearch.org/tabid/198/Default.aspx.
17. Murray DM. *Design and Analysis of Group-Randomized Trials.* USA: Oxford University Press; 1998.
18. Mallick U, Bakhai A, Wang D, Flather M. Cluster randomized trials. In: *Clinical Trials: A Practical Guide to Design, Analysis and Reporting.* London: Remedica Medical Education & Publishing; 2006. p. 141–51.

19. Brown CA, Lilford RJ. The stepped wedge trial design: A systematic review. *BMC Med Res Methodol* 2006;6(1):54.
20. Mdege ND, Man M-S, Taylor nee Brown CA, Torgerson DJ. Systematic review of stepped wedge cluster randomized trials shows that design is particularly used to evaluate interventions during routine implementation. *J Clin Epidemiol* 2011;64(9):936–48.
21. Hussey MA, Hughes JP. Design and analysis of stepped wedge cluster randomized trials. *Contemp Clin Trials* 2007;28(2):182–91.
22. Hemming K, Haines TP, Chilton PJ, Girling AJ, Lilford RJ. The stepped wedge cluster randomised trial: Rationale, design, analysis, and reporting. *BMJ: Br Med J* 2015;350(h391):1–8.
23. Power and Sample Size. powerandsamplesize.com. http://powerandsamplesize.com/Calculators/Compare-2-Means/2-Sample-Equality.
24. Woertman W, de Hoop E, Moerbeek M, Zuidema SU, Gerritsen DL, Teerenstra S. Stepped wedge designs could reduce the required sample size in cluster randomized trials. *J Clin Epidemiol* 2013;66(7):752–8.
25. Ioannidis JP, Haidich AB, Pappa M et al. Comparison of evidence of treatment effects in randomized and nonrandomized studies. *JAMA* 2001;286(7):821–30.
26. Spieth PM, Kubasch AS, Penzlin AI, Illigens BM, Barlinn K, Siepmann T. Randomized controlled trials – a matter of design. *Neuropsychiatr Dis Treat* 2016;12:1341.

CHAPTER 22

Grounded theory

David R. Thomas

Grounded theory is one of the common strategies used for qualitative research in primary care. Its focus is on the analysis of qualitative data. Effective use of grounded theory, as for most qualitative research strategies, requires that the raw data to be analysed (such as transcribed interviews) has considerable detail, sometimes described as 'rich' or 'thick' data.

The initial book written by Glaser and Strauss,[1] *The Discovery of Grounded Theory*, was published in 1967. Subsequently, the two authors developed somewhat different versions of grounded theory, with Glaser emphasising a less-structured approach. Strauss and Corbin co-authored a revised version of grounded theory, published as *Basics of Qualitative Research*,[2] for which there are now several editions. Another approach to grounded theory has been published by Charmaz.[3] A review of four varieties of grounded theory[4] distinguished these approaches in terms of (1) the specificity of procedures used during data analysis and the extent to which the theory constructed is reported as a distinct model (Strauss and Corbin) versus (2) a more textual narrative account (Glaser, Charmaz).

Grounded theory is one of several qualitative analysis strategies commonly used in qualitative research in primary health care. Table 22.1 provides a comparison of four strategies: Grounded theory, thematic or general inductive approaches, discourse analysis and phenomenology.

Grounded theory is similar to thematic or general inductive approaches. However, it explicitly distinguishes open coding and axial coding. Discourse analysis typically provides a detailed account of the perspectives and rhetorical devices evident in a sample of text. Phenomenology seeks to understand the lived experience among people who have had a common experience (e.g. living with cancer) and to write a coherent account of the meaning of those experiences. Several articles have compared specific strategies for qualitative

TABLE 22.1 Comparison of qualitative analysis strategies

	Grounded theory	**Thematic or general inductive approaches**	**Discourse analysis**	**Phenomenology**
Analytic strategies and questions	To generate or discover theory using open and axial coding with theoretical sampling	Identify core themes or categories in the text, relevant to the research objectives	Concerned with talk and texts as social practices and their rhetorical or argumentative organisation	Seeks to uncover the meaning that lives within experience and to convey felt understanding in words
Outcome of analysis	A theory or model that includes key themes or categories	A model including themes or categories most relevant to the research objectives	Multiple meanings of language and text identified and described	A description of the lived experience reported by participants
Presentation of findings	Description of theory that includes core themes	Description of most important themes	Narrative account covering multiple meanings evident in text	A coherent story or narrative about the experience

data analysis.[5-7] These provide insights into the similarities and differences among common qualitative analysis strategies.

The key procedures and concepts relevant to grounded theory are outlined in Table 22.2.[8] Grounded theory uses 'inductive analysis', which refers to analysis starting with detailed readings of raw data from which the researcher derives concepts, themes or a model. This model consists of interpretations made by the researchers. Because it is inductive, it is not appropriate to write hypotheses for grounded theory research, or for any other inductive qualitative research.

The researcher (or data analyst) starts with the raw data, which is often in the form of transcribed interviews. However, any type of textual data can be used. In the initial phase, referred to as open coding, key ideas or themes are constructed. These are sometimes referred to as 'codes' or categories (see example in Box 22.1). There are likely to be many specific themes at this stage. During the open coding phase, the researcher typically starts linking specific themes or categories either in a hierarchical relationship or merges multiple themes into a single category where they represent specific components within a more general category. This emerging phase is referred to as axial coding. Part of the process of axial coding is making theoretical comparisons

TABLE 22.2 Grounded theory: Key processes

Process	Description
Open coding	Initial coding involving close reading of the text data to identify concepts in text data and create initial categories to represent these concepts
Axial coding	Refining and combining categories developed during open coding into an emerging framework or model that includes higher level categories and subcategories
Making theoretical comparisons	Making comparisons among emerging categories and concepts to identify underling processes and to create more abstract or general concepts; identifying gaps in the emerging categories to identify further interview questions or observations
Selective coding and development of theory	Creating and refining a model or framework that represents the researchers view about the most important processes and categories evident in the text data
Memos and diagrams	Notes and conceptual maps created by the researcher to record insights and emerging ideas during the data analysis process to assist development of a theory or model
Theoretical sampling	Sampling to select diverse cases to enhance comparison of emerging concepts for similarities and differences
Data saturation	Conducting data collection (e.g. interviews) until no new themes or ideas are evident during the data analysis

BOX 22.1   EXAMPLE OF A SPECIFIC CATEGORY— RECOGNITION OF DEPRESSION BY GPs[9]

Researcher description: Most GPs reported that patients with depression could present in several ways, with different symptoms. The most common signs of depression were disclosure of depression directly by the patient, the patient reporting symptoms that were commonly associated with depression and, less commonly, the use of screening questions or a checklist to assess depression.

Text coded from GP interviews
   … sometimes the patient will be saying that they just don't have enthusiasm for things. They might use the phrases about being down, or wanting to give up, things like that.
   … other times it would be a patient who's younger and seems to have a lack of enthusiasm either for work, or hobbies, or relationships, things like that. Other times patients are tearful.

(referred to as 'constant comparison' in some versions of grounded theory) to develop emerging categories and concepts at a more general level and to identify underling processes.

During the data analysis process, researchers typically keep notes or memos about their thoughts on emerging categories and their implication. The process of writing memos is an important part of the analytic process and is a skill that should be developed by qualitative researchers. Memos will help identify any gaps in the information available. These might lead to additional questions or prompts in subsequent interviews or data collection.

Modification of interview topics during the process of interviewing and preliminary analysis is an advantage in grounded theory research. For grounded theory, interviews do not use a standard set of interview questions; rather the topics or prompts used are adapted during each interview to elicit insights about topics or experiences from interviewees.

In a later phase of the analysis, the researcher uses selective coding to aid the development of a theory or model. Decisions are made about which categories or themes are most important given the purposes of the research. How are the themes to be assembled into an overall model or framework which captures the key processes the research has identified during the data analysis?

Two other processes are part of a grounded theory process: Theoretical sampling and data saturation. Theoretical sampling refers to the selection of additional cases during data gathering to ensure that there are a wide range of experiences represented in the data.[10] For example, cases may be selected to ensure inclusion of both men and women and people who have had extensive experience with the phenomena of interest as well as those with less experience.

Data saturation refers to the process of adding new cases (e.g. more interviews) during the data analysis and finding that few or no new themes or categories are emerging from the added cases. Note that the use of theoretical sampling and data saturation require that the data analysis begins while the data gathering is in process. Thus, the data gathering and analysis are concurrent. This contrasts with quantitative research, where the data collection is typically completed before the data analysis begins.

Grounded theory findings result from multiple interpretations made from the raw data by the researcher(s) who carry out the data analysis. Inevitably, the findings are shaped by the assumptions and experiences of the researchers. During the data analysis, researchers must make decisions about what is more important and less important in the data. Researchers who are not used to this process may find it difficult to make decisions about what is important in the data.

WRITING THE FINDINGS

For researchers not familiar with qualitative research, writing the findings from a grounded theory research project is often difficult. When writing findings, there should be a clear presentation of over-arching categories or themes which are integrated into a coherent model or framework. A common mistake is to present a series of quotes from raw text without a coherent framework. Grounded theory is not content analysis. The key outcomes are concepts, experiences or processes and are not based on the number of times specific words were mentioned.

GROUNDED THEORY IN CONTEXT

Grounded theory is not easy; many researchers struggle to come to grips with the underlying assumptions and procedures required to conduct a grounded theory study.[11] However, the insights from a well-conducted grounded theory study are well worth the effort. There are several examples in primary health care which illustrate how to carry out a grounded theory analysis[12,13] and how to write the findings.[14] Some of the key concepts from grounded theory, such as theoretical sampling and data saturation, have been adopted by other approaches to qualitative research.[15]

REFERENCES

1. Glaser BG, Strauss AL. *The Discovery of Grounded Theory: Strategies for Qualitative Research*. Chicago: Aldine; 1967.
2. Strauss A, Corbin J. *Basics of Qualitative Research: Techniques and Procedures for Developing Grounded Theory*, 3rd ed. Newbury Park: Sage; 2007.
3. Charmaz K. *Constructing Grounded Theory*, 2nd ed. Thousand Oaks, CA: Sage; 2014.
4. Apramian T, Cristancho S, Watling C, Lingard L. (Re)Grounding grounded theory: A close reading of theory in four schools. *Qualitative Research* 2017;17(4):359–76.
5. Frost N, Nolas SM, Brooks-Gordon B et al. Pluralism in qualitative research: The impact of different researchers and qualitative approaches on the analysis of qualitative data. *Qualitative Research* 2010;10(4):441–60.
6. Slaughter S, Dean Y, Knight H et al. The inevitable pull of the River's current: Interpretations derived from a single text using multiple research traditions. *Qual Health Res* 2007;17(4):548–61.
7. Starks H, Brown Trinidad S. Choose your method: A comparison of phenomenology, discourse analysis, and grounded theory. *Qual Health Res* 2007;17(10):1372–80.
8. Strauss A, Corbin J. *Basics of Qualitative Research: Techniques and Procedures for Developing Grounded Theory*, 2nd ed. Thousand Oaks, CA: Sage; 1998.
9. Thomas DR, Arlidge B, Arroll B, Elder H. General practitioners' views about diagnosing and treating depression in Māori and non-Māori patients. *J Prim Health Care* 2010;2(3):208–16.
10. Draucker CB, Martsolf DS, Ross R, Rusk TB. Theoretical sampling and category development in grounded theory. *Qual Health Res* 2007;17(8):1137–48.
11. Suddaby R. From the editors: What grounded theory is not. *Acad Manage J* 2006;49(4):633–42.

12. Dunn PJ, Margaritis V, Anderson CL. Understanding health literacy skills in patients with cardiovascular disease and diabetes. *The Qualitative Report* 2017;22(1):197–212.
13. Sbaraini A, Carter S, Evans R, Blinkhorn A. How to do a grounded theory study: A worked example of a study of dental practices. *BMC Med Res Methodol* 2011;11(1):128.
14. Williams AM, Irurita IF. Therapeutically conducive relationships between nurses and patients: An important component of quality nursing care. *Aust J Adv Nurs* 1998;16(2):36–44.
15. Bowen GA. Naturalistic inquiry and the saturation concept: A research note. *Qual Res* 2008;8(1):137–52.

CHAPTER 23

Doing interpretive phenomenological primary care research

Valerie A. Wright-St Clair

INTRODUCTION

This chapter sets out to do three things. Firstly, it discusses how phenomenological research can serve the primary care practice agenda. Secondly, it describes how to design and conduct robust primary care research using a phenomenological methodology. Thirdly, it invites the reader's engagement by using writing activity boxes. Applications from the field provide primary care practitioners, including general practitioners, family doctors, practice nurses and community pharmacists, with practical examples of doing phenomenological primary care research. Links to further readings are provided for practitioners who want to delve into phenomenology's philosophical underpinnings (Box 23.1).

Phenomenological primary care research is taken as being meaningful to and 'done in a primary care context'.[1] Because 'primary care clinicians, including family doctors, encounter health problems less frequently seen or managed in other sectors of health care',[1] phenomenological primary care research findings have the potential to inform relevant clinical research questions, understand patients' worlds and guide improvements in primary care delivery. *'We gather other people's experiences because they allow us to become more experienced ourselves'*[2] in practice matters.

From a philosophical point of view, phenomenology is a meaning-giving method of inquiry.[3] Therefore, primary care researchers choose phenomenological methods when they seek to understand the meaning of people's everyday realities.[3] The way to understanding is by researching people's lived experiences of phenomena related to matters of everyday life, health, well-being and health services. Designing research to explore a pre-reflective nature of experiencing phenomena, rather than as they are thought about,[4] is what makes phenomenological research a useful 'tool' in the primary care practitioner's toolkit. Pragmatic examples of phenomenology's distinguishing features are illustrated in the following sections and show how it is a discrete form of qualitative research.

BOX 23.1   FURTHER READING ABOUT PHENOMENOLOGY

van Manen's[3] book on the 'phenomenology of practice' is a good choice for primary care practitioners who want to reflect more deeply on how understanding lived meaning can inform practice for, and with, those they serve. His earlier book on researching lived experience is staple reading for researchers using a phenomenological approach.[2]

Groenewald[5] situates his descriptive phenomenological study of teaching and learning practice within a wider, yet succinct, illustration of phenomenology for the novice researcher. It moves from philosophical and historical roots to a step-wise case example of how descriptive, or Husserlian, phenomenology was applied. Note that descriptive phenomenology differs from interpretive phenomenology in two fundamental ways: It aims for rich descriptions of experiences rather than interpreting meaning, and a key assumption is that the researcher's pre-understandings can be bracketed, or put aside.

IDENTIFYING THE TOPIC OF INTEREST

In general, phenomenological research is useful for exploring topics related to people's experiences of things when little is known about the phenomenon, when understanding is taken-for-granted, or when it is concealed in some way (Box 23.2).[4] Topic examples are understanding primary care patients' experiences of life transitions,[6] living with particular conditions,[7] patient-practitioner encounters,[8] primary care interventions[9] and service processes.[10] From the perspective of being a primary care practitioner, topic examples are understanding practitioners' experiences of professional relationships,[11] practicing in particular settings[12] and doing primary care research in practice.[13]

BOX 23.2   IDENTIFYING THE TOPIC OF INTEREST

Identify a topic related to primary care patient or practitioner experience you would like to explore.

ASKING A PHENOMENOLOGICAL QUESTION

Interpretive and descriptive phenomenological research questions seek to understand lived experiences by asking 'what' the experience is, or 'how' it is experienced (Box 23.3).[4] For example, Grace and Higgs[9] asked what contribution integrative medicine (IM) made 'to the quality of primary care practices from the perspectives of consumers and providers of IM'?[9] Tarlier et al.'s second question, 'how are practical knowledge and clinical wisdom revealed in the practice narratives of experienced outpost nurses?',[14] is a good phenomenological question. However, their first question, 'how do experienced outpost nurses perceive and enact their role?'[14] is not a good fit, as perception is a psychological process rather than a pre-reflective experience. This question could be addressed using a different methodology such as a general inductive approach. A methodologically congruent question would be 'how do skilled outpost nurses experience their day-to-day practice?'

BOX 23.3 ASKING A PHENOMENOLOGICAL QUESTION

Write a phenomenological question to explore the primary care practice topic you wrote down in practice Box 23.2.

DETERMINING THE INCLUSION CRITERIA

Because phenomenological primary care research aims to understand people's experiences of a phenomenon, research participants need to have some experience of the thing of interest.[4] Including people who have a little to a lot of experience of the thing can be revealing (Box 23.4). Tarlier et al.[14] identify clear, appropriate inclusion criteria for their study. Australian practitioners with a minimum of 'five years nursing practice ... three years outpost experience ... eight months spent in one community [and] outpost experience within the past two years' were eligible for inclusion.[14] Importantly, the inclusion criteria clearly fit with the aim of understanding *experienced outpost nurses'* practices.

BOX 23.4 DETERMINING THE INCLUSION CRITERIA

List the inclusion criteria for participants in your proposed primary care research. Be specific. Justify each inclusion criterion in respect to your research question.

RECRUITING PARTICIPANTS

Purposive, or purposeful, recruitment is a suitable method for locating participants for phenomenological research. This is because researchers need to identify and invite people who have at least some experience of the phenomenon of interest. Recruiting a representative sample is not the aim. A snowball recruitment method can be useful for locating 'hard to find' participants (Box 23.5).[5] Handley et al.[7] give a good description of how they located adults with type 2 diabetes as prospective participants. They introduced the study at a primary care practitioners' staff meeting, provided written information sheets, used third party methods to identify potential participants who met the inclusion criteria and used methods to minimise the risk of coercion and power relationships to gain written informed consent.

BOX 23.5   RECRUITING PARTICIPANTS

Write down how you might locate and recruit participants for your proposed study.

GATHERING PHENOMENOLOGICAL DATA

Phenomenology's distinguishing features as qualitative research become particularly evident at the data gathering stage. As a phenomenological researcher, it is important to start by making overt one's presuppositions, assumptions and biases in relation to the phenomenon of interest. This can be done by writing down one's reflections of relevant personal history and practice experiences or by being interviewed by a colleague (Box 23.6). Existing understandings would be used by researchers using descriptive phenomenology to 'bracket' or put aside 'one's knowledge of the topic'.[15] Researchers using interpretive phenomenology would use such pre-understandings to take 'account of them as best as possible when gathering and analysing data'[4] in order to see 'through the presumptions and suppositions that shape our understandings of the world and understanding life'.[3]

BOX 23.6   GATHERING PHENOMENOLOGICAL DATA

Consider what you 'already know' about the phenomenon of interest from your life history and practice experiences.

Semi-structured individual interviews[7,14,16,17] are a primary data gathering method because they allow for deep, rich exploration of each participant's experiences. Two of the interpretive phenomenology examples in this chapter used individual and focus-group interviews[9,12] and one used focus groups only.[11] Conversational-style interviews are used to explore participants' lived experiences openly by inviting accounts of 'living through' particular situations or 'moments of pre-reflective, pre-predicative experience'[3] before they had interpreted, or theorised about, them. After all, 'lived experience cannot be captured in conceptual abstractions'.[2] In other words, participants are asked to recount particular situations or moments in which the thing of interest might appear. Accordingly, the lived-through, phenomenological nature of the data is influenced directly by the nature of the interview questions (Box 23.7). Interviews are typically audio-recorded and transcribed verbatim.

Of the interpretive phenomenology examples in this chapter, the most methodologically congruent interview question is reported by Tarlier et al.[14] They asked participants to 'share stories from their practice describing situations that had in some way been significant, memorable, or meaningful enough to influence their practice'.[14] Notice how the question invites stories about particular practice moments and events. Conger and Plager's[12] main questions are not phenomenological in nature as they seek ontic or factual data, such as 'What is your role in managing the health-illness continuum of clients … ?'[12] However, the probing questions invite ontological or phenomenological data, such as 'please tell us some specific examples from your practice'[12] Other authors state the interview topic areas only[11,17] or give no indication of topic areas or questions.[7,9,16] This means the reader has no way to discern the methodological congruence of the interview questions.

BOX 23.7   INTERVIEW QUESTIONS

List the interview questions you might use to elicit your participants' stories of lived moments of the phenomenon.

DOING PHENOMENOLOGICAL DATA ANALYSIS

Coherent stories describing lived-through situations or moments make good phenomenological data for analysis. One of the best illustrations in this chapter's examples begins, I 'went to numerous doctors, … . The first doctor was an infectious diseases specialist who took vials of blood but couldn't find anything wrong. Then I came here, and, as soon as I started treatment, I started getting better …'[9] How this participant experienced the significance of integrative medicine, the phenomenon of interest, begins to show itself in the data. Generalised stories of 'how things usually are' make poor phenomenological data. One example, from a different study, is a direct quote from a general practitioner who said 'I think that they [pharmacists] are probably more businessmen than we are, probably more motivated by the business side of things than we [GPs] tend to be'.[11] The story describes the participant's assumptions rather than his or her experience of barriers to working inter-professionally, the phenomenon of interest.

Data analysis is an iterative process of writing reflectively to clarify and make the structures of the experience explicit.[2] It is interpretive, going behind the words themselves to elucidate meaning. Analysis is done alongside data gathering. Rather than work with verbatim transcripts, a method of drawing coherent, 'lived-moment' stories from the data is methodologically sound.[4] The collected stories, rather than the transcripts themselves, would be returned to participants for verification. Van Manen's[2] descriptions of identifying thematic statements by using a whole text, selected sentences, or a line-by-line approach are helpful for the novice researcher. Grace and Higgs'[9] succinct description of their analysis methods shows good integrity: 'repeated reading of the data enabled ... higher-order themes to be identified. Emerging themes were refined, expanded, or discarded .... Ultimately, the findings from all phases of the research were fused to form metathemes'.[9] They report using a qualitative research software package for data management; however, phenomenological data analysis suits iterative writing methods.

'Phenomenology orients to the meanings that arise in experiences'.[3] That means the phenomenological primary care researcher is called on to interpret across participants' stories of lived situations and moments to describe what they mean, from the participants' perspectives. None of the example articles used in this chapter offered an explicit interpretation of meaning. Handley et al.[7] hinted at 'the meaning' of adults' day-to-day experience of living with type 2 diabetes as implicitly or explicitly holding 'an underlying wish or need to control their condition'.[7]

CONCLUSION

Phenomenological primary care research looks to be easy from the outside. Yet, the seeming simplicity arises from its nuanced complexity. Each step in the whole of the research process, from wording the question, to gathering and analysing participants' experiential 'as-lived' stories, to interpreting the meaning of the hidden phenomenon, contribute equally to making it phenomenological, rather than generally 'qualitative,' research. The examples drawn on in this chapter show how phenomenology has its place in exploring primary care practice questions.

REFERENCES

1. Beasley JW, Dovey S, Geffen LN et al. The contribution of family doctors to primary care research: A global perspective from the International Federation of Primary Care Research Networks (IFPCRN). *Prim Health Care Res Dev* 2004;5:307–16.
2. van Manen M. *Researching Lived Experience: Human Science for an Action Sensitive Pedagogy.* 2nd ed. London, Ontario: The Althouse Press, 2001.
3. van Manen M. Phenomenology of practice. *Phenomenol Pract* 2007;1(1):11–30.

4. Wright-St Clair VA. Doing (interpretive) phenomenology. In: Nayar S, Stanley M, eds. *Qualitative Research Methodologies for Occupational Science and Therapy*. New York, NY: Routledge, 2015:53–69.

5. Groenewald T. A phenomenological research design illustrated. *Int J Qual Methods* 2004;3(1):42–55.

6. Scannell-Desch EA. Prebereavement and postbereavement struggles and triumphs of midlife widows. *J Hosp Palliat Nurs* 2005;7(1):15–22.

7. Handley J, Pullon S, Gifford H. Living with type 2 diabetes: 'Putting the person in the pilots' seat.' *Aust J Adv Nurs* 2010;27(3):12–19.

8. Williams-Barnard CL, Mendoza DC, Shippee-Rice RV. The lived experience of college student lesbians' encounters with health care providers: A preliminary investigation. *J Holist Nurs* 2001;19(2):127–42.

9. Grace S, Higgs J. Integrative medicine: Enhancing quality in primary health care. *J Altern Complement Med* 2010;16(9):945–50.

10. Juliani C, MacPhee M, spiri W. Brazilian specialists' perspectives on the patient referral process. *Healthcare (Basel, Switzerland)* 2017;5(1):4. DOI: 10.3390/healthcare5010004.

11. Hughes CM, McCann S. Perceived interprofessional barriers between community pharmacists and general practitioners: A qualitative assessment. *Br J Gen Pract* 2003;53(493):600–06.

12. Conger MM, Plager KA. Advanced nursing practice in rural areas: Connectedness versus disconnectedness. *Online J Rural Nurs Health Care* 2008;8(1):24–38.

13. Hange D, Bjorkelund C, Kivi M et al. Experiences of staff members participating in primary care research activities: A qualitative study. *Int J Gen Med* 2015;8:143–48.

14. Tarlier DS, Johnson JL, Whyte NB. Voices from the wilderness: An interpretive study describing the role and practice of outpost nurses. *Can J Public Health* 2003;94(3):180–84.

15. Meadows LM, Verdi AJ, Crabtree BF. Keeping up appearances: Using qualitative research to enhance knowledge of dental practice. *J Dent Educ* 2003;67(9):981–90.

16. Pirie ZM, Fox NJ, Mathers NJ. Delivering shiatsu in a primary care setting: Benefits and challenges. *Complement Ther Clin Pract* 2012;18(1):37–42.

17. Rapport F, Maggs C. Measuring care: The case of district nursing. *J Adv Nurs* 1997;25(4):673–80.

CHAPTER 24

Why ethnography is an important part of primary care research and how it is done

Carissa van den Berk-Clark

The Student-Physician (1957)[1] and *Boys in White* (1965),[2] two famous qualitative studies, reveal the process of socialisation that medical students acquire as they strive to become doctors. *The Student-Physician* evaluated a model of learning that was popular at the time, referred to as the Cornell Comprehensive Care and Teaching Program. On the surface, this teaching model was designed to help with medical knowledge comprehension; however, the model had a second goal – to help students develop the appropriate values and attitudes needed for the medical profession as they relate to patients and colleagues. *Boys in White* went further, by studying a group of young male university students. The researcher studied how they lived, their schedules, their efforts to conform to professors' expectations, their culture and their assimilation into medical values both through peer and professor pressure.

Both studies were powerful at the time, because they helped outsiders gain an insider's view of the actions, interactions and behaviours of medical students and the ways that medical students, medical professionals and patients interpreted these actions, interactions and behaviours. These studies also influenced medical education because, for the first time, medical educators were able to see themselves from a different perspective. The authors of these studies were able to influence both groups through their use of ethnographic methods, a unique methodology which represents a preference for fieldwork over armchair theorisation.

As Figure 24.1 shows, the ethnographic approach differs from other qualitative methods because it is grounded in a commitment to first-hand experience via participant observation. Rather than directing data collection, researchers participate by 'hanging around' in the setting of interest and recruiting gatekeeper 'informants' or 'co-researchers' who act as a guide to the inner workings of those settings. Ethnography literately means, 'writing about people'.

The context and real life of being a primary care physician is quite relevant in *Boys in White*, which very clearly illustrates the world of 1960s medicine, where white male physicians commonly operated in self-governing practices. Today, about 50% of physicians are female, and people from all over the world are attracted to US medical schools. The medical profession also has seen what has been referred to as 'hyper-specialisation', and because of complexities inherent to US payer systems, layers of administration make it much more difficult for doctors or groups of doctors to be entirely self-governing. Rather than coming from within organisations, standards are developed through relations with other organisations, including private health insurance companies, medical associations and public institutions such as health and human services. The ethnographic method offers enormous potential for studying these large organisations and networks and understanding the roles and routines of medical professionals, administrative staff, stakeholders and patients. It also helps us understand why some interventions work in some settings but not others.

Implementation research is a growing area of research in primary care focused on strategies needed to deliver new interventions, especially as it relates to quality improvement, which relies heavily on ethnographic methodology. Implementation is vital to primary care research because it is necessary to be able to provide answers about the implementation process, why some interventions are successful while others are not and why some interventions work only in certain settings. Take, for example, an ethnographer who wants to examine one aspect of implementation such as how physicians make decisions about whether to provide an opioid prescription after the CDC released medical guidelines about opioid prescribing practices. It needs to be shown how these guidelines not only affect what the physicians did but how they

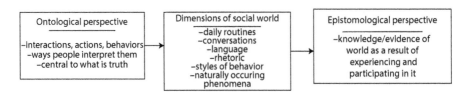

FIGURE 24.1 How ethnography contributes to scientific knowledge.

felt and talked about the guidelines, how the guidelines changed relationship hierarchies and workflows and whether or not these guidelines were met with resistance, compromise and/or the establishment of workarounds. This type of evidence is derived mostly through direct observation, a hallmark of ethnography.

STANDARD TRICKS OF THE TRADE

Sources of data

- People (these can be individuals, groups and collectives)
- Organisations, institutions and entities
- Texts (these can be published or unpublished; in the case of medicine, these can include charts and other types of administrative records collected by health organisations)
- Settings and environment (these can be material, visual and virtual, that is information about the setting or environment that is found on a web site)
- Objects, artefacts and media products
- Events

Sampling

When you consider data sources, consider the 'sampling frame.' The focus is on a strategic, not a representational, sample. It includes questions such as

- What are you interested in?
- Where is the data located?
- Do they match the ontological (e.g. what is reality?) and epistemological (e.g. what is truth?) perspective of ethnography (see Figure 24.1)?
- How practical and ethical is it for me to get data from these sources?

Sampling methods can include snowball sampling (a form of convenience sampling where informants introduce the researcher to new participants), theoretical construct sampling (sampling based on a theoretical model) and typical or extreme instance sampling.

Observation and negotiating access

Ethnographic methodology has the capacity to capture interactions involving large groups of people and to capture data available through other sources because it involves phenomena difficult to articulate. However, in order to be able to observe actions and interactions, especially those taking place in environments that are not completely open to the public, such as health organisations, you must first be able to negotiate access through some type of gatekeeper. Difficulty in negotiating access can vary depending on the organisation, which likely had policies in place or standing committees to review these requests. In less formal settings, such as small public health non-profits or federally qualified health centres (US government subsidised safety net health clinics), the process for being able to observe the organisation is much less formal. However, you need approval to do research more than the organisation needs research done most of the time. Thus, it is a good idea to study the group or organisation to get a sense of their needs, to design the proposal to fit well with the needs of the organisation. You should also be willing to consult with and ask permission from multiple parties. It is at this time that you will need to clarify a commitment between yourself and the organisation, and put in place a list of ground rules you will promise to follow.

Once you have the necessary permission, the setting requires that you prepare yourself for observing. To get past the gatekeeper and begin finding informants, you will need to manage and orchestrate social interactions by essentially hanging out and participating in the day-to-day life of the organisation.

Conversations with purpose

Stricter forms of ethnography do not use structured interviews but instead engage in conversations that are indistinguishable from interaction and dialogue that is naturally occurring. These are 'conversations with a purpose' and can occur through one-on-one interactions or through group discussions and can be done face-to-face, over the phone or on the internet. The fluidity of these conversations is fundamental and necessary to develop unexpected themes and detailed descriptions, integrate multiple perspectives, describe the process of an event or other phenomena, bridge inter-subjectivity, identify variables and frame hypotheses. These interactions also need to be meaningful to participants. Just as in any other social interaction in the real world, you must be able to have empathy and relate to the research participants' experiences.

Writing field notes

Because much of ethnographic data collection occurs as the researcher becomes part of the environment, which makes it difficult for them to get recordings of formal conversations, the researcher must develop a strategy to retain the information that is collected. Field notes, therefore, take a number of forms depending on the setting and type of data.[4] Notes can be a running log written at the end of each day or information organised in sets, which is separated from sequential notes. Some researchers will write elaborate notes after witnessing relevant events while others will write less detailed handwritten notes, and then, in the evening, fill in the rest of the details. Generally, at the end of each entry, it is customary to write an interpretive in-process memorandum to provide first impressions of the observations, to make connections with other field notes, to interpret member meanings or to relate to evolving or existing theoretical frameworks.

Establishing a thematic narrative

Qualitative data analysis usually involves first reading and re-reading transcripts or field notes, generating codes to organise the data and then grouping the codes into themes. What distinguishes ethnographic methodology from other qualitative methods is that coding is usually organised around analytic points, and analytic points are organised into themes and themes are organised into a coherent 'story' about life. Analytic points are organised into excerpt-commentary units which essentially facilitate transposing field notes into ethnographic texts. These units include the analytic point (an argument you are trying to make), orientating information (i.e. the context of the excerpt) and the excerpt itself. The researcher than orders the excerpt commentary units within a section (i.e. the theme), and then creates a narrative story which connects all the themes.

How do you make this research 'robust'?

There are six well-known strategies[3] for enhancing rigour in qualitative research, also applicable to ethnography. These are important to consider because they differ greatly from the methods used by quantitative researchers to ensure rigour.

1. *Prolonged exposure*: Improves reactivity and respondent bias—spending long periods of time in the field and getting accepted or at least tolerated by participants
2. *Triangulation*: Improves reactivity, researcher bias and respondent bias— relying on multiple sources (people, setting, documents) for information
3. *Peer debriefing/support*: Improves researcher and respondent bias— meeting with research team members or 'peers' to get and give feedback about fieldwork and data analysis as it proceeds
4. *Member checking*: Improves reactivity, researcher and respondent bias— returning to the field and asking participants about your impressions of data to ensure you are on the right track
5. *Negative case analysis*: Reduces researcher bias—focusing on events and situations which negate your main theories
6. *Audit trail*: Reduces researcher bias—documenting each step of your data collection and analysis so that others can reproduce your findings

REFERENCES

1. Merton, R.K., Reader, G., Kendall, P.L. 1957. *The Student-Physician: Introductory Studies in the Sociology of Medical Education.* Boston, MA: Harvard University Press.
2. Becker, H.S., Geer, B., Hughes, E.C., & Strauss, A.L. 1965. *Boys in White: Student Culture in Medical School.* NY: Transaction Publishers.
3. Padgett, D.K. 1998. *Qualitative Methods in Social Work Research: Challenges and Rewards.* Thousand Oaks, CA: Sage.
4. Emerson, R.M., Fretz, R.I., & Shaw, L.L. 1995. *Writing Ethnographic Field Notes.* Chicago, IL: University of Chicago.

CHAPTER 25

Case study

Robin Ray, Judy Taylor
and Robyn Preston

WHAT IS CASE STUDY DESIGN?

Case study is a research design linked with mixed methods and qualitative approaches to research that enables a rich, in-depth exploration of the phenomena of interest within a recognisable boundary such as a person, community, institution or diagnostic group. As a design, it defines what will be studied more than how the phenomena will be studied.[1] Case study research involves a detailed understanding of the complexities of a single case or multiple cases as they occur in the context of real life over time. Methods already discussed in this book, including observation/ethnography, interviews, surveys and clinical audits, are used in case study research.

When considering the reason for using a case study design, Stake[2] takes a qualitative, constructivist perspective, seeking to make sense of what is happening rather than applying statistical methods to identify causal factors.[3] From this subjective standpoint, three types of case study can be considered; intrinsic, instrumental and collective.

- An intrinsic case study examines the case itself because that case embodies a particular problem or characteristic of interest (a patient with a unique disease presentation), rather than contributing data to answer a wider question.
- Similarly, an instrumental case study draws on a particular case (e.g. Alcoholics Anonymous group) to provide insight into a specific issue (alcohol abstinence) to support existing evidence.
- Alternatively, a multiple or collective case study design considers a number of especially selected cases chosen to represent a population

or general condition when a deeper understanding or theorising is required (for example, a collective of individual cases comprising social networks that support a person with a degenerative life-limiting illness in an attempt to theorise the social impact of community-based care).

Yin concurs that case studies can be single or multiple, but takes a more positivist approach, establishing causal relationships and generating theories and hypotheses usually from a mixed-methods approach.[4] A single case study of an organisation such as a medical practice or a health service may include studying several operations or programmes within that organisation, creating cases in themselves. This is referred to as an embedded design (see Type 2 Figure 25.1). Similarly, a multiple case study may be relevant when testing a theory across a number of comparable cases. This design provides scope for implementing an intervention across a number of cases, evaluating the outcome then comparing results to determine if the impact differs or is the

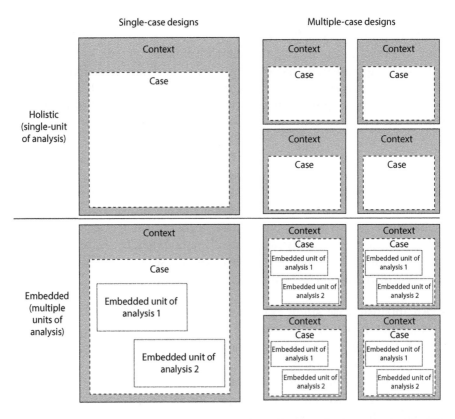

FIGURE 25.1 Basic types of case studies. (From Cosmos Corporation in Yin RK. *Case Study Research: Design and Methods.* 5th ed. Thousand Oaks, USA: Sage Publications, 2014.)

same across cases. Yin suggests that the outcomes may indicate a need to reconsider the original theoretical proposition of the study and case selection.

While generalisability is not an expected outcome from case study research, the lack of generalisability is a criticism of single case studies. Researching or reviewing a number of case studies with similar or contrasting characteristics improves the validity of the research and should be considered when adopting this design.[5] Therefore, it is important that the purpose of the case study and the expected outcomes are carefully considered when planning this research design.

WHAT IS A CASE?

> *Your case study is defined not so much by the methods that you are using to do the study, but the edges you put around your case – the direction and extent to which you want your case to go.*[6]

In case study design the boundaries of the case must be defined at the outset. Researchers need to define the case in order to replicate data collection and conduct a sampling strategy, see examples in Box 25.1. Case studies as a research design are distinguished from case series or case reports used in epidemiological research.

BOX 25.1 EXAMPLES OF CASE STUDY RESEARCH IN PRIMARY CARE

A person

Research question: How do older people see themselves and how do their caregivers see them in relation to maintaining their autonomy?[7]

Definition of case: An older individual – Mr Powell was 91.

Sampling: In this study, 11 individuals living in a residential setting in the south of The Netherlands, whose stories might have 'learning potential', were selected. Mr Powell was not necessarily the most representative of the group, but he demonstrated a need to stay independent and the researchers were interested to know why this was.

A general/primary health care practice

Research question: How is repeat prescribing accomplished in general practice, and what are the contributors and barriers to quality and safety?[8]

Definition of case: A general practice system related to repeat prescribing including doctors, receptionists and administrative staff.

Sampling: Purposive sampling of four urban UK general practices varying in demographic and organisational characteristics. The sample favoured 'opportunity to learn' over 'typicality'.

A general practice

Research question: To understand how practitioners in different nursing roles work with patients in primary care practices in New Zealand.[9]

Definition of case: A NZ primary care system where nursing roles include nurse practitioners, physician's assistants, primary care enrolled nurses and primary care practice assistants.

Sampling: Three dissimilar primary care practice systems in NZ navigating expanded nursing roles, responsibilities and scopes of practice.[8]

A diagnostic group

Research question: To explore effects of shame and stigma on female caregivers of people living with AIDS in southern Thailand.[10]

Definition of case: A household including a person with a diagnosis of AIDS and a family member or other significant person who acted as a carer who lived in the same house.

Sampling: Ten cases (families) were selected who were knowledgeable about the topic and who could reflect on and provide detailed experiential information and who were involved in the main caregiving tasks. The key informant needed to speak Thai or the southern Thai dialect.

A care system

Research question: What are the ways to improve transfer of care to tertiary hospitals for rural consumers with a serious mental illness?[11]

Definition of case: A primary mental health care system including the patient, carers, clinicians and those involved in transporting the patient.

Sampling: Six primary mental health care settings in rural, remote and regional South Australia were purposively sampled on the basis that each of the six patient participants involved agreed to participate in the research and had been admitted for acute mental health care to a city hospital from the location.

A partnership

Research question: How do communities and the health sector work together on primary prevention in regional communities?[12]

Definition of case: 'A partnership between a community based non-governmental organisation (NGO), volunteers and/or citizens, and paid public or private health sector employers based in a regional community of place'.[12]

Sampling: Eight cases were purposively selected to demonstrate health sector and community groups working together in primary prevention of chronic illness. Four were selected in regional communities in South Australia and four in North Queensland.

HOW TO DO CASE STUDY RESEARCH

Case study research involves analysing changing multi-levelled and complex phenomena. To handle this complexity, a case study protocol is important, see Box 25.2.

The protocol will assist in producing consistent types of data if there is more than one case involved. It is strongly advised that preliminary visits are made to study potential cases prior to sampling. This is not to pre-empt data collection, but to ensure that this case is likely to provide information to answer the research questions.

Types of data

Usually multiple sources of quantitative and qualitative data are collected appropriate to answering the research questions, see Box 25.3. Multiple

---

BOX 25.2   CASE STUDY PROTOCOL

- Defining case boundaries.
- Establishing inclusion and exclusion criteria for selecting case.
- Dates and locations for preliminary case assessment.
- Case data collection.
- Types of data.
- Sequence and dates of data collection.
- How field notes will be recorded.
- What will be observed through non-participant observation?
- How feedback and communication to people and organisations involved in the case will be maintained about the progress of the case study.

BOX 25.3 TYPES OF DATA USED IN CASE STUDY DESIGN

- Surveys or questionnaires of groups of people who have information about the case.
- Clinical audits.
- Interviews with individual participants who meet selection criteria.
- Focused group interviews when it is thought that information about the case is best obtained through group discussion.
- Non-participant observation, such as attendance at meetings, should be structured and carefully recorded into appropriate categories.
- Field notes taken about the case can supplement data and assist with methodological issues, including reflexivity.
- Documents such as annual reports, published articles or books, newspaper or online commentary, historical records, photo-voice products and other visual records.

data sets enable triangulation, a strategy for justifying and underpinning knowledge by gaining additional knowledge.

DATA COLLECTION

Replicating the types and process of data collection in each case is essential. Ideally, data collection proceeds one case at a time so that the researcher becomes immersed and can build up a picture of the case. If field visits to dispersed locations are required, then it makes sense to collect all the data in one location at one time as much as possible. If there are multiple cases, a decision must be made about the sequence of data collection. Researchers might prefer to commence data collection in a more familiar location. Relationships are very important in conducting case study research because they enable access to the phenomena of interest. However, they must be carefully managed, particularly if the researcher is examining phenomena that they have some connection with, for example, their own workplace.

TIPS FOR DATA ANALYSIS

In case study research, data analysis occurs as soon as data collection commences, as the researcher is immersed in these data *in situ*. Gaining distance from these data is also essential, and having read transcripts and documents or analysed health-systems data, it is advisable to enter data into a

---

BOX 25.4   CASE ANALYSIS

Within-case analysis
- Coding qualitative material involves using defined categories from theory or literature, or enabling codes to emerge, or a bit of both.
- Similar material in codes are amalgamated up into themes. The themes might be deduced from the material or they might relate back to relevant literature or theory. They are all related to the research questions.
- These themes are triangulated with field observations, documents and non-participative observation.
- Material is integrated and a within-case analysis is produced.

Across-case analysis
- Across-case analysis involves comparing themes across cases using some type of matrix format.
- From this comparison, related and unrelated themes across cases will emerge. Each of the themes are re-examined to account for different nuances from each case. It is these merged and integrated themes that answer the research questions in some manner.

software programme. This is a useful way to manage these data and integrate different types of data and puts the researcher somewhat at arms-length. Box 25.4 outlines some steps in data analysis.

Usually, cases are quite unique and so using theory to relate to themes can help with transferability of findings.

RESEARCH TRANSLATION

As soon as possible, a report for each case should be provided. Only deidentified data should be included, and sometimes this is difficult if it is a small data set. It is inevitable then that some data might be lost. For example, in a small community, there might be only one GP, so these data will have to be carefully handled in order to maintain confidentiality. Translation should include novel means of dissemination, such as posters or digital translation. Generally, relationships have been established between people in the research team and the people who were part of the cases, and there is an ownership and sharing of the findings. So the opportunity of joint translation of findings is an exciting one. This might involve joint workshops with participants who are interested in the results or joint conference presentations. These activities provide opportunities to reflect on results and plan further translation efforts.

REFERENCES

1. Flyvjerg B. Case study. In: Denzin NK, Lincoln YS, eds. *The Sage Handbook of Qualitative Research.* 4th ed. Thousand Oaks California: Sage, 2011:301–16.
2. Stake RE. Qualitative case studies. In: Denzin NK, Lincoln YS, eds. *Strategies of Qualitative Inquiry.* Thousand Oaks California: Sage, 2008, pp. 119–149.
3. Boblin SL, Ireland S, Kirkpatrick H et al. Using stake's qualitative case study approach to explore implementation of evidence-based practice. *Qualitative Health Research* 2013;23(9):1267–75.
4. Yin RK. *Case Study Research: Design and Methods.* 5th ed. Thousand Oaks, USA: Sage Publications, 2014.
5. Miles MB, Huberman M. *Qualitative Data Analysis: An Expanded Sourcebook.* CA: Sage Publications Inc., 1994.
6. Thomas G. *How to Do Your Case Study: A Guide for Students and Researchers.* London: Sage Publications Inc., 2011.
7. Abma TA, Stake RE. Science of the particular: An advocacy of naturalistic case study in health research. *Qualitative Health Research* 2014;24(8):1150–61.
8. Swinglehurst D, Greenhalgh T, Russell J et al. Receptionist input to quality and safety in repeat prescribing in UK general practice: ethnographic case study. *BMJ: British Medical Journal* 2011;343:d6788.
9. Walker L, Clendon J, Nelson K. Nursing roles and responsibilities in general practice: Three case studies. *Journal of Primary Health Care* 2015;7(3):236–43. [published online: 06 October 2015]
10. Kittikorn N, Street AF, Blackford J. Managing shame and stigma: Case studies of female carers of people with AIDS in Southern Thailand. *Qualitative Health Research* 2006;16(9):1286–301.

11. Taylor J, Edwards J, Kelly F et al. Improving transfer of mental health care for rural and remote consumers in South Australia. *Health & Social Care in the Community* 2009;17(2):216–24.
12. Taylor J, Braunack-Mayer A, Cargo M et al. A role for communities in primary prevention of chronic illness? Case studies in Regional Australia. *Qualitative Health Research* 2013;23(8):1103–13.

Interactional analysis of primary care consultations

Maria Stubbe, Anthony Dowell, Kevin Dew and Lindsay Macdonald

WHY USE INTERACTIONAL ANALYSIS?

Audio-visual recordings offer a unique window into the 'black box' of how people actually interact with one another, unlike more mainstream research methods that rely on reported data from interviews or surveys. In a primary care context, recordings make it possible to directly observe the ways patients and providers interact with one another in real-life consultations and to tease out specific practices that foster or hinder effective communication and improved outcomes. The value of this kind of direct observation has been recognised by primary care researchers and educators since the early days of portable recording technology. An influential example is Byrne and Long's foundational 1976 study of clinical decision making, *Doctors Talking to Patients*.[1] They analysed audio recordings of 2,500 consultations with 71 British GPs, using a standardised coding scheme to identify the phases of interaction and evaluate the degree of empathy and patient-centeredness displayed by the doctors. More recent developments of this approach include the Roter Interaction Analysis System (RIAS),[2-4] and the Verona Coding Definitions of Emotional Sequences (VR-CoDES).[5-7]

While coding methods can provide a statistically reliable overview of high-level communication patterns in recorded consultations, the specific details of how an interaction unfolds in a particular context are of necessity 'washed out' in this type of analysis.[8] Additionally, many coding studies use recordings of 'standardised' (simulated or analogue) consultations rather than naturally occurring routine health encounters,[9,10] which limits their direct applicability to practice.[11,12] By contrast, micro-analytic approaches to health care discourse, such as interactional sociolinguistics and conversation analysis, offer much more nuanced insights into the mechanics of how provider-patient communication actually works.[13] Researchers using interactional methods pay very close attention to the fine detail of how talk is co-constructed turn-by-turn as a consultation proceeds, and they use recordings of real consultations as their primary data rather than relying on simulations or the retrospective accounts and perceptions of research participants.

This chapter provides a practical overview of what is involved in conducting robust and ethical research using recorded health interactions, focusing in particular on the collection, transcription and analysis of data. Examples from recent research in the primary care setting illustrate some ways interactional methods can be incorporated into a multidisciplinary and/or mixed-methods study design. We conclude with a brief discussion of what can be learned from studying the fine detail of health encounters and how the findings can be used to positively influence primary care practice and outcomes.

HOW MIGHT YOU GO ABOUT IT?
Methods of data collection and analysis

The key requirement for an interactional analysis of primary care consultations is to ethically obtain good quality recordings, preferably on video (see Box 26.1 for an example of a data collection checklist). The talk is then transcribed in detail to capture how participants structure the interaction (e.g. turns at talk, overlaps, transitions) and the finer nuances of how the talk is produced (e.g. hesitations and pauses, intonation, changes in speed or volume, laughter, grammatical structure, word choice, non-verbal cues etc.). A typical transcript excerpt is shown in Box 26.2, with a key to the symbols used shown in Box 26.3. Transcribing at this level of detail facilitates an in-depth grounded analysis, not just of the content of a consultation (i.e. *what* is *said*), but also of the social or institutional actions being performed by means of the talk (i.e. what is being *done* and *how*). Analysts also pay close attention to the sequential structure of the interaction and how this is progressively built up.

The analysis usually proceeds iteratively in data sessions involving discussions amongst multiple researchers who all view the data. Using recordings supported by detailed transcripts slows down the action for repeated analysis—this provides opportunities to identify important features of the interaction that we cannot pick up in real time. Analysis involves repeated hearings/viewings of each relevant focus excerpt in the collection until a consensus on interpretation is reached and no new observations emerge.

Analysis and interpretation must be based on observable evidence in the data; namely, the way the interaction unfolds turn-by-turn in its local context, and not the analysts' pre-existing assumptions or common-sense attributions. For example, an utterance that is formulated as a question might look on the surface like a simple request for information, but a close analysis of the way it is produced and/or responded to may indicate that it is actually being treated as an indirect disagreement or resistance to advice.[14] Similarly, the manner in

BOX 26.1 DATA COLLECTION CHECKLIST

The checklist below is based on the methodology for collecting and archiving interactional data in New Zealand primary care, developed by the Applied Research on Communication in Health (ARCH) Group.[40,41]

Data collection
Protocols and documentation
- Establish robust methodological/technical protocols and documentation templates for every stage of the research journey. (Participant recruitment and informed consent through to the collection, processing, secure storage and management of data and feedback to participants).
- Obtain approval from the appropriate institutional ethics committee/board for the planned project (as required for observational health research involving participants in their capacity as patients). Ethical matters to be addressed include obtaining informed consent; participants' rights over how their data is used; avoiding coercion and exploitation; ensuring data privacy, confidentiality and security and restricting access to or dissemination of identifiable (non-anonymized) or potentially re-identifiable personal information.
- Seek separate consent and ethical approval for the archiving and unspecified future use of project data.

Recruitment of participants
- Recruit practices/clinics and gain consent from participating health practitioners/other staff.
- Liaise with practice team to devise a suitable strategy for identifying, approaching and gaining consent from potential patient participants.

Technical preparation
- Obtain a compact video camera capable of HD recording in a standard format (e.g. MPEG), and suitable tripod or pole, plus a separate digital voice recorder as backup.
- Familiarisation with equipment controls and settings. (Training from an experienced videographer is very helpful).
- If possible, visit the recording site to assess positioning of recorders and other technical considerations and conduct a dry run.

Site logistics
- Devise and pilot a workable data-collection process with the practice team.
- Set up the recording equipment in the consultation room.
- Once patient consent is confirmed, ask each research participant to fill out a standard demographic form, and arrange for completion of any other questionnaires or interviews included in the research protocol. (Assign a unique identifier to each participant and code all completed/ signed documents with this.)
- For each patient to be recorded, enter the consultation room to turn recorders on, depart the consulting room and return at end of consultation to turn off, *or* leave recorders running and ask the health professional to verbally record a code number after confirming patient has consented. (Avoid asking the health provider to deal with recording equipment. Provide a cloth to cover the camera lens during a physical examination if applicable, and offer to delete all or part of the recording straight after the consultation if participants request this.)
- Arrange a time to collect and code any agreed additional documentation for each recording (e.g. consultation notes, referral letters from the practice).

Data processing and archiving
It is desirable to set up standardised processes and documentation for data collection and processing. In the ARCH Corpus, these integrate seamlessly with an administrative database and archiving system:
- Project information sheets and consent forms are tailored to each project, but share a common format which includes a set of graduated options for consent.
- Participants can choose to agree to the collection of different types of data (e.g. recordings, consultation records), whether or not the data may be permanently archived or must only be used for the current project, what data formats may be used for research presentation or teaching purposes (e.g. anonymised versus original video and audio or anonymised transcript only) and whether they are willing to be contacted again.
- Free-text field observations, including site information and technical data, are recorded onto templates.
- Upload and catalogue all recordings as soon as possible post-recording, assign pseudonyms, enter demographic information and link to any related documents on file.
- A research nurse then creates a lay synopsis and timed content log of the video file (including explanation/glossing of clinical content and terminology) for each recorded interaction prior to transcription. These allow for rapid searching and location of key content within recordings.
- Trained research assistants create base transcriptions onto a standard template. These can be readily converted to Jeffersonian (CA) transcripts, or used for automated searching.

BOX 26.2   SAMPLE TRANSCRIPT: EXCERPT OF LIFESTYLE ADVICE FROM A GP CONSULTATION

ARCH IS-GP01-03

1	GP:	.hhh um hhh ↑alcohol you- (.) regular drinker, or
2	PT:	yes to be (.) honest. [um]
3	GP:	[yeah]
4	PT:	reasonable yes no not [(too)] regular.
5	GP:	[so::]
6	GP:	ho:w >how many times a week would you< (.)
7		go out (0.3) most most days
8	PT:	yeah quite a bit (.) on my way home [(for)]
9	GP:	[°yep°]
10	PT:	It's bec-it's like a habit [it's like]=
11	GP:	[sure]
12	PT:	=on coronation street i suppose
13	GP:	yea(h) h (h) okay
14	PT:	little ↑clubs not pubs generally
15	GP:	yep
16	PT:	little clubs for a couple of hours (.) go home
		for tea
17	GP:	right okay=
18	PT:	=(um) that's it
19	GP:	so what would you do (0.2) three four, four
		five, or
20	PT:	wh<u>at</u> [hah hah hah]
21	GP:	[hah hah hah]
22	GP:	drinks
23	PT:	yes but measure?
24	GP:	um [you tell me]
		((lines omitted))
42	PT:	yeah pints basi[cally]
43	GP:	[yeah ok]ay (and what are we
		talking)=
44	PT:	=oh
45	GP:	three or four
46	PT:	yeah
47	GP:	okay ((nods))
48	PT:	<maybe lavishly six>
49	GP:	right
50	PT:	that's abou- that's about it
51	GP:	yeah

BOX 26.3 TRANSCRIPTION CONVENTIONS

General points

- The symbols shown are based on the standard conversation analysis (CA) transcription system.[42]
- Transcripts generally include line numbers.
- All names and other identifying details are replaced with pseudonyms.
- Standard punctuation and capitalisation are not used.
- When transcribing, it is usual to use a non-proportional font (such as Courier New) to preserve the alignment of overlapping talk.

Key to symbols:

WHAT WAS SAID	(word)	Transcriber's best guess at what might have been said
	( )	Unclear or indecipherable talk
NON-SPEECH SOUNDS	hh	In-breath (*note the preceding full strop*)
	.hh	Out-breath (*aspiration*)
	hah hah hah	Laughter tokens
	sto(h)p i (h)t	(h) signals laughter 'bubbling' within speech
	((coughs))	Transcriber's description (*of a sound or gesture*)
	A: word [word] B: [word]	Start and end of overlapping talk
TIMING	(.)	A micro-pause
		(just noticeable - hearable but too short to measure)
	(3) (0.2)	A timed pause
	A: word=	(number of seconds / tenths of seconds - '*one thousand and one*')
	B:=word	No discernible gap between turns or word
HOW IT WAS SAID (PRODUCED) Pitch, speed, volume compared to surrounding talk	.	Utterance-final intonation
	,	List intonation
	?	Strong rising ('questioning') intonation (*irrespective of grammar*)
	word WORD	Underline sounds are louder, capitals louder still (compared to surrounding talk)
	wo::rd	Colons denote stretching of the immediately prior sound
	wo-	Dash marks a sharp cut-off of the preceding sound
	↑word ↓word	Arrows denote noticeable rise or fall in pitch
	>word word<	Inwards arrows show faster speech
	<word word>	Outwards arrows show slower speech
	°word°	Degree marks denote talk that is noticeably quieter

which an utterance is produced can indicate a degree of interactional difficulty or delicacy.[15,16] Examples include hesitations, cut-off utterances, and the use of hedges (mitigating words) or laughter which can all work to soften the impact of what is said. By looking in very close detail at such features of the talk as they occur, it is possible to identify empirically what communicative actions are being oriented to by the participants themselves (why this utterance or response, in this way, at this point?).

Research design

Analysis of clinical interactions can be incorporated into a research design in a number of different ways, depending on the study aims and research questions and also on the expertise of the researcher(s) involved. In much of the health-interaction research published to date, conversation analysis and related methods were used as the primary methodology by researchers with specialised training. Such studies typically involve close analysis of how the talk-in-interaction unfolds in relatively small purposefully chosen samples that focus on a clinically relevant topic (e.g. lifestyle behaviour talk[17]) or a collection of excerpts relating to a routine consultation activity from a much larger number of consultations (e.g. the opening of a consultation,[18] candidate diagnoses[19]).

However, interactional analysis at varying levels of detail is increasingly being built into more applied clinically focused studies, often combined with other qualitative methods, such as thematic analysis of interview data and document analysis, to build in-depth comparative or longitudinal case studies. Some researchers have also successfully used conversation analysis within larger-scale mixed-methods studies, including RCTs and international studies.[20,21] Applied studies such as these typically involve multidisciplinary teams that include both clinical researchers and team members with specialist training in interactional methods. See Box 26.4 for examples of health-interaction studies involving different designs and sampling strategies.

Collecting and processing authentic recordings of health interactions is resource-intensive, and the feasibility of identifying and collecting an appropriate sample within the required timeframe needs careful thought at the design stage. Prospective designs in primary care research tend to work best where the research question lends itself to recording a number of routine consultations in a finite period of time. This is most likely to be the case where the research relates to a specific clinical topic or activity that arises regularly in primary care consultations or where the inclusion is based on specific patient characteristics.[8,22,23]

Designing a field methodology that will yield enough data of a more-specific type is often more challenging, though it can be achieved under the right circumstances. For example, our research group was interested

BOX 26.4   EXAMPLES OF RESEARCH DESIGNS INCORPORATING INTERACTION ANALYSIS

A. Prospective studies

Example 1: Communication in routinely occurring consultation activities

Collins et al. 2005: 'Unilateral' and 'bilateral' practitioner approaches in decision-making about treatment.[43] This study used conversation analysis to look in detail at how UK doctors talk about and enact treatment decisions, comparing primary care diabetes consultations with interactions in ENT oncology clinics. Video recordings of 168 consultations were collected, representing a diverse range of practice cultures and views about patient participation in decisions about their care. The researchers reviewed these data for overall patterns in how individual practitioners approached decision making with their patients. They then transcribed decision-making sequences in a subset of 80 consultations for closer analysis of their verbal and nonverbal features, focusing on 45 in particular detail (22 from primary care). Participants were also interviewed individually.

Example 2: Communication as an aspect of complex case studies

Dowell et al. 2018: A longitudinal study of interactions between health professionals and people with newly diagnosed diabetes.[31] This analysis was part of a large qualitative mixed-methods study, *Understanding Diabetes Management in Primary Care*. A multidisciplinary research team observed in detail all interactions involving 32 patients newly diagnosed with diabetes over a 6-month period in 10 general practices. The aim was to identify key points where challenges to effective communication occurred. Data included video recordings of consultations with all health professionals involved in each patient's care (e.g. GPs, nurses, dietitians) and ethnographic data (field observations, clinical notes, educational materials, exit interviews with patients and focus groups with practice teams using trigger clips and transcripts from the video data).

B. Sampling existing data sets – secondary analysis

Example 3: Communication in routinely occurring consultation activities

Barnes (2017): Preliminaries to Treatment Recommendations in UK Primary Care: A Vehicle for Shared Decision Making?[25] This study analysed a large collection of 'pre-recommendations,' where GPs request information from patients about previous medications prior to making a treatment recommendation (e.g. 'what've you tried taking'). Analysis of two existing UK datasets (N = 590) of audio-recorded consultations collected between 2004 and 2015 identified 393 instances of physician-initiated recommendations for new medications, of which 57 included pre-recommendation sequences. Conversation analysis of these cases was used to explore precisely how doctors deployed pre-recommendations and whether or not these reduced patient resistance and/or encouraged mutual participation in decision making.

Example 4: Consultation talk relating to a specific clinical issue

Morris et al. (2016): 'It's complicated'-talking about gout medicines in primary care consultations.[28] This exploratory study analysed patterns of communication about gout during routine primary care consultations in New Zealand. The sample comprised video recordings of 31 health care consultations between patients and a range of primary care practitioners (including GPs, practice nurses, podiatrists and dietitians) from the ARCH Corpus. Consultations that included any discussion about gout were included. Consultation transcripts were analysed using a qualitative inductive approach from clinical and linguistic perspectives supplemented with visual observation of the interactions.

C. Intervention studies

Example 1: Randomised controlled trial

Heritage et al. (2007): Reducing patients' unmet concerns in primary care: The difference one word can make.[20] This study tested the hypothesis that by training physicians to ask 'Is there something else you want to address in the visit today?' (SOME condition), rather than 'Is there anything else you want to address in the visit today?' (ANY condition), this would reduce the incidence of patients' unmet concerns (defined as concerns that patients identified in pre-visit surveys but not raised by patients or physicians). Acute-care visits involving 20 physicians and 80 patients were videotaped and transcribed, followed by a cross-sectional comparison of the two experimental questions. The study concluded that unmet concerns can be dramatically reduced by a simple inquiry in the SOME format, without increasing consultation length.

Example 2: Designing a brief opportunistic intervention

Gray et al. (2018): A Taboo topic? How General Practitioners talk about overweight and obesity in New Zealand.[27] This study aimed to systematically examine how GPs successfully broached the topic of weight and weight management in routine consultations. A secondary analysis using content and interactional analysis was conducted of 36 video-recorded consultations in New Zealand general practices (selected from an existing database of 205 consultations in the ARCH Corpus). This confirmed that engaging in opportunistic discussions about being overweight is often interactionally delicate for both doctor and patient, but also identified a number of effective communication strategies; these subsequently formed the basis of a brief intervention for weight management in primary care.

in tracking the process of decision making when patients were referred to a specialist. However, referrals of this type are not especially frequent in general practice, nor is it possible to predict in advance when they will occur. To obtain our target of six to eight cases where a patient was referred to a specialist, we had to collect 125 routine GP consultations. The subsequent 22 specialist consultations were far more straightforward to record, as we had already identified and obtained consent from the patients concerned. Fortunately, we had built this additional data collection into our research protocol and funding bid, and the larger data set allowed us to explore other interesting aspects of primary-care consultation processes.[24]

The reuse of interactional data held in formal or informal archives can be a useful alternative where a suitable collection of data already exists and is available for reuse, especially for smaller studies where time is limited. Such collections offer cost-effective opportunities for secondary analysis of health communication and often allow researchers to access larger and more varied collections than would be possible if collecting data *de novo*.[25,26] Existing data can also be useful as a test bed for designing a more targeted study or intervention, or to engage in comparative or collaborative research, while at the same time reducing the burden on participant groups.[27,28] Box 26.5

BOX 26.5   EXAMPLES OF HEALTH COMMUNICATION DATA ARCHIVES

One in a Million Primary Care Consultations Archive
A restricted access database managed by Bristol University. It comprises 300 video-recorded GP consultations along with verbatim transcripts and a range of associated data including demographics, consultation records and standardised questionnaires. The consultations were recorded in 12 general practices in the West of England in 2014–2015, with permission from participants for future reuse in research and education.[44]

http://www.bristol.ac.uk/primaryhealthcare/researchthemes/one-in-a-million

Carolinas Conversations Collection
A restricted access digital collection of transcribed audio and video recordings of conversations about health held at the Medical University of South Carolina Library. It has two cohorts: 125 unimpaired multi-ethnic older speakers with a chronic condition and a longitudinal set of 400 conversations with 125 persons with dementia. It includes information about health literacy, health status and cognitive function.[45]

http://carolinaconversations.musc.edu/about/collection

Nottingham Health Communication Corpus
500,000 words of health language data in a range of different settings including a range of practitioner–patient exchanges and patient/service-user narratives. The NHCC is maintained by an interdisciplinary health language research group (HLRG) at Nottingham University and incorporates multiple data sources, from both computer-mediated communication and from spoken texts.[26]

http://www.nottingham.ac.uk/research/groups/hlrg/index.aspx

ARCH Corpus of Health Interactions
The ARCH Corpus is a restricted access collection of approximately 500 digitised video/audio-recorded health encounters and 250 interviews, along with related ethnographic and demographic data collected in New Zealand since 2003. This material is permanently archived at the University of Otago for approved future use in research and education.[41]

http://www.otago.ac.nz/wellington/research/arch/corpus

---

provides information about four such electronic archives of English-language health-communication data from the UK, US and New Zealand.

WHAT CAN WE LEARN FROM STUDYING HEALTH INTERACTIONS?
Interaction analysis is now a well-established approach in studies of health communication and related aspects of service provision in primary health care. Researchers have used these methods to document in fine detail the

communicative processes and structures that occur routinely in many primary care settings, including consultations with GPs, nurses, physiotherapists, pharmacists and other allied health professionals, and to explore important topics such as clinical decision making, agenda setting, prescribing talk and lifestyle advice, amongst many others.[8,20–22,29–31] The findings from this basic research are now starting to inform pre-service training and professional development for health professionals,[32,33] with a small but growing body of published work that reports on the development and evaluation of communication interventions based on evidence from health-interaction research.[27,34–36] The use of interactional methods has recently also started to expand into new domains of primary care research. These include exploration of how health-informatics technologies and multi-modal (non-verbal) aspects of interaction influence communication in consultations.[37–39]

For those interested in learning more, Box 26.6 lists details of some general readings and links to open-access resources, in addition to the references already provided.

BOX 26.6 ADDITIONAL RESOURCES

Hamilton HE, Chou W-yS, editors. *Routledge Handbook of Language and Health Communication. Routledge Handbooks in Applied Linguistics*: Florence, KY, USA: Taylor and Francis; 2014.

Harvey K, & Koteyko N. *Exploring Health Communication. Language in Action*. London, New York: Routledge; 2013.

Hepburn A, Bolden G. Transcribing for Social Research. UK: Sage; 2017.

Heritage J, Maynard DW (Eds). *Communication in Medical Care: Interaction Between Primary Care Physicians and Patients*. Cambridge: Cambridge University Press; 2006.

Heritage, J. *Conversation Analysis*. e-Source Behavioral & Social Sciences Research http://www.esourceresearch.org/eSourceBook/Conversat ionAnalysis/1LearningObjectives/tabid/382/Default.aspx (Accessed February 2018). *Guided reading exercise: Describes the main dimensions of conversation analytic research in medical practice and some key findings of conversation analysis in the context of primary care.*

Rapley B. *Doing Conversatiion, Discourse and Document Analysis*. London: Sage; 2007.

Sidnell J, Stivers T. *The Handbook of Conversation Analysis*. John Wiley & Sons; 2012.

Stokoe, E. *'The science of analyzing conversations, second by second'* TEDxBermuda https://www.youtube.com/watch?v=MtOG5PK8xDA. (Accessed February 2018).

Ten Have P. *Doing Conversation Analysis. A Practical Guide*. 2nd ed. London: Sage 2007.

REFERENCES

1. Byrne PS, Long B. Doctors talking to patients. *A Study of the Verbal Behaviour of General Practitioners Consulting in Their Surgeries.* London: Her Majesty's Stationary Office; 1976.
2. Roter D, Hall J. *Giving and Withholding Information: The Special Case of Informative Talk in the Medical Visit. Doctors Talking with Patients/Patients Talking with Doctors: Improving Communication in Medical Visits* 2nd ed. Westport, CT: Praeger; 2006. p. 127–40.
3. Roter DL, Hall JA, Blanch-Hartigan D, Larson S, Frankel RM. Slicing it thin: New methods for brief sampling analysis using RIAS-coded medical dialogue. *Patient Education and Counseling.* 2011;82(3):410–9.
4. Wolff JL, Clayman ML, Rabins P, Cook MA, Roter DL. An exploration of patient and family engagement in routine primary care visits. *Health Expectations.* 2015;18(2):188–98.
5. De Maesschalck S, Deveugele M, Willems S. Language, culture and emotions: Exploring ethnic minority patients' emotional expressions in primary healthcare consultations. *Patient Education and Counseling.* 2011;84(3):406–12.
6. Riley R, Weiss MC, Platt J, Taylor G, Horrocks S, Taylor A. A comparison of GP, pharmacist and nurse prescriber responses to patients' emotional cues and concerns in primary care consultations. *Patient Education and Counseling.* 2013;91(1):65–71.
7. Zimmermann C, Del Piccolo L, Bensing J et al. Coding patient emotional cues and concerns in medical consultations: The Verona coding definitions of emotional sequences (VR-CoDES). *Patient Education and Counseling.* 2011;82(2):141–8.
8. Heritage J, Maynard DW, editors. *Communication in Medical Care: Interaction Between Primary Care Physicians and Patients.* Cambridge: Cambridge University Press; 2006.
9. Mazzi MA, Bensing J, Rimondini M et al. How do lay people assess the quality of physicians' communicative responses to patients' emotional cues and concerns? An international multicentre study based on videotaped medical consultations. *Patient Education and Counseling.* 2013;90(3):347–53.
10. Roter DL, Erby LH, Adams A et al. Talking about depression: An analogue study of physician gender and communication style on patient disclosures. *Patient Education and Counseling.* 2014;96(3):339–45.
11. Stokoe E. The (in) authenticity of simulated talk: Comparing role-played and actual interaction and the implications for communication training. *Research on Language and Social Interaction.* 2013;46(2):165–85.
12. White SJ, Casey M. Understanding differences between actual and simulated surgical consultations: A scoping study. *Australian Journal of Linguistics.* 2016;36(2):257–72.
13. Drew P, Chatwin J, Collins S. Conversation analysis: A method for research into interactions between patients and health care professionals. *Health Expectations.* 2001;4(1):58–70.
14. Barton J, Dew K, Dowell A et al. Patient resistance as a resource: Candidate obstacles in diabetes consultations. *Sociology of Health & Illness.* 2016;38(7):1151–66.
15. Haakana M. Laughter as a patient's resource: Dealing with delicate aspects of medical interaction. *Text–Interdisciplinary Journal for the Study of Discourse.* 2001;21(1–2):187–219.
16. Moriarty HJ, Stubbe MH, Chen L et al. Challenges to alcohol and other drug discussions in the general practice consultation. *Family Practice* 2011;29(2):213–22.
17. Sorjonen M-L, Raevaara L, Haakana M, Tammi T, Perakyla A. Lifestyle discussions in medical interviews. In: Heritage J, Maynard DW, editors. *Communication in Medical Care: Interaction between Primary Care Physician and Patients. Studies in Interactional Sociolinguistics.* Cambridge, New York, Melbourne, Madrid, Capetown, Singapore & Sao Paulo: Cambridge University Press; 2006. p. 340–77.

18. Gafaranga J, Britten N. 'Fire away': The opening sequence in general practice consultations. *Family Practice*. 2003;20(3):242–7.
19. Gill VT, Maynard DW. Explaining illness: Patients' proposals and physicians' responses. In: Heritage J, Maynard DW, editors. *Communication in Medical Care: Interaction between Primary Care Physicians and Patients*. Cambridge: Cambridge University Press; 2006. p. 115–50.
20. Heritage J, Robinson JD, Elliott MN, Beckett M, Wilkes M. Reducing patients' unmet concerns in primary care: The difference one word can make. *Journal of General Internal Medicine*. 2007;22(10):1429–33.
21. Stivers T, Heritage J, Barnes RK, McCabe R, Thompson L, Toerien M. Treatment recommendations as actions. *Health Communication*. 2017:1–10. DOI: 10.1080/10410236.2017.1350913
22. Pilnick A, Coleman T. 'Do your best for me': The difficulties of finding a clinically effective endpoint in smoking cessation consultations in primary care. *Health*. 2010;14(1):57.
23. Stivers T. Non-antibiotic treatment recommendations: Delivery formats and implications for parent resistance. *Social Science & Medicine*. 2005;60(5):949–64.
24. Dew K, Dowell A, Macdonald L, Stubbe M. Using conversation analysis, Part 3, techniques of social research. In: Davidson C, Tolich M, editors. *Social Science Research in New Zealand*. Auckland: Auckland University Press; 2018 (forthcoming, August 2018).
25. Barnes RK. Preliminaries to Treatment Recommendations in UK Primary Care: A Vehicle for Shared Decision Making? *Health Communication*. 2017;1–11. DOI: 10.1080/10410236.2017.1350915.
26. Crawford P, Brown B, Harvey K. Corpus linguistics and evidence-based health communication. In: Hamilton H, Chou WS, editors. *The Routledge Handbook of Language and Health Communication*. 2nd ed. London; New York: Routledge, Taylor & Francis Group; 2014. p. 75–90.
27. Gray L, Stubbe M, Macdonald L, Tester R, Hilder J, Dowell T. A Taboo topic? How General Practitioners talk about overweight and obesity in New Zealand. *Journal of Primary Health Care*. 2018;10(2). DOI: 10.1071/HC17075.
28. Morris C, Macdonald L, Stubbe M, Dowell A. 'It's complicated'-talking about gout medicines in primary care consultations: A qualitative study. *BMC Family Practice*. 2016;17(1):114.
29. Land V, Parry RH, Jane S. Communication practices that encourage and constrain shared decision making in health care encounters: Systematic review of conversation analytic research. *Health Expectations*. 2017;20(6):1228–1247. DOI:10.1111/hex.12557.
30. Robinson JD, Tate A, Heritage J. Agenda-setting revisited: When and how do primary-care physicians solicit patients' additional concerns? *Patient Education and Counseling*. 2016;99(5):718–23.
31. Dowell A, Stubbe M, Macdonald L et al. A longitudinal study f interactions between health professionals and people with newly diagnosed diabetes. *The Annals of Family Medicine*. 2018;16(1):37–44.
32. Barnes R. Conversation analysis: A practical resource in the health care setting. *Medical Education*. 2005;39(1):113–5.
33. Tsai M, Lu F, Frankel RM. Teaching medical students to become discourse analysts. In: Hamilton H, Chou WS, editors. *The Routledge Handbook of Language and Health Communication*. New York: Routledge; 2014. p. 327–43.
34. Antaki C, editor. Six kinds of applied conversation analysis. *Applied Conversation Analysis: Intervention and Change in Institutional Talk*. London, UK: Palgrave Macmillan.
35. Robinson JD, Heritage J. Intervening with conversation analysis: The case of medicine. *Research on Language and Social Interaction*. 2014;47(3):201–18.

36. Stokoe E. The Conversation Analytic Role-play Method (CARM): A method for training communication skills as an alternative to simulated role-play. *Research on Language and Social Interaction*. 2014;47(3):255–65.

37. Dowell A, Stubbe M, Scott-Dowell K, Macdonald L, Dew K. Talking with the alien: Interaction with computers in the GP consultation. *Australian Journal of Primary Health*. 2013;29:275–82.

38. Sikveland R.O., Stokoe E. Enquiry calls to GP surgeries in the United Kingdom: Expressions of incomplete service and dissatisfaction in closing sequences. *Discourse Studies*. 2017:1461445617706999.

39. Swinglehurst D, Roberts C, Li S, Weber O, Singy P. Beyond the 'dyad': A qualitative re-evaluation of the changing clinical consultation. *BMJ Open*. 2014;4(9):e006017. DOI:10.1136/bmjopen-2014-006017.

40. Stubbe M. Evolution by design: Building a New Zealand Corpus of health interactions. In: Marra M, Warren P, editors. *Linguist at Work: Festschrift for Janet Holmes*. Wellington: Victoria University Press; 2017. p. 196–214.

41. ARCH Group. ARCH Corpus of Health Interactions: University of Otago; 2017 [Available from: http://www.otago.ac.nz/wellington/research/arch/].

42. Hepburn A, Bolden G. *Transcribing for Social Research*. UK: Sage; 2017.

43. Collins S, Drew P, Watt I, Entwistle V. 'Unilateral' and 'bilateral' practitioner approaches in decision-making about treatment. *Social Science & Medicine*. 2005;61(12):2611–27.

44. Jepson M, Salisbury C, Ridd MJ, Metcalfe C, Garside L, Barnes RK. The 'One in a Million' study: Creating a database of UK primary care consultations. *The British Journal of General Practice*. 2017;67(658):e345–e51.

45. Pope C, Davis BH. Finding a balance: The Carolinas conversations collection. *Corpus Linguistics and Linguistic Theory*. 2011;7(1):143–61.

SECTION V

How to disseminate your research

CHAPTER 27

How to write and how to publish

Felicity Goodyear-Smith and Katharine A. Wallis

Communication with, and dissemination to, others is an integral part of research. Written communication is necessary throughout the research process, from seeking funding to making known what we have found. Research is about creating new knowledge, and the new knowledge you have generated needs to be shared. Researchers need to know how to write and how to publish their research in peer-reviewed journals. This chapter explains the common structure of scientific writing and offers some generic writing tips and guidance on how to publish.

TIPS ON SCIENTIFIC WRITING

All medical research writing follows the same basic structure. Generic principles apply regardless of whether you are writing a research proposal, an ethics application, a report, thesis or article for publication. They also apply to poster presentations. You need to be answering the questions who, when, where, what and how. In the words of Rudyard Kipling:

> *I keep six honest serving men*
> *(They taught me all I knew);*
> *Their names are What and Why and When*
> *And How and Where and Who.*

> *– The Elephant's Child, Just So Stories, 1902*

This is often called IMRaD, which stands for **I**ntroduction (what do you already know and why you did this study), **M**ethods (what you did and how you did it where, when and with whom), **R**esults (what you found) **a**nd **D**iscussion (So what?). Within these broad headings, you will cover different components, sometimes using subheadings (such as those in the words underlined below). Note that for a research proposal and an ethics application, you will only have introduction and methods sections, and you will be writing what you plan to do, not what you have done.

Introduction

This section explains why you have done your study. You need to present the rationale for your research – why does knowing more in this area matter, what is the justification for your study? You also need to have a background, which explains what was already known about this topic. This might be a scoping or even a systematic review of the existing literature. This section will need to reference the articles and other literature you discuss. Having identified what was already known and what is not, the aim of your research is to fill a knowledge gap. Your research question is what you wished to find out, and you may have a hypothesis that you wished to test. You may have had some specific objectives about what you planned to achieve and how this was to be accomplished.

Methodology and methods

This section covers what you did and how you did it. This book has already described many different research approaches and methodologies. Also refer Box 27.1 for guides on how to conduct and report on specific types of research. Sometimes you may wish to discuss the reasons why you chose a particular approach, and you may reference key works here. However, in general, references belong in the introduction and discussion sections, but less so in the methods and not at all in the results. First describe your study design – what sort of study did you do? You need to explain your setting – where and when did your study take place? Your study population needs to be defined. Who (or what) were your participants? They may be individuals (for example, patients of health care professionals) or groups such as clinics. You need to describe how you sampled these – consecutive patients or a random selection, for example. What were your criteria for inclusion in, and exclusion from, the study? You then outline what you measured. You may have some baseline measurements, some interim ones taken during your study and outcome ones at the end. Regardless of whether your study is quantitative or qualitative, you generated some data and this is where you explain how you did this, and what your data consist of. Finally you explain how you went about your analyses of these data. Usually in your methods section you will also declare that you have received <u>ethical approval</u> for doing this research, citing the ethical approval or institutional review body and reference number or explaining why ethics approval was not necessary or waived.

Results or findings

Often the heading Results is used for quantitative and Findings for qualitative studies. Regardless, this section is about what you found. First you <u>describe your sample</u> – who were they, what were their characteristics? You may need to include the <u>response rate</u>. How many did you invite who declined? How many were ineligible? Sometimes you may have some data on non-responders, and you can compare these with responder details to see if there were any significant biases in your final sample. Then you report the findings of your analyses. You may choose to do this in text, or in tables and figures. The latter is often a good way to present detailed results succinctly. However, do not duplicate. If you use tables and figures, then only highlight some key findings in the text and then say 'see table'. Do not copy and paste your analysis direct into the results. Extract the results you need and construct your own tables or figures in line with the journal guidelines. Usually you present descriptive results first and then bivariate/multivariate analyses. Remember that results do not have to be positive. What you find may not be what you had expected. It is still important to report on negative findings. It is important that people know an intervention has no measurable effect, for example. Not reporting this can contribute to a publication bias.

For qualitative findings, your interpretations in your own words are the key findings, not the quotes. The quotes are there to support the validity of your interpretation. One quote per main point is usually sufficient.

Discussion

This is the section where you explain the meaning of your findings, the 'So what?'. Here you get to interpret. You summarise your key findings and explain how this fits in to what is already known. Does it confirm findings from other settings? If not, why might this be? You identify the strengths of your study and the weaknesses and limitations. All studies have both. You discuss the implications of what you have found for future practice, policy and/or further research. You may make recommendations, and you finish with a conclusion.

GUIDE TO WRITING ORGANISATION AND STYLE

You need to make time to write. You can either set aside a block of time ('pressure cooker' approach) or work on it slowly over time (the 'slow cooker'

BOX 27.1   GUIDELINES FOR SPECIFIC METHODS

Guidelines for specific methods

There are a number of guides for conducting and reporting on different types of research, which provide statements and sometimes checklists and flowcharts.

- *Systematic reviews and meta-analyses*: PRISMA (Preferred Reporting Items for Systematic Reviews & Meta-Analyses), http://www.prisma-statement.org/
- *Randomised trials*: CONSORT (Consolidated Standards of Reporting Trials), http://www.consort-statement.org/
- *Observational studies*: STROBE (STrengthening the Reporting of OBservational studies in Epidemiology) Statements for cohort, case-control, & cross-sectional studies, https://www.strobe-statement.org/index.php?id=strobe-home
- *Statistical reporting*: SAMPL (Statistical Analyses & Methods in Published Literature), http://www.equator-network.org/wp-content/uploads/2013/03/SAMPL-Guidelines-3-13-13.pdf

---

tactic), where you keep picking it up and deal with a small amount at a time. Either way, you need to be organised. Have everything you need available and easily accessible, ideally in folders and subfolders on your computer. This may include grant proposals, your ethics application, reports, dataset and bibliography library (using software such as Endnote, RefWorks or Mendeley). There will be considerable material, especially on your background and methods sections, that you can cut, paste and then rewrite.

Check that you put your text in the correct place, for example, no introduction in methods and no discussion in results. Have a logical flow from one part to the next to make it easy to read. The clearest writing is simple and direct. Have one idea per sentence; several short, simple sentences are usually much clearer than one long sentence with subclauses. Paragraphs help to order your thoughts. There should be one topic per paragraph. The first sentence introduces the topic, and transitions relate one idea to the next. Keep paragraphs short, between two and six sentences.

Flowery language does not belong in scientific writing; stay away from metaphors, similes and clichés. Use everyday English, with minimal use of foreign phrases, scientific words and jargon. Avoid colloquialisms, for example, use *Did not* instead of *Didn't*. Use short words in preference to long words, and fewer words in preference to more. For example, *The cow jumped over the moon* is much easier to read and understand than *The attempt made by the female bovine adult to discontinuously traverse the Earth's lunar body was not unsuccessful.* Beware of nominalisations. These are nouns formed from other parts of speech such as adjectives or verbs, by adding a suffix or ending such as -ism, -ity, -tion or -ment. Turn nominalised nouns back into verbs, for example:

> *Take into consideration* becomes *Consider*
> *We undertook an investigation* becomes *We investigated*
> *There was a group agreement* becomes *The group agreed*

The following sentence contains seven nominalisations: *The proliferation of nominalisations in a discursive formation may be an indication of a tendency toward pomposity and abstraction.* What this actually means is that *writers who overload their sentences with nominalisations tend to sound pompous and abstract.*

Use the active voice in writing, as this is clearer and more concise than the passive voice. The active voice follows the sentence construction subject – verb – object. For example, *The dog ate the meat* has a more logical flow and is easier to understand than *The meat was eaten by the dog.*

Limit your use of upper case (capital letters) to the beginning of sentences and proper nouns (names of specific people, places and things). For example, Doctor John Smith has capitals, because the title is capitalised as part of his name, but if you ask, *Is there a doctor in the house?* this is not a specific person so 'doctor' is in lower case. Similarly, you would say that *There are sailboats on Lake Geneva*, but *There are sailboats on many lakes in Switzerland.* Thus, words such as 'general practitioner' should be in lower case.

Many people use apostrophes incorrectly. They may soon become obsolete, but in the meantime you need to get them right. They have two uses. The first is to show possession (that something belongs to the subject). For example, *the cow's tail*, or *the farmers' market.* The other use is to show that a word is contracted, that there is a missing letter or letters e.g. *It's* (it is) *cold today* and *It doesn't* (does not) *matter.* An apostrophe should not be used to denote plural – for example *Three GPs work together* is correct, while *Three GP's work together* is incorrect.

It is important to be consistent in your writing. Set your proofing language, for example to UK English or US English, and ensure your spelling always matches – for example, analyse and paediatric or analyze and pediatric. Be consistent with your tenses. You will use the future tense in your proposal (*we will do this*), but the present (*we find that*) or past (*we found that*) tense in your report or paper. Similarly, decide if you are writing in the first (I, we) or third (the researcher[s], he, she or they) person, and whether this is singular (I or we) or plural (he/she or they).

You must also be consistent with your formatting. Ensure that you are consistent with your font type and size, your alignment (left or justified), your word spacing (usually a single space between words and between sentences) and your line spacing (e.g. single, 1.5 lines, or double). Use the space bar to separate words, line break (Enter) to separate paragraphs (not multiple spaces) and page breaks to start a new page (not multiple line breaks). Switch on the paragraph mark symbol (¶) in Microsoft Word, which makes it easy to check that you have consistent spacing. Headings and subheadings may be different font to your text, but choose your style and use it consistently. If you are writing a journal article, download and read the journal's 'Instructions to authors' and follow the instructions regarding font and formatting.

WRITING AN ARTICLE FOR JOURNAL PUBLICATION
Choosing a journal

Before you start writing, choose your journal. You want to have one that is indexed in the databases (e.g. PubMed), so that it will be found by others conducting literature searches and ideally with an impact factor. You should check the journal's aim, scope and readership to ensure that your article fits with what they publish and will reach your target audience. Balance appropriate readership with a realistic impact factor.

Other ways to choose a journal are to look where relevant articles have been published in your reference list, and ask colleagues where they have published. Check journal estimated review, decision and publication times and their acceptance rates. For example, the *New England Medical Journal* has an acceptance rate of 5%, *BMJ* 7%, *BMJ Open* 50%, *PLOS ONE* 69% and the overall average for journals on health is 46%. Aim high, but be realistic about the chance of a top journal publishing your work. Sometimes reviewer comments will be helpful in revising your article.

Consider the type of journal you wish to publish in: National, pertaining to your region, or international. If the latter, consider whether you want more of a UK/European or North American focus. Is it suitable for a general medical or primary care journal or possibly a sub-specialty? Think laterally – perhaps there is a particular aspect you can focus on, and therefore select a journal dealing, for example, in health informatics, or ethnicity issues.

Consider Open-Access journals, which often have rapid review times and may be free for your audience to access, although you will need to pay the publishing fee. Beware the increasing number of predatory journals. You have to pay to publish in these, they provide poor or no peer review, have no impact factor and are not reputable places to publish. See also Box 27.2 on how to check if a journal is reputable, and for other useful resources.

Writing your journal article

Download the instructions for authors for your chosen journal and follow carefully. It can be helpful to prepare a template using the specified font

BOX 27.2   USEFUL RESOURCES

Check if your chosen journal is trusted; see http://thinkchecksubmit.org/check/.

International Committee of Medical Journal Editors (ICMJE): You can download Recommendations for the conduct, reporting, editing and publication of scholarly work in medical journals, and the ICMJE Form for Disclosure of potential conflicts of interest (generate a disclosure statement for your manuscript) is available at http://www.icmje.org.

Author Aid: Support developing-country researchers in publishing their work (rovides a large number of useful resources), http://www. authoraid.info/en/resources/.

Medical Subject Headings (MeSH) terms: https://www.nlm.nih.gov/mesh/ MBrowser.html

type and size, line spacing, page numbers, proofing language, headings and subheadings. Set your bibliography software to the style they require for their references. Note the maximum word count for the abstract and the text. You can have a look at articles in the journal and chose an exemplary one as a model (but ensure you do not plagiarise). Follow instructions for all sections and aspects of your manuscript.

If you have collaborators, determine who your co-authors are and reach an agreement about author order at the outset. Authors must make a substantial contribution to the conception and design or analysis and interpretation of data and drafting of the article or revising it critically for important intellectual content. Be as inclusive as possible but participation solely in the acquisition of funding or collection of the data does not justify authorship.

You can cut and paste sections from ethics applications, research proposal and reports into your template under the appropriate headings and then rewrite them. You may need to change future to present or past tense.

Your title is usually a distilled description. Include information that will make electronic retrieval sensitive and specific. The journal may want information about your study design and may also specify the maximum number of words or characters.

The title page usually contains the names, degrees and institutional affiliations of the authors and contact details for the corresponding author.

You are usually asked for key words. Keep to the designated number (may range from 3 to 10). These are important because they help others find your work. Use Medical Subject Headings (MeSH) terms https://www.ncbi.nlm. nih.gov/mesh wherever possible because these are the words used for indexing PubMed. Key words that are also in your title and abstract will increase the chances of your article being found in literature searches.

Your <u>abstract</u> is very important. Sometimes it may be the only part of your article that is read. It needs to be a clear and accurate summary. Keep to the specified word count and, if specified, the stipulated headings. Abstracts do not contain references. It is usually easier to write your abstract after you have written the article.

The <u>main body</u> of your text follows the scientific structure outlined earlier. Keep to the word count. Use bibliography software to insert your references, compiling as you go. Import these from databases wherever possible and check their accuracy. Format in the style designated by the journal.

You need to acknowledge funders, study participants and sometimes colleagues who have assisted but who are not eligible for authorship. Some journals require their written permission to name them. There may be other sections required, such as declarations of conflicts of interest, an outline of the contribution of each author, copyright statements, or summaries such as *How this fits in* or *What gap this fills*.

Once you have a draft, you need input from your co-authors. Sometimes this is easier one at a time, so that you do not get too confused by several different track-changes versions. Make sure the process does not stall at this point. Set co-authors a time limit in which to respond.

You will need to do a final edit and proofread. You want your manuscript to be clear and not too wordy. Usually. there will be text you need to cut out at this stage. Check that your spelling, punctuation and grammar are correct. You may ask a colleague, or even a layperson, to read who can give you feedback on comprehension and readability. You need to recirculate to your co-authors who all must approve the final version. You can use the default that no response within a specified time limit indicates approval.

You may need to prepare a cover letter that explains why the editor should publish your work: How it fits with the journal's aim and scope, the perceived value to their journal audience, your study's relationship of study to the existing body of work and what your research adds to what is already known.

Now you are ready to submit. Make sure you have all the documents ready, including signed conflict of interest and copyright forms when required. You may also need the names and contact details of suitable reviewers. Authors of articles you have cited can be helpful here. You may be asked to anonymise your manuscript, or submit tables and figures separately. Read and follow the journal instructions!

Your paper may be returned without review, or rejected after reports from the referees have come in. Do not put your article away in the drawer at this point, never to be visited again. Ask yourself whether this was a suitable journal (right aim and scope). Carefully consider feedback from the editor and/or the reviewers. Choose a new journal and, using the constructive comments, revise and improve your article. Make sure you follow the new journal instructions and tailor your article to fit. Include previous submissions, rejections and reviews in your cover letter. You may have to repeat this process several times, but unless your research was fatally flawed, you should be able to find a home for your article, even if it is not in the top-ranking journal you initially hoped for.

CHAPTER 28

How to create an effective poster: Keep it simple, keep it visual, keep it clear

Katharine A. Wallis

A poster presentation session is an opportunity for you to present your work, engage colleagues in discussion, and receive feedback about your research. A poster is a conversation starter; it is not an opportunity to present your entire research project. Unlike a journal article, a poster is transient.

A conference poster session is often in a crowded room with people milling about, chatting, eating and drinking. You will need to stand by your poster for the duration of the session, usually for about an hour and try to engage colleagues in discussion. It helps if you smile and wear your name badge, so people can see who you are. You may want to have business cards or handouts to share.

DESIGNING YOUR POSTER

A poster is a visual communication tool. Design your poster to convey one key message in a visually appealing way. A picture paints a thousand words: Use simple images to convey your message and show your story, instead of words to tell your story. For example, use graphs rather than tables. Remember to label your images. Use plenty of space and use colour, but avoid going crazy with colour or writing in a colour that is difficult to read.

Use only minimal text. A poster need only present the highlights or main points of your research project, not every detail. The structure of your poster should emphasise your message or the main points. State your key message in the title, and show your message through headings and graphics.

The layout of your poster should be logical and easy to follow, guiding the viewer from beginning to middle to end. If your poster is in landscape format, using columns will make it easier to read, for example, three columns.

The most effective posters follow the mantra: Keep it simple, keep it visual, keep it clear.

- *Keep it simple*: Focus on one key message. Consider a results-oriented message, for example: 'Smoking kills'. Keep the focus of the poster on your message.
- *Keep it visual*: Use simple images, such as graphs or pictures, to tell the story. Keep words to a minimum. Choose the layout and colour of the poster to reflect the story you want to tell. For example, a green might help convey an environmental message.
- *Keep it clear*: Use an obvious and well-ordered structure that is easy for the eye to follow. Make it easy for your colleagues to read and understand at a glance the message you are trying to convey.

CREATING YOUR POSTER

It takes time and work to create a simple, effective poster. Start preparing your poster well in advance of the conference; allow time to step back and reflect and to get others to proof read your poster. Read and follow the conference poster presentation instructions. Keep a copy of the instructions handy so you can refer back to them as you create your poster. Create your poster according to the specified size and format, such as portrait or landscape. Get your poster to the printer in good time. When travelling to present your poster, it is often easier to have it printed on fabric, so it can be folded into a suitcase rather than rolled and carried separately.

When creating your poster, you first need to identify your key message. Sketching out your flow of ideas on paper or in a Word document may help you to identify and fine tune your message. Once you have identified your message, start creating your poster. You can create your images and boxes of text and then join them together to create your poster. A commonly used tool for creating posters is Microsoft PowerPoint, but there are alternative software options for creating posters, such as OpenOffice Impress (https://www.openoffice.org/product/impress.html) and Omnigraffle (https://www.omnigroup.com/omnigraffle). You can create your graphics in Microsoft Excel and export them to PowerPoint. Adobe Photoshop can be good for images.

POSTER COMPONENTS

Title: Your title should convey your message and be designed to attract the attention of colleagues. Do not use all capitals in your title; words are easier to read when written in sentence case. Your title should be in a large font, for example, 72.

Authors: List the authors and affiliations and your contact details.

Text: Use minimal text; aim for no more than 500–1000 words. Use a font size of no less than 24, to ensure that your poster is easily visible from two metres. Use plain language, and avoid using jargon and acronyms. Avoid long sentences and paragraphs, instead use bullet points and boxes. There is usually a brief introduction, followed by methods, results and then conclusions. The conclusions section is where you interpret your results; you may reiterate key information but avoid simply repeating your results. You may want to suggest future work as this may prompt questions and discussion with colleagues. Posters do not need an abstract.

Acknowledgements: Acknowledge your funders and include key icons that are often a contractual requirement. It can be helpful to include your email address should people want to contact you afterwards and details of any publications or web sites linked to the research that people can find later should they be interested.

COMMON MISTAKES

A common mistake is to include too much information on your poster. Fewer words in a larger font and an image will more effectively convey your message than using too much text in a font that is too small to read easily from a distance. Think, for example, of the very effective poster: *'Your country needs you'*.

Another common mistake is to have the key message obscured and no clear conclusion. It is not easy to pare back your research project to one essential key message, but this is essential to creating an effective poster. An effective poster makes it easy for the audience to find the main point.

Another mistake is for posters to be poorly designed, with no obvious flow of ideas. Try and organise the flow of information in a logical and organised fashion; from brief introduction, to methods, results and then to your conclusion. Some posters make the mistake of being visually unappealing and confusing. Try and keep your graphs simple and the design and choice of colours pleasing to the eye.

Remember, an effective poster conveys a simple message in a visual medium: Keep it simple, keep it visual and keep it clear.

CHAPTER 29

Using social media to disseminate primary care research

Charilaos Lygidakis and Raquel Gómez Bravo

Social media are a powerful means of communication among health care professionals, patients and the public. Their use has been increasing steadily globally, transforming the way that people exchange information, interact and collaborate. Physicians are using more and more social networks to connect with broader audiences, communicate with their patients and their colleagues and build a network of trustworthy peers.[1] Researchers are also leveraging social media, capitalising on the velocity with which the messages can spread and the ability to disseminate them to the general public in addition to research communities, thus attracting more attention and increasing the influence and impact of their work.[2]

DEVELOPING A STRATEGY

First, social media should be considered as tools. As such, and before setting off to use them professionally, it is of utmost importance to study and understand the full extent of their potential and the implications of their use (Box 29.1). Familiarising oneself with one's own institutional social media policy or guidelines is a necessary first step.

An online presence is a reflection of who a person is, and expresses individual beliefs, values and priorities. According to the policy on professionalism in the use of social media of the American Medical Association: *'Physicians must recognize that actions online and content posted may negatively affect their reputations among patients and colleagues, may*

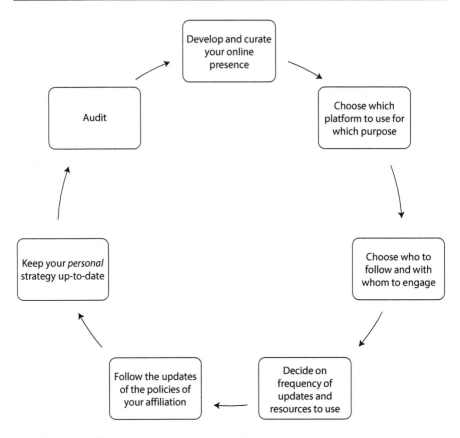

FIGURE 29.1 Elements of a personal social media strategy.

have consequences for their medical careers, and can undermine public trust in the medical profession.'[3] The Mayo Clinic summarised its Social Media Policy in 12 words: 'don't lie, don't pry, don't cheat, can't delete, don't steal and don't reveal'.[4]

Second, it is important to develop and maintain a proper personal strategy by meticulously establishing an online profile, carefully separating personal and professional aspects, being consistent in the posted messages and the proper interactions and auditing the online presence on a regular basis (Figure 29.1).

DISSEMINATION AS PART OF THE RESEARCH WORK
Maintain an online presence and networking

Maintaining an up-to-date online profile can increase the influence and impact of one's work, and eventually strengthen one's reputation. It is also important to consider carefully who to follow and with whom to engage on

BOX 29.1   KEY RECOMMENDATIONS

- Social media should be considered as a tool. As such, read the manual first!
- Become familiar with the terms and conditions of the networks you employ, learn how to use the privacy and profile settings and be aware that confidentiality is difficult to be guaranteed.
- You don't need to use every network; critically choose the platform that suits your personality and type of work.
- Your online presence is a reflection of your personality, so it is important to keep conversations authentic, expressing yourself openly, but always with respect and contributing with the proper expertise and experience.
- It is recommended to act as though any information that is posted will remain forever online, and might be distributed, commented or shared by anyone— even if the conversation takes place within a private group or network.
- Respect copyrights, familiarise yourself with the different licences, and share content giving credit appropriately.
- Evaluate whether or not what you write can be perceived as just a personal message or the position of your institution; even if a disclaimer is present (e.g. *'These tweets represent my personal views'*), you are always representing your institution or discipline online, even indirectly.
- Google yourself and regularly audit your profile pages, assess how people who do not know you will perceive what you write.

social platforms. Moreover, the researcher must determine which one of the social networks offers the most appropriate platform for the dissemination of his/her work. There are a variety of networks, ranging from those used by the public (e.g. *Facebook, Twitter*) and professionals (e.g. *LinkedIn*) to more closed communities dedicated to health care professionals (e.g. *Doximity*) and researchers (e.g. *ResearchGate, Academia*).

Blogging and microblogging

The demanding workload of researchers, whether it is inside academia or in the clinical setting, becomes the driving force behind blogging, offering the opportunity to reflect on one's work and life, share ideas, interact with an audience of peers and the general public and, ultimately, stay inspired (Box 29.2). There are two specific forms particularly useful for disseminating the work of researchers: *blogging* and *microblogging*.

Blogs are one of the oldest and most established forms of social media, which has been used in medicine since 2004.[5] They can reach wide audiences, include large amounts of information in different media (text, video, audio) and provide a platform for the readers to interact with the authors and share the content of it in other platforms. Maintaining a blog implies a high commitment to keep the audience interested and engaged, provide regular updates and an active participation in the conversations with readers.

In addition to dedicated, popular and free platforms, like *Blogger* and *Wordpress*, two other networks offer the possibility to post updates about one's ongoing work: *LinkedIn* with its blogging feature *Pulse*, and *ResearchGate* within the *Projects*. Posting on these networks offers the opportunity to target the specific audiences that access them, thus maximising the impact of one's work within the academic and professional community. Linking these updates on the profile page of these networks will also provide unique insight into one's work, skills and personality and complement the online presence.

When an article is published, it is highly recommended that the authors create different summaries of the publication, each one targeted to different audiences (for instance, one for physicians and one for the general public), with an outline of the key objectives, methods and outcomes. Videos can be an even more effective way to reach the general public.

BOX 29.2   BOOST THE IMPACT OF YOUR WORK

- When blogging, make frequent posts.
- Post tweets about your ongoing work—not only your publication.
- Create multimedia content, such as summary videos and podcasts. Photos, videos and other material from your fieldwork may drive curiosity and enable your peers to understand the background and context of your research better.
- Similarly, presentations from scientific communications can be an effective way to summarise your work. You can share them on such platforms as *Slideshare* and *ResearchGate*.
- Post a blog update with a summary of your publication tailored according to the audience that you target.
- Encourage your affiliated institution or scientific association, and your colleagues to post on their blogs and with their *Twitter* accounts.
- Take advantage of social citation. Share your publication in reference managers, such as *Zotero* and *Mendeley*, and academic networks, such as *ResearchGate* and *Academia*. If you hold the appropriate licence, upload a copy of your work for prompt sharing.
- Explore the opportunities to reach broader audiences with the help of a press specialist or the communications office of your affiliation.
- Identify podcasts relevant to your research and contact their producers to inform them about your work.
- React promptly when someone comments on your post or mentions you directly in a conversation.[6]

Microblogging is a more dynamic and perhaps concise form of information exchange, with which it is possible to share brief content and hold conversations with followers, typically in a rapid manner, thus easily establishing communities of practice. *Twitter*, with its 280-character *tweets*, is the most used microblogging platform. The messages can include a range of media (e.g. photos and videos) and hyperlinks and can be labelled with *hashtags* – a type of metadata, which constitutes an informal taxonomy for indexing information and enabling users to discover content by carrying out thematic or context-based searches. Two interesting applications of the *hashtags* are their use during conferences to facilitate conversations between attendees and augmenting the experience of the event, and online journal clubs, in which articles are commented openly on using *Twitter*.

MEASURING THE IMPACT: ALTMETRICS

Altmetrics, such as the *Altmetric* score, the *Article-Level Metrics* in *PLOS*, and *Impactstory*, can measure the impact of dissemination on social networks rapidly, offering an alternative and complementary way for the evaluation of how researchers and the general public perceive and engage with publications (Figure 29.2). In addition to articles, other research-related outputs, such as

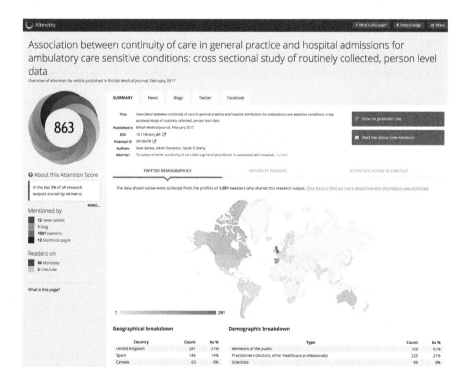

FIGURE 29.2 An example of the metrics of an article provided by *Altmetric*.

presentations and data sets, can be assessed. The advantages of *Altmetrics* stem from the wide range of sources that can be assessed in nearly real-time: The information gathered comes from citations on blogs and *Wikipedia* articles; mentions on social networks, including *Facebook*, *Twitter*, and *LinkedIn*; communities, such as *Reddit* and records on the reference managers, such as *Mendeley*, as well as coverage in the more traditional news outlets.

REFERENCES

1. Jain SH. Practicing medicine in the age of Facebook. *N Engl J Med* 2009;361(7):649–51.
2. Rowlands I, Nicholas D, Russell B, Canty N, Watkinson A. Social media use in the research workflow. *Learn Publ* 2011;24(3):183–95.
3. American Medical Association. Professionalism in the Use of Social Media. 2010.
4. Leibtag A. A 12-Word Social Media Policy [Internet]. Mayo Clinic Social Media Network. 2012 [cited 9 January 2018]. Available from: https://socialmedia.mayoclinic.org/2012/04/05/a-twelve-word-social-media-policy/
5. Grajales FJ, Sheps S, Ho K, Novak-Lauscher H, Eysenbach G. Social media: A review and tutorial of applications in medicine and health care. *J Med Internet Res.* 2014;16(2):e13.
6. Carroll CL, Ramachandran P. The intelligent use of digital tools and social media in practice management. *Chest* 2014;145(4):896–902.

CHAPTER 30

Reaching decision-makers and achieving social impact with your research

Bob Mash, Nasreen Jessani and Liesl Nicol

Publishing in a scientific journal is the most common way for researchers in the health sciences to disseminate their findings. Publication, however, does not guarantee that the knowledge will translate into influencing policymakers and other stakeholders or achieve social impact. Furthermore, any one study, including yours, may be one amongst several other perhaps complementary or contradictory research studies on the topic. The synthesis of this body of research in order to reach conclusions on the evidence available can be conducted through a systematic review (see Chapter 15). There is often a substantial gap between what is known (evidence) and what is done (policy and clinical practice). In recent years, there has been growing interest in the concept of knowledge translation and how one can bridge this 'know-do gap'.

Knowledge translation has been defined as 'the exchange, synthesis and effective communication of reliable and relevant research results. The focus is on promoting interaction among the producers and users of research, removing the barriers to research use and tailoring information to different target audiences so that effective interventions are used more widely'.[1] This definition implies that the research agenda requires involvement of researchers as well as research users alike.

Although we might aspire to a world where policy formation is entirely evidence-based, this is far from the complex reality. The concept of evidence-informed decision making recognises the existence of other factors that influence policy. These might include political ideology, social or cultural norms, economic constraints, relative cost-effectiveness of different options under consideration, operational feasibility, competing priorities, influence of other lobbyists or stakeholders and appraisal of a range of different types of evidence.[2] Evidence from research may have different purposes within policy making such as proving the existence or the magnitude of a problem, comparing the effectiveness of different policy options, legitimising existing policy or enabling the formulation of new policy.

STAKEHOLDER ANALYSIS

Knowledge translation starts with an analysis of your stakeholders. Stakeholders are people, groups or organisations that have a concern or interest in the topic of your research.[3] Stakeholders might use your research in decisions, policy or practice or be affected by the implementation of such decisions, policy or change in practice. If you were to brainstorm a list of stakeholders with your research team you might then analyse them in terms of attributes relevant to your research or initiative. For example, you could place them on a matrix in terms of their power or interest. Power refers to their level of influence with respect to the success or failure of your research, project, intervention, programme or initiative. Interest refers to their level of interest in your issue or topic. You can then tailor your communication with different stakeholders according to their relative power and interest as shown in Figure 30.1.[4] Other key aspects to consider in relation to each stakeholder

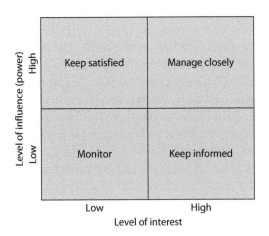

FIGURE 30.1 Matrix of power and interest for stakeholders. (From Stakeholder power/interest analysis. Available from https://requirementstechniques. wordpress.com/stakeholder-analysis/stakeholder-powerinterest-analysis/ [Accessed 8 February 2018].)

are what is important to this stakeholder, how might they contribute to the use of your research or block the use of your research.[5]

ENGAGEMENT STRATEGY

Having identified and analysed your stakeholders, the next step would be to develop an appropriate engagement strategy for each one. Such a strategy should consider the following questions:[2]

- What is the purpose of your engagement?
- What is/are the key message(s)?
- What is the best medium(s) to convey this message?
- Who is the most effective messenger(s)?
- When would be the best time to engage?
- What resources are needed to support this engagement?

Being clear about the purpose implies having a clear goal for your engagement with this stakeholder.[6] Are you, for example, trying to raise awareness and interest, provide new knowledge and information or change current policy and practice?

Given the purpose of your engagement with this stakeholder, it would make sense to clarify the key message(s) that you want to convey. The message should command attention, be clear and consistent, communicate a benefit, appeal to the head (i.e. statistical information) as well as the heart (i.e. stories), create trust and build relationships, as well as call to action if this is appropriate.[3] The message should of course make the connections to the stakeholder's existing interests and priorities, avoid results which are very uncertain and be clear about the benefits versus risks.

The message can be conveyed in a wide variety of formats.[2,3] Printed material such as research articles, newsletters, policy briefs, editorials, reports or issue briefs may be used. Visual or oral media may be useful in some situations, for example, infographics, video clips on *YouTube*, radio or television spots, drama, music or even sermons. Face-to-face communication may include presentations at conferences, workshops or targeted meetings. Social media is emerging as another important way to communicate your message (see Chapter 29), as well as electronic networks dedicated to research or family medicine. Usually, a multifaceted and targeted approach to disseminating your findings to relevant stakeholders will be required.

One should also consider who is the best person to convey the message, as this may not always be yourself as the researcher. The message may be better conveyed via other senior researchers or faculty, community members, funders, journalists or another intermediary.[3]

Finally, consider the best timing for your engagement. There may be particular times of the year that dovetail with budgetary or decision-making cycles within the department of health or with a clinical guideline development and revision process. There may be particular events or opportunities for engagement. There may be a particular sequence to your types of engagement or frequency with which you want to engage.

Having considered all of these factors in relation to your stakeholders, you should be able to identify all the resources that you need to support your engagement. Resources may be human (e.g. graphic designer, administrative), material (e.g. printing of policy briefs) or operational (e.g. travel and accommodation). You will need to prepare a budget for your knowledge translation strategy and identify sources of funding.[3]

EVALUATION

While we hope that the knowledge translation strategy will have the desired impact, a semblance of a monitoring and evaluation impact assessment will provide you with some insight regarding the extent to which this has occurred. Although the ultimate impact of your research may relate to the effect on society, health, policy or clinical practice, this outcome or impact evaluation is more focused on the success of your knowledge translation strategy. For example, did you reach all your stakeholders and achieve your engagement goals? Apart from evaluating the effectiveness of the engagement strategy, such an evaluation may help to justify the resources used and to improve future knowledge translation strategies. As with all project evaluation, it is best to design the monitoring and evaluation at the same time that you plan the project itself and to evaluate the outcomes throughout the life cycle of the project.

Evaluation for specific stakeholders should be aligned with the engagement goal that you set and should measure the activities that were planned or development of resources to achieve that goal, for example:[7]

- *Policy makers*: Number of face-to-face meetings, use of research in policy
- *Health professionals*: Change in clinical practice or quality of care
- *Public*: Media coverage of research findings, change in public attitudes or awareness
- *Researchers*: Number of conference presentations, citations, requests for collaboration
- *Media*: Newspaper, magazine, radio or TV coverage and social media presence

Different types of qualitative findings or quantitative indicators can be used:[8]

- *Reach indicators*: To what extent has the information been disseminated, downloaded, requested or looked at? e.g. *Altmetrics* tracks the reach of your work on a wide variety of media platforms such as news outlets, blogs, references, *Wikipedia, Facebook.*
- *Usefulness indicators*: Did the stakeholder read it, find it relevant, feel satisfied with the engagement, gain new knowledge, change their attitudes or views?
- *Use indicators*: Did the stakeholder intend to use the information; have they adapted the information; have they used the information in policy, guidelines, curriculum or research or have they used the information to change clinical practice?
- *Relationship indicators*: Has the information supported the development of new collaborations or partnerships or built capacity in others?

This chapter has briefly outlined a systematic approach for knowledge translation to more consciously plan for the impact of your research on key stakeholders. This phase of the research journey is often neglected, unfunded and undocumented. You can change that.

REFERENCES

1. World Health Organization. *World Report on Knowledge for Better Health: Strengthening Health Systems.* Geneva: WHO, 2004. Available from http://www.who.int/rpc/meetings/wr2004/en/index8.html (Accessed 8 February 2018)
2. Jessani, N, Nicol L. Evidence-Informed Decision making: The Art, Science and Complexity of Knowledge Translation. Stellenbosch University, Cape Town, S. Africa. 26–28 September 2017. Lecture.
3. Bennett G, Jessani N. (eds). 2011. *The Knowledge Translation Toolkit: Bridging the Know-Do Gap: A Resource for Researchers.* Delhi, India: IDRC/SAGE. Available from https://www.idrc.ca/en/book/knowledge-translation-toolkit-bridging-know-do-gap-resource-researchers (Accessed 8 February 2018)
4. Stakeholder power/interest analysis. Available from https://requirementstechniques.wordpress.com/stakeholder-analysis/stakeholder-powerinterest-analysis/ (Accessed 8 February 2018)
5. Stakeholder analysis matrix template. Available from http://www.tools4dev.org/resources/stakeholder-analysis-matrix-template/ (Accessed 8 February 2018)
6. Harmworth S, Turpin S. 2001. Creating an Effective Dissemination Strategy. An Expanded Interactive Workbook for Educational Development Projects. http://www.innovations.ac.uk/btg/resources/publications/dissemination.pdf (Accessed 8 February 2018)
7. Ohkubo S, Sullivan T, Harlan S, Timmons B, Strachan M. *Guide to Monitoring and Evaluating Knowledge Management in Global Health Programs.* Baltimore, MD: Center for Communication Programs, Johns Hopkins Bloomberg School of Public Health, 2013. https://www.globalhealthknowledge.org/sites/ghkc/files/km-monitoring-and-eval-guide.pdf (Accessed 8 February 2018)
8. Barwick M. Getting to Impact: Why Knowledge Translation Matters for Researchers with Melanie Barwick. Available from https://www.youtube.com/watch?v=xzmLrUIkONs (Accessed 14 February 2018)

SECTION VI

Building research capacity

CHAPTER 31

How to supervise and mentor a less-experienced or novice researcher

Elizabeth Sturgiss and Lena Sanci

All relationships are a two-way street, and supervision and mentorship in primary care research are no different. This chapter has tips for both senior and junior researchers, and is based on the literature on mentorship, blogs and writing from academics in social media and the experience of both authors (Box 31.1).

There are opportunities within primary care research supervision for both parties to grow and develop regardless of the stage of academic career. Primary care promotes lifelong learning to clinical students, and this advice is relevant in the research arena. Primary care research is strengthened through the nurturing of novice researchers to create a welcoming and vibrant community. We offer points for reflection and tips to prepare for a successful mentoring or supervision partnership.

MENTORSHIP AND SUPERVISION: WHAT IS THE DIFFERENCE?

Supervision is usually seen as a task-orientated process, and mentorship is more concerned with the overall development of the person being mentored (the 'mentee').[1] Supervision is often associated with some kind of evaluation or assessment of the junior researcher's performance, for example, within a higher degree research setting or as the junior researcher's boss. The common most definitions of mentoring suggest that the mentor should not be involved in assessment, and instead aim to provide a holistic supporting role for the mentee's personal and career development.[2]

BOX 31.1   A SERENDIPITOUS, CROSS-INSTITUTION, MENTORING RELATIONSHIP

Associate Professor Lena Sanci and Dr Liz Sturgiss have had an informal mentoring arrangement since late 2015. Liz was introduced to Lena by Prof. Alastair Hay from Bristol University after they met at the 2015 NAPCRG conference in Cancun. Alastair and Lena are colleagues through the Oxford Primary Care Leadership Program, and he suggested that Liz would benefit from a mentoring relationship with Lena. With this side introduction to Lena, Liz emailed Lena and asked if she would consider being a mentor. They agreed that they would have a telephone meeting to discuss the options. This first call lasted one hour and they agreed telephone meetings would work well. Liz sets up meetings via Lena's personal assistant whenever she has questions that she would like to ask. They generally meet on the phone every couple of months for about 30–45 minutes. Lena and Liz first met in person about one year into the mentoring relationship at a general practice conference in Perth. It was great to share a cup of tea together after all that time. Their mentoring relationship is the result of serendipity, following up on invitations and a willingness to share experiences.

A supervisor may provide some of the functions of a mentor, but if they are involved in assessment and performance review processes, they cannot fulfil the same function. Junior researchers should be encouraged to consider having mentors that are separate to their workplace or research supervision settings. Often junior researchers will need more than one person to support all their personal and career needs, and this should be endorsed.

A mentor also experiences benefits.[3] In an academic setting where there are strong and supported mentoring relationships, there is less staff turnover, better work satisfaction and better workplace productivity. Mentors often describe feeling refreshed and energised by mentorship relationships that are working smoothly.

As this chapter covers both supervision and mentorship of novice researchers, we have used the terms 'partnership' and 'relationship' where the tips are applicable to both settings. When the tip is more applicable to supervision or mentorship, this is indicated in the text.

HOW TO BE A HELPFUL SUPERVISOR AND MENTOR
How to attract novice researchers to your team

The key ingredient behind any excellent research is an excellent team. A group of people who enjoy working together on challenging research questions makes academia worthwhile at every stage of career. Attracting new researchers to primary care academia can be challenging. Primary care research is often not well-funded, there are no certainties for ongoing work, as is common in many areas of scientific endeavour. It is even more challenging to attract clinician researchers who have the option of work that is better paid with more certainty.[4]

We can look to economics for the key features that can attract and retain new researchers. Any person will perform better and be retained in a specific job if they have a sense of autonomy and meaning in their work, and feel that they have mastered something.[5] Admittedly, as a new researcher, these endeavours can be difficult, if not impossible. To the three ingredients, we add 'appreciation.' A novice researcher who feels appreciated is more likely to have the confidence to carry on.[6]

A number of factors are helpful for new academics:

1. Nurture curiosity and build a culture that supports risk taking in research.
2. Support in academic writing, particularly for grant writing.
3. Offer longer term contracts.
4. Exposure to top-performing academics.
5. Encourage interdisciplinary interest and study.
6. Support to join academic organisations in their community.
7. A supportive workplace culture that encourages mentoring.[4]

Finding time can be a challenge for the mentoring relationship, but the rewards and mutual benefit for mentors and mentees make it worthwhile. Some choose to catch up over breakfast, lunch, by phone, or by email. There is no set frequency for meetings needed for a good outcome. The mentee is usually responsible for scheduling the meetings, driving the relationship and following up on any actions.

Determining the kind of help your novice researcher needs

Novice researchers in primary care come from a wide variety of backgrounds with varying degrees of previous research experience. Many novice researchers will seek out more than one person to mentor them during their early career, and this should be encouraged. It is unlikely that one senior researcher can meet all the needs of a new researcher.

Tailoring the type of support to the new researcher's needs is the first important step. This is only possible following a discussion that outlines what you are able to offer in terms of expertise, as well as what the researcher is hoping to gain from the partnership. It is better to start with clear expectations for what you both anticipate for the frequency, length and mode of communication. All good relationships start with clear expectations and continue with clear communication; this situation is no exception to the rule. The type of assistance and amount of support a new researcher needs changes over time. Reviewing where things are going with your research student is always helpful, to keep both parties on the same page.

Being cognisant of gender-related issues for your mentee can start to break down barriers related to gender[7] in the primary care research space. Traditionally, men have held more senior positions in academia, although in the primary care research world, men may be less prominent, due to the predominance of women in the allied health fields. Issues to be aware of include:

- Carer-related responsibilities for both men and women; this might include children, aging parents or unwell family members; do not assume that only women have caring duties, or that women are the primary carer in their family; tailor your discussions to the needs of the mentee.
- Assess your mentee for signs of 'imposter syndrome',[8] a pattern of thinking that makes the mentee feel like a 'non-expert' in the field that will soon be exposed, which may occur more commonly in women.
- Assess the need for 'sponsorship', which describes when a senior person in the field introduces a junior mentee to influential others;[9] purportedly more frequent by men for junior men and a possible reason why women rise less quickly to leadership positions.

Mentors also have a duty of care to mentees. If the mentor becomes aware of a course of action that may have potentially serious consequences for the mentee, mentors should share their concerns or help them become aware of risks.

Goal setting

In formal research supervision settings, formal goal setting may be required and even occur naturally, for example, with PhD milestone reporting. In informal mentorship partnerships, goal setting is not generally considered to be part of the role, but it may provide a framework for determining the needs of the researcher. Not all new researchers will want to make goals, or some may even want to keep these private. All of these options are okay and should be respected if it is helpful for the mentee.

Breaking seemingly insurmountable problems into small achievable goals is a way forward when the researcher is needing assistance. As is usual in goal setting, the 'SMART' principles (Specific, Measurable, Achievable, Realistic, Time based) are important to increase the likelihood of change. As a mentor, helping a new researcher be 'Realistic' about their goals from your experience is an invaluable asset. Following up with your mentee on how they are progressing with their goals is a way to stay on track.

Relationship is key

Excellent supervision and mentorship of junior researchers are built on solid relationships.[10] Respectful engagement, the ability to ask questions considerately and listen without reproach, and to give criticism constructively, have been highlighted as qualities of an excellent mentor.[11] These factors are much more possible when care and consideration of the mentee as a person with goals and aspirations is considered. The mentor must be a trusted confidante with whom the mentee can share issues, goals and dreams. Mentors need to be non-judgmental, be active listeners and withhold advice unless asked, to assist mentees to problem solve and reflect on pros and cons of various options for their own circumstances.

We all live in a busy world with a multitude of activities vying for time and attention. It can be difficult to maintain nurturing relationships with junior researchers whom we supervise, especially if feeling stressed or overburdened. Without respectful relationships as a starting point, supervision and mentorship will never be helpful for anyone.

When things do not progress as expected

Sometimes relationships do not work out, perhaps because of personal incompatibility, a mismatch in expectations, or needs being unmet. It is usually helpful to negotiate a review of how the relationship is going early on, and agree that if either person wants to end mentorship for any reason at any time, then they can do so without recrimination.

Sometimes problems arise when mentorship is used for something it was not intended. While mentoring augments the development of the researcher, it is not a replacement for formal supervision, nor for organisational management. While personal life circumstances are often discussed during mentoring relationships, with a view to sharing tips on managing life and career, mentoring is not a replacement for formal therapy, nor assistance with personal issues.

For problems between supervisors and students, and in formal mentorship programmes, there is usually an independent academic coordinator who can be consulted for assistance, who may help with finding an alternative mentor or supervisor if necessary. Problems have a better chance of being solved if caught early and discussed.

HOW TO GET THE MOST FROM A SUPERVISION/MENTORSHIP RELATIONSHIP FOR THE NEW RESEARCHER
How to find a mentor

Often junior researchers will have formal supervisors who are part of their study programme or head of department, if working in a university.

Universities may also offer formal 'mentorship programmes', matching junior with senior researchers.

It may be useful for a junior researcher to seek support and advice from an experienced person from outside their institution or workplace for support for issues such as:

- Career advice
- Expertise in specific methodology
- Negotiating contracts
- Workplace culture
- Research ethical issues
- Family life and academic work
- The culture shock of the academic world
- Balancing work, life and self-care
- The list is endless!

There are always opportunities to seek out further support and mentorship through less formal channels. Being introduced by a colleague, or meeting new people at conferences, are common examples. Telephone and web-conference calls are all possible ways to have meetings with a mentor located remotely.

Meeting people at conferences is often intimidating, especially if you are new on the scene. If possible, scan the attendees list prior to see if there are researchers who share your interests. You can attend their talks and then wait afterwards to say hello. Asking positively framed questions of presenters is a great way to indicate your interest in their work – this can be quite challenging in front of a large audience! Approaching people at social events or tea breaks is a great way to break the ice. A simple business card can assist confidence in approaching new people.

What to expect from a mentor and how to get what you need

At the beginning of the relationship, be clear about each party's expectations. The junior researcher can direct this discussion. Features to negotiate include:

- Opportunity to meet face-to-face? If so, how frequently, where and for how long will each meeting occur?
- Communication via email or telephone? As needed, or on a regular basis?
- Does the mentor have a personal assistant or administration officer with whom to make appointments?
- How long will the relationship last? Is it open-ended? Or to be reviewed after a time period?

- What topics are for discussion at meetings? Any areas that mentee or mentor wish not to discuss?
- Any conflicts of interest to be discussed (such as job network or supervision issues)?
- Both agree to maintain the confidentiality of the conversations or to speak together if sharing something with an outside party, for example, introducing the mentee to other academics to assist with future goals.

It may be important to negotiate these items formally, or the relationship may develop naturally with just discussion about how and when to meet.

An agenda, or at least a list of questions, for each meeting can help a junior researcher get the best out of the relationship. This is even more important in a formal supervision situation. Sending an agenda, preferably a couple of days prior to the meeting, is ideal. This helps the mentor consider the issues in advance and add to the agenda as needed.

After a meeting, consider sending a quick email outlining the main points of the meeting. This gives another opportunity to clarify any issues of contention. Always end the email with the time and date of the next meeting and ensure administration staff who need to diarise this are aware too.

Goal setting and problem solving

At times, the world of research can feel like a never-ending rollercoaster ride without a clear destination. Trying to stay on top of current projects, complete previous projects, and keep looking to future projects can be overwhelming. Goal setting can help when research problems loom large. A mentor can help with keeping goals realistic. Mentors can draw on their own experience to make suggestions. They are usually helpful for knowing alternative research methodologies, reference sources or other experts in the field to give a whole new outlook on the issues being faced.

What to do when things do not progress as expected

Invariably there are times when a supervision or mentorship relationship does not go to plan. This may result from beginning the relationship with ambiguous expectations or expectations that are not clearly communicated to the other party. Sometimes even with the best intentions, plans do not work out. Depending on the situation, a number of options are available to the mentee:

- Discuss with another trusted senior colleague, or a peer.
- Arrange a meeting with the supervisor outlining the issues, alongside ways to move forward.

> ## BOX 31.2   FREELY AVAILABLE RESOURCES
>
> *ThinkWell*: Resources for academia and PhD students, http://www.ithinkwell.com.au/resources
> *The Thesis Whisperer*: Online blog and resources for thesis writing and academia generally, https://thesiswhisperer.com/about/
> *Research whisperer*: https://theresearchwhisperer.wordpress.com/
> *Mind tools*: https://www.mindtools.com/

- In an informal arrangement, sometimes the maximum benefit from the relationship has been derived and there is no need to continue. Although difficult, there is no need to continue informal partnerships that are no longer helpful.[12]
- All research institutions have formal policies for handling grievances in situations that cannot be resolved, or that involve serious breaches of trust, including harassment.

CONCLUSION

There are many online resources for learning more about mentorship and supervision. Some of our favourites are listed in Box 31.2 - we hope that you are inspired to explore, learn and discover more about this essential part of being a primary care researcher. The nurturing of junior researchers is an essential part of being a senior researcher in primary care. Our primary care research community cannot thrive without the addition of new, interested and enthusiastic researchers. It is a privileged position to supervise or mentor another person, and the rewards for both can be enormous. A well supported junior researcher will thrive and develop quickly and will be more likely to stick with the career path. A supportive and welcoming research community will best do the job of answering questions that will better the health of our patients and communities.

REFERENCES

1. Acker S. Advising and mentoring graduate students. In: Bank B, editor. *Gender and Higher Education*. Baltimore, MD: Johns Hopkins University Press; 2011, p. 330–36.
2. Harper J, Sawicka T. Academic mentoring: A pilot success at Victoria University of Wellington. In: Hall C, editor. *Nga Taumata Matauranga O Aotearoa/Higher Education in New Zealand: Occasional Paper Series*. Wellington, New Zealand: Syndicate of Educational Development Centres of New Zealand Universities, 2001.
3. Nick JM, Delahoyde TM, Prato DD et al. Best practices in academic mentoring: A model for excellence. *Nurs Res Pract* 2012;2012:937906.
4. Aronson JK. How to attract, retain and nurture young academic clinicians. *JRSM* 2011;104(1):6–14.

5. Pink D. The surprising truth about what motivates us. Secondary The surprising truth about what motivates us 2010. https://www.youtube.com/watch?v=u6XAPnuFjJc

6. Steele MM, Fisman S, Davidson B. Mentoring and role models in recruitment and retention: A study of junior medical faculty perceptions. *Med Teach* 2013;35(5):e1130–8.

7. Crabb A. *The Wife Drought: Why Women Need Wives, and Men Need Lives.* Sydney: Penguin Random House Australia, 2014.

8. Clance PR, Imes S. The imposter phenomenon in high achieving women: Dynamics and therapeutic intervention. *Psychother Theory, Res Pract* 1978;15(3):1–8.

9. Ibarra H, Carter NM, Silva C. Why men still get more promotions than women. *HBR* 2010;88(9):80–5, 126.

10. Miller E. The second supervision rule: Foster psychological safety. In: Mewburn I, Miller E, editors. *The Supervision Whisperers*, 2017. https://thesupervisionwhisperers. wordpress.com/2017/03/14/the-second-supervision-rule-foster-psychological-safety/

11. Lee A, Dennis C, Campbell P. Nature's guide for mentors. *Nature* 2007;447(7146):791–97.

12. O'Hara C. How to break up with your mentor. *HBR*, 2014. https://hbr.org/2014/05/ how-to-break-up-with-your-mentor.

CHAPTER 32

Creating the right environment for mentoring to flourish

Amanda Howe

Mentorship is recommended in many business and professional settings to help people develop the appropriate skills for their careers, give guidance on what will help them to improve their performance, and support them to understand the context, opportunities and expectations that may operate in their particular setting. This chapter addresses mentorship in the context of academic family medicine, which is usually in the setting of a university or regional health-service institution. It focuses on three aspects of this 'system': The academic trainee (AT), who might be doing a postgraduate degree or be employed as a lecturer or other early career grade; the academic mentor (AM), who is likely to be a more senior member of staff in the same institution and the academic department (AD), which is the setting where the mentoring relationship occurs.

In any academic setting, one purpose of mentorship is about the needs of the AT – helping them to apply new academic competencies in their teaching and research, identifying and working through any concerns and guiding them about training needs and opportunities. For the AD, the main aim is building capacity and getting outputs – new teachers, new publications, the next generation of research active staff – and thus strengthening the profile of the institution through these successes. So the AM often has both a formative supportive role, but also a summative delivery role: Is this AT reaching their goals? Are they progressing in their PhD? Publishing? Getting work accepted at conferences? And are they giving and getting good feedback? So much rests on making this mentoring relationship an effective one for both mentee and mentor.

An AD which creates a successful culture for effective mentorship needs to have training in place for the mentors, which will mean most of the academic staff-and this role should be included in their job description. New staff need an induction into both the principles of mentorship and the department's particular needs – which can vary across the staff spectrum. The rationale for, and the values and skills which drive effective mentorship, need to be reflected both in the training and in the ongoing expectations of the mentorship role. Broadly, mentors need interpersonal skills to build trusting relationships; effective communication skills, asking the right questions in a helpful way; a genuine commitment to the AT's development and an understanding of the context in which they are working and will work. They also need time, personal availability and an ability to make good judgements about how things are going. Humility and respect in a mentor are important, as well as authority and confidence.

Most academic organisations encourage more than one type of mentorship – for example, a new lecturer may have a senior lecturer as their line manager and core institutional mentor, but also be encouraged to join a 'peer mentorship' group of other lecturers who can share career challenges and experiences. A third type of mentorship is the classic supervisory role, where mentoring focuses on particular research projects and scholarly pursuits. Beyond this, many academics find aspects of mentorship through broader academic networks in national and international professional bodies – for example, the author has often used colleagues in the Society of Academic Primary Care (see www.sapc.ac.uk), the Royal College of GPs and the World Organization of Family Doctors (see www.globalfamilydoctor.com) for specific advice, new professional opportunities and identification of other academics with work in similar fields. It is part of the job of an AD to introduce their ATs to the relevant professional networks, journals and best academic conferences for their discipline – so that they get experience of the academic community and the broader academic culture of family medicine. Having these different 'types' of mentorship in an AD allows, for example, an AT to have an academic supervisor from one background and a research supervisor from another who, together, bring different academic and professional context and skills into the relationship – which may be valuable in a department where senior personnel are limited.

From the perspective of the AT, there needs to be clarity both about who does what and who is available. A degree of choice in a mentoring relationship is important, though not always easy where a team is small; in an academic setting, there is often some additional choice through a postgraduate director or the human resources or pastoral care team, and these can also be used if a learner has a particular need or if primary mentorship relationships break down. Structures such as monthly appointments with the named academic mentor ensure that the relationship can be established through regular contacts, and goal setting and achievement kept under review. Having an 'annual appraisal' is a common model in professional settings and allows a more formal stocktake of progress. A programme of supportive activities such as shared seminars, training modules and social contacts allows ATs to see the work of others and to find additional 'go-to' people – for example, to test ideas on promotion with peers before formal discussions with the AM. A departmental culture that ensures that all staff and trainees feel free to ask, experiment and learn through different work relationships and opportunities will be one where mentorship thrives; similarly, working in isolation with a rigid mentorship allocation and few other contacts may risk a narrow career vision and a lack of overall development.

A final important component of institutional mentorship is governance and safeguarding. Relationships can break down, become collusive or even abusive and the need to set out professional behaviours and boundaries is essential to protect both ATs and AMs. Key issues include how to avoid emotional dependency, recognise cultural difference, seek help on a confidential basis if problems arise and being open and transparent about any conflicts between personal support and performance management. A 'good' system will include third party expertise which is outside the department and its interests, where either party can seek advice. If the relationship is part of formal institutional arrangements, then it should be routinely evaluated and changes made as needed. Issues such as equity – for example, ensuring access for both men and women ATs to academic opportunities – can also be monitored, and this can detect unconscious bias in mentors which favour some over others.

Much of the chapter to date is not speciality specific: So, does academic family medicine (FM) mentorship have specific challenges? In some countries, FM is a new speciality, and there may be few ATs who may feel rather isolated in the larger medical community. If FM is seen as an 'odd' choice, or of low status, AMs may need to address the uncertainties which can be caused for their ATs by such prejudices. Indeed, active mentorship may be needed *before* an academic FM post is chosen, to raise awareness of the new speciality with junior doctors and senior medical students as they begin to choose their career posts, to raise the profile of a new academic department in a medical school, and to persuade funders and other faculty to invest in academic capacity building for FM.

One 'golden opportunity' for active mentorship that can lead to a positive choice of academic FM is the identification of suitable students during their placements in basic medical training and early career posts. Some host practices who teach for the author's university create 'alumni' networks where they systematically keep in touch with students who express interest in, and seem suitable for, FM. This type of mentorship both makes students feel recognised and valued and also allows 'direct-to-student' adverts of training posts and career options. Similarly, offering research projects, intercalated degrees and elective attachments in FM academic departments allows students to start early contact with the academic community and can bring them into firm commitments later – all such placements will have a named supervisor or mentor, and provide another aspect to academic capacity building for FM. Finally, ensuring that FM ADs offer everything that other specialities offer – prizes, bursaries to present at conferences, project presentations and involvement with clinical and academic activities on an equal footing to ATs working in other specialities – is a key step towards making sure that the outputs of effective mentoring get seen and respected by others.

In conclusion, family medicine mentorship may bring people with strong interpersonal and professional skills together in the academic setting, but other aspects may be dictated by the organisation and its basic aim of attracting students, high performing academics and research grants. The need to balance personal support with career progression and an introduction to the wider academic world is the role of both individuals and departments or institutions. Developing an academic career needs a variety of opportunities over time, and a single institutional mentor should be supplemented by the broader networks accessible through organisations such as WONCA, where ATs can gain international contacts and broaden their thinking around where research fits into the needs of health patients and systems. Being an AM can be a very satisfying role because it leaves a legacy – the next generation of FM researchers! Making mentorship happen is a key role for growing our discipline.

CHAPTER 33

A systems approach to building research capacity: Individuals, networks and culture

Grant Russell

At its heart, *How to Do Primary Care Research* is a book about increasing an individual's capacity to become a part of the primary care research world. It is aimed at those practitioners who wonder how to make a start in research and to those who have made that start, but are now beginning to explore new research worlds. Earlier chapters have shown how to ask an answerable question and of how to hone the method to fit the question. Section V shows some novel ways to get the results to a wider audience and shows how to make that difficult transition from your first project to a career in primary care research.

Yet, when I hear primary care academics speaking of the challenges of primary care research, they don't ponder how to ask the best question, or (thankfully) debate the pros and cons of qualitative versus quantitative designs. No, it's not long before the talk turns to research capacity.

The primary care research community holds a deep anxiety about sustainability in an increasingly uncertain and fragile academic world. Ironically this comes at a time when governments are convinced of the contribution of primary care to equity and improved outcomes[1] and expect the sector to narrow the gap between knowledge and practice.

Deans, departmental chairs and research directors are desperate for primary care academic departments to be more research active. Professional colleges struggle to embed an academic culture amongst members whose main priority is delivering quality patient care. And early career researchers worry about building a research career in a time where funds are short and much of the glamour goes to their hospital colleagues.

In this chapter, I broaden the concept of capacity in primary care research from an individual to a systems level, resurrect a decade-old model of research capacity building and outline ways in which capacity can be built at a time when challenges seem to come from everywhere.

DELIVERING PRIMARY CARE RESEARCH: HOW ARE WE PERFORMING?

Research output is growing within primary care disciplines.[2] While barely a handful of primary care-relevant articles were published in the late 1960s, by the turn of the twenty-first century, 12,000 academic primary care articles were being published each year in Australia, Canada, Germany, the Netherlands, the UK, and the US.[3] However, the capacity to sustain this output is fragile. Many primary care academics are frustrated as to how hard it is to secure mainstream research funding. In 2012, family medicine departments in the US received around $157 million of dedicated internal and external research funding—impressive until we understand that figure is only 0.13% of all US medical-research funding ($117 billion).[3] Australia's main research funding body, the National Health and Medical Research Council, has for many years allocated barely 1% of its total allocations towards primary care.[4]

In some nations, a difficult situation is getting worse. In 2015, Australia experienced a substantial withdrawal of federal support for primary care research. Funding ceased for the nation's PHC funding and knowledge translation organisation, the Australian Primary Health Care Research Institute (APHCRI). Activities of the admired Primary Health Care Research and Information Service (PHCRIS) (http://www.phcris.org.au/index.php) were cutback and the Australian primary care Research Network (APCReN) (http://www.apcren.org.au) was mothballed.

I had personal insights into some of these challenges while head of a School of Primary and Allied Health Care in a large Australian University (https://www.monash.edu/medicine/spahc). The school comprised a range of primary care relevant disciplines including general practice, occupational therapy, physiotherapy, social work and paramedic practice.

School academics were passionate about building their emerging disciplines. We had several research champions, but few research teams, and most publication output related to health professional education. School departments were geographically dispersed, overwhelmed by teaching demands and often found it difficult to collaborate with other disciplines. Many junior academics spent a great deal of time writing grant applications, the overwhelming majority of which were unsuccessful.

The enthusiasm of the members of our school and frustrations in moving a research agenda forward are reflected internationally. In 1997, a national working group conducted a major review of the primary care research capacity in the UK's National Health Service. The resulting Mant report identified the lack of evidence behind much of the organisation and delivery of primary care. The report's recommendations were aimed at addressing the small critical mass of primary care researchers, limited research funding, poor methodological quality, minimal leadership and what they called 'a failure to recruit enough of the most able individuals from all health professional groups and related disciplines to primary care research'.[5] A similar evaluation of research capacity in primary health care in Canada in 2007 viewed the problems similarly. In addition, despite Canada's undoubted international leadership in knowledge transfer and exchange, its ability to improve policy and practice was limited by sparse funding, no 'common vision for PHC research' and minimal support for both clinician and research scientists.[6]

It is not that there isn't anyone fostering research capacity in primary care. The last decade has seen a range of initiatives directed at improving research capacity in primary care. Box 33.1 gives details of three current capacity-building initiatives.

All of these programmes have a focus on up-skilling enthusiastic individuals, many of whom are destined to be leaders of the future. While necessary, all of this activity is insufficient without attention to the environment where graduates and other enthusiasts are going to work.

SYSTEMS THINKING AND RESEARCH CAPACITY

There is an increasing interest in systems-based approaches to solve challenging questions in health care. In the last two decades, the principles of complexity science have percolated into health care delivery, management and education.[7] I believe that a similar systems approach can help us move to a more sustainable primary care research future.

In 2005, Cooke proposed a systems-based roadmap of research capacity in health sciences.[8] She saw research capacity building in health sciences as having six 'overarching principles'. Four of these (skills and confidence, dissemination, infrastructure and sustainability) are common to other literature on health research capacity building. Two principles (partnerships and the idea of conducting research close to practice) have additional importance in the applied disciplines that go to make up primary care.

Importantly, she also showed how these principles had relevance in developmental activity aimed at four different levels: Individuals, teams, organisations and inter-organisational networks. She contended that the levels interact and that 'one level can have an impact on capacity development at another level, and could potentially have a synergistic or detrimental effect on the other'.[8,9]

BOX 33.1 SELECTED PRIMARY CARE RESEARCH CAPACITY BUILDING INITIATIVES

Transdisciplinary Understanding and Training on Research in Primary Health Care (TUTOR-PHC): TUTOR PHC is a Canadian multi-university collaboration that has, since 2003, been led by the University of Western Ontario. With a focus on collaborative interdisciplinary primary care research, TUTOR has delivered training to mid-career health professionals and or participants in graduate programs within disciplines such as family medicine, epidemiology nursing, psychology and social work. TUTOR's one-year certificate program uses online and face-to-face approaches to teach primary health care research skills and interdisciplinary theory and processes. http://www.uwo.ca/fammed/csfm/tutor-phc//

The Oxford International PC Research Leadership programme: Results from a long collaboration between University Departments from eight countries (England, Scotland, Northern Ireland, The Netherlands, Germany, Australia, US and Canada). Its two-year program has a similar online and face-to-face peer learning approach to TUTOR and is designed to build leadership, connections and academic skills in primary care research. http://www.oxfordleadershipprogramme.com

The Grant Generating Project of the North American Primary Care Research Group (NAPCRG):

NAPCRG runs a number of programs for North American junior family medicine faculty. Their Grant Generating Project http://www.napcrg.org/Programs/GrantGeneratingProject(GGP) provides a 'fellowship without walls' for family practice researchers, particularly those who have minimal access to capacity support in their home environments. Since 1995, the GGP has trained close to 200 fellows and produced over 1,000 grant proposals yielding more than $1 billion in grants to Departments of Family of Medicine.

Taken another way, skills and confidence aren't just relevant to the individual but also to teams and networks; partnerships are important to organisations but also to individuals and research teams. Some recent activity in capacity development has embraced these principles. Holden contended that the principal *motivators* for research are intrinsic to the individual, while the principal *barriers* are organisational. He used the theory in developing an intervention study of the impact of a complex team oriented research capacity building intervention.[10]

What follows are some thoughts as to some capacity approaches that may have surprising success, taken at the level of the individual, the team, and within and between organisations. Taken together they may make life easier for department heads, research directors and those leading professional and/or government organisations who together are faced with pervasive challenges in sustaining primary care research capacity. Box 33.2 gives examples of two

---

BOX 33.2   TWO NATIONAL LEVEL PRIMARY CARE
RESEARCH CAPACITY BUILDING INITIATIVES

The Netherlands School of Primary Care Research (CaRe): CaRe has operated as a research school since 1995. Supported by the Government of the Netherlands, CaRe has a close affiliation with NIVEL, the national institute for health services. CaRe has had a major focus on primary care PhD training and acts as a catalyst for collaboration between a number of primary care research institutes. http://www.researchschoolcare.nl

The Scottish School of Primary Care (SSPC): Since 2000, SSPC has used a broad strategy to develop high-quality research to address important issues in Scotland, to increase recruitment to clinical trials and to ensure higher-level career-development opportunities. The School manages the Scottish Primary Care Research Network (SPCRN) whose focus is to improve access to patients for trials and to reduce research burden on primary care practices. The SSPC has a wide inter-organisational network with other national primary care research organisations, in particular with CaRe and the Oxford Leadership initiative. http://www.sspc.ac.uk

---

nations who have used a systems approach to energise their primary care research enterprise.

BUILDING A RESEARCH ACTIVE DEPARTMENT

There are few more complex jobs in a University than being the chair of a clinical department. Budgets need to be balanced, undergraduate students taught, postgraduates inspired and faculty members supervised, while continuing the balancing act of being the person sitting behind the desk where the 'buck stops'. The chair is often the main advocate of the discipline to both the broader university and clinicians at the coal face. And of course, s/he is the person held responsible when research output is falling.

A 2006 survey of 134 US departments of family medicine found that 40% had minimal or no research capacity. Only one in 30 of the Departments were said to have an extensive or 'replicating' capacity.[2] The situation is little better in developing economies. A survey of 139 academic family physicians from eight Arab countries showed that while three in four academics were required to conduct research, less than one-half had authored one publication.[11]

So does a systems approach to research-capacity building have anything to offer the beleaguered chair? I'd suggest that if departmental research is sluggish, then instead of bemoaning the state of research funding for primary care in the nation, or blaming faculty members for their disinterest, that chairs should think of addressing the individual, organisational and contextual barriers within their control. Table 33.1 provides some suggestions along these

TABLE 33.1 A non-comprehensive series of strategies for building research capacity for academic departments

	Individuals	Teams	Organisations	Inter-organisational networks
Skills and confidence	Providing clinical educators with training in research methods within defined learning plans	Investing in quality team processes (i.e. deliberative dialogue)[25]	Participation and/or leadership of mentor programmes	Active invitations for external experts to visit
Research close to practice	Giving non-clinician researchers opportunities to experience the clinical setting	Including clinicians and practice staff in design and reporting of quality-improvement interventions	Articulation of the link between research and practice/policy in all research endeavours	Fostering Practice Based Research Networks
Linkages and collaborations	Support for research conference attendance for students and junior staff	Implementing high quality efficient communications between dispersed team members	Seed research funding directed at building links between different parts of the organisation	Building regional partnerships between policymakers and academia
Appropriate Dissemination	Organise writing skills workshops and internal 'research rounds' to build skills	Academic writing retreats incorporated into research grant funding applications	Investing in quality web sites and social media to promote departmental activities	Participation in endeavours like 'How to Do Primary Care Research'.
Infrastructure	Access to libraries for PBRN clinicians	Quality communication technology	Funding for a departmental research manager	Contributing to profession wide capacity development schemes
Continuity and Sustainability	Actively supporting junior and mid-career academics in fellowship applications	Prioritising applications for longer term team funding initiatives	Use of an active strategic plan for the research operations in the organisation	Incorporating support for the PBRN in relevant project funding applications

Source: Hogg W et al. *Can Fam Physician* 2009;55(10):e35–40.

lines by showing a matrix of capacity-building activities in a hypothetical academic department of primary care.

Much of it is about creating a culture within the department that supports and encourages practitioners to participate in research activities. Low-cost options would include framing a mentor programme for junior staff and establishing research as a core expectation of job roles and as a key criterion for recruitment of educators.[8,12] Simply running regular research grand rounds (preferably in collaboration with other primary care and community health disciplines) can have a substantial effect on changing a culture.

Isolation in research doesn't just affect individuals. It acts at the organisational level as well. I have seen a number of smaller departments make exponential improvements in research capacity by using Cooke's principle of partnerships as a way to increase their links with the broader primary care community. These partnerships can be through interdepartmental visits, shared supervision, collaborative grant proposals and collaborating in either formal research networks or, primary care's version of a learning community: the practice based research network (see Chapter 7). William Hogg and colleagues have published a detailed description of their road to development of their own research centre within the University of Ottawa.[13]

THE FORGOTTEN INDIVIDUAL: THE NON-CLINICIAN RESEARCHER

Health-professional disciplines like family medicine, nursing and physiotherapy will always prioritise, value and reward those who are 'card-carrying professionals'. Professional organisations want to give academic skills to clinicians, while primary care Departments will always prioritise those who can teach clinical skills.

However, it has been my experience that the most successful research teams are reliant on a contribution from non-clinician researchers. Many of the greats in primary care research over the last few decades have been non-clinicians: Moira Stewart (an epidemiologist) led the articulation of the patient centred clinical method;[14] Benjamin Crabtree (an anthropologist) conducted seminal investigations of the patient centred medical home;[15] and, more recently, health economist Carl May has championed one of the key approaches to implementation science: Normalisation Process Theory.[16]

Non-clinician researchers bring much to the table. Their research training is robust and invariably theoretically bound. They bring insights and approaches that are often not well developed in clinician scientists. However, the Mant report emphasised the complex disincentives that discourage young non-clinical researchers to become involved in primary care research and development.[17] They follow a more traditional academic career path than their clinician colleagues and are particularly plagued by postdoctoral career uncertainty. Lacking the security of a clinical income, and often unable to teach, career stability is dependent on the annual cycle of grant and fellowship income. I have seen many talented, passionate young social scientists reluctantly leave primary care for other disciplines with more security.

While departments have little leverage on national funding streams, one of the early priorities of departments seeking to build capacity in research would be to strengthen their methodological expertise by collaborating with and helping build the careers of social scientists. Although they may need support in building networks and gaining understanding of the primary care context, huge benefits can come from fostering the careers of the right person.

TEAMS: A NICE IDEA, SO LET'S SUPPORT THEM

Family medicine has a long tradition of solo researchers. Many founders of the primary care disciplines were clinicians intrigued by clinical questions in their own practices or communities. James McKenzie spent 29 years methodically cataloguing a wealth of cardiac conditions as a GP in Lancashire. In Australia, Max Kamien illuminated the lives of indigenous communities in Bourke NSW, and Charles Bridges Webb paved the road to the International Classification of Primary Care through his careful practice-based observations in rural New South Wales.

It's a sign of the complexity of modern medicine and health-services delivery that there are hardly any stories like this being written anymore. Multidisciplinary teams deliver health services and also the vast majority of health care research. Funding agencies have accelerated this trend. Over the last decade or so, Australia and the UK have supported Centres of Excellence in primary care research, while Canada has spent over $30 million to support 14 Community Based Primary Health Care research teams.

Teams are becoming more complex as well. They are often geographically dispersed, are working across different time zones and are more and more reliant on technology to communicate. As part of several large research teams, I have become acutely aware of the challenges of researching at a distance. Across national and provincial borders, ethics regulations can be mismatched, data storage challenging and quality communication sometimes overwhelming.

Departments, universities and jurisdictions could make it easier for researchers to collaborate in multidisciplinary teams. Our lessons from the understanding of teams within small organisations[18] can help us answer questions such as, how can we develop and lead a widely dispersed research team? How should we communicate? How can we make expectations clear? And, how do we deal with members who aren't pulling their weight?

Furthermore, there is a need for better technology for collaboration and for data storage. Many research teams I have been a part of have spent precious time trying to negotiate communication platforms and discover secure means of storing data. Despite the potential of virtual communication, I am convinced that funding bodies need to acknowledge the value of face-to-face communication at critical times of project design, analysis and dissemination.

BUILDING PRACTICE RELEVANT NETWORKS: GETTING RESEARCH CLOSE TO PRACTICE

Most are familiar with the caricature of the expert sitting at an academic institution making pronouncements about a world he or she rarely experiences. Primary care research has learned how to breach the walls of the ivory tower in some intriguing ways, ways that fit well with the principle of doing research close to practice. One of the signature initiatives of the last couple of decades within the discipline of family practice has been the growth in popularity of Practice-Based Research Networks (PBRNs). These are sustained collaborations between practitioners and academics dedicated to developing relevant research questions, working together on study design and conduct, and translating new knowledge into practice.[19]

PBRNs first developed over 50 years ago in the UK and the US. They have steadily increased in popularity since then and have been promoted as 'research laboratories' and learning communities of primary health care.[20] Comprising a network of research-interested family medicine practices and an academic department, they have found support from professional bodies,[21] university departments or, sometimes, from teaching hospitals keen to reach into the community.[22] It is a popular model: The 28 PBRNs in the US in 1994 expanded to over 140 in 2011.[23]

Several nations have developed national PBRN networks. Several of these commenced as part of influenza surveillance and have expanded their work to other projects involving chronic disease. Some have been of great interest to governments keen to collaborate with the pharmaceutical trial industry. The concept of 'bottom up' PBRNs have been long championed by the North American Primary Care Research Group, which sponsors an annual PBRN conference with the support of the Agency for Health care Research and Quality (http://www.napcrg.org/ICPF).

While it can be daunting for academic departments to set up a PBRN, one easy way to start would be to make an approach to either teaching practices, or practices that have already shown an interest in research.

CONCLUSION

Research can be an isolating process. Fortunately, the sense of discovery, the feeling that one may be making a difference and, for most of us, the friends we make along the way, make it all worthwhile. Although individuals have a personal responsibility for excellence, the idea of research capacity as a system responsibility opens the door to a more sustainable future if we take the additional responsibility of helping promote system improvement.

It is not a new message and resonates in a seminal paper published many years ago by the acclaimed Canadian primary care academic Martin Bass. He wrote of the subtle, system-wide forces of disconnected specialists, Big Pharma and the lure of technology, that, while well-meaning, foster learned helplessness from both clinicians and primary care researchers. He saw office-based research as fundamental to throwing off the 'yoke of learned dependence'. He challenged the research community to develop 'research networks that involve physicians who, by themselves, might not have the opportunity to engage in research. We can involve others in our research. We can publish research papers that are readable and clinically relevant. Finally we can identify and oppose the forces that foster our dependence and we can foster those endeavours that tend towards the expansion of our areas of interest and expertise'.[24]

It is not a bad note to conclude on. I wish you well on the journey.

ACKNOWLEDGEMENT

Acknowledging the vision of Dr William Hogg and others at the CT Lamont Primary Care Research Centre in Ottawa for the detail of many of these strategies. The team's approach to capacity building is described in a 2009 article in the Canadian Family Physician.

REFERENCES

1. Starfield B, Shi L, Macinko J. Contribution of primary care to health systems and health. *Milbank Q* 2005;83(3):457–502.
2. Ewigman B, Davis A, Vansaghi T et al. Building Research & Scholarship capacity in departments of family medicine: A new joint Adfm-Napcrg initiative. *Ann Fam Med* 2016;14(1):82–3.
3. Glanville J, Kendrick T, McNally R et al. Research output on primary care in Australia, Canada, Germany, the Netherlands, the United Kingdom, and the United States: Bibliometric analysis. *BMJ* 2011;342:d1028.
4. McIntyre EL, Mazza D, Harris NP. NHMRC funding for primary health care research, 2000–2008. *Med J Aust* 2011;195(4):230 [published online: 17 August 2011].
5. Mant D. R&D in Primary Care. *National Working Group Report.* London: Central Research and Development Committee, National Health Service, 1997. p. 71.
6. Russell G, Geneau R, Johnston S et al. *Mapping the Future of Primary Health Care Research in Canada: A Report to the Canadian Health Services Research Foundation.* Ottawa: Canadian Health Services Research Foundation, 2007. p. 1–52.
7. Plsek PE, Greenhalgh T. Complexity science: The challenge of complexity in health care. *BMJ* 2001;323(7313):625–8.
8. Cooke J. A framework to evaluate research capacity building in health care. *BMC Fam Pract* 2005;6:44.
9. Golenko X, Pager S, Holden L. A thematic analysis of the role of the organisation in building allied health research capacity: A senior managers' perspective. *BMC Health Serv Res* 2012;12:276.

10. Holden L, Pager S, Golenko X et al. Evaluating a team-based approach to research capacity building using a matched-pairs study design. *BMC Fam Pract* 2012;13:16.
11. Romani MH, Hamadeh GN, Mahmassani DM et al. Opportunities and barriers to enhance research capacity and outputs among academic family physicians in the Arab world. *Prim Health Care Res Dev* 2016;17(1):98–104.
12. Jones ML, Cifu DX, Backus D et al. Instilling a research culture in an applied clinical setting. *Arch Phys Med Rehabil* 2013;94(1 Suppl.):S49–54.
13. Hogg W, Donskov M, Russell G et al. Riding the wave of primary care research: Development of a primary health care research centre. *Can Fam Physician* 2009;55(10):e35–40. [pii] [published online: 15 October 2009].
14. Stewart M. Towards a global definition of patient centred care. The patient should be the judge of patient centred care. *BMJ* 2001;322(7284):444–5.
15. Crabtree BF, Nutting PA, Miller WL et al. Primary care practice transformation is hard work: Insights from a 15-year developmental programme of research. *Med Care* 2011;49(Suppl.):S28–35. [published online: 22 September 2010].
16. May CR, Mair F, Finch T et al. Development of a theory of implementation and integration: Normalization process theory. *Implement Sci* 2009;4:29. [published online: 23 May 2009].
17. Mant D. *National Working Party on R&D in Primary Care*. Final Report. London: NHSE South and West; 1997.
18. Tannenbaum SI, Mathieu JE, Salas E et al. Teams are changing: Are research and practice evolving fast enough? *Ind Organ Psychol* 2015;5(01):2–24.
19. Pearce C, Phillips C, Hall S et al. Following the funding trail: Financing, nurses and teamwork in Australian general practice. *BMC Health Serv Res* 2011;11:38.
20. Mold JW, Peterson KA. Primary care practice-based research networks: Working at the interface between research and quality improvement. *Ann Fam Med* 2005;3(Suppl. 1):S12–20.
21. The College of Family Physicians of Canada. CFPC Research Initiatives. http://www.cfpc.ca/Research_Initiatives/. Accessed May 15 2018.
22. Drummond N. North Toronto Primary Care Research and Development Network (Nortren). 2002 [28 August]. Department of Family Medicine. About Utopian. Available from https://www.dfcm.utoronto.ca/about-utopian. Accessed May 15 2018.
23. Peterson KA, Lipman PD, Lange CJ et al. Supporting better science in primary care: A description of practice-based research networks (PBRNs) in 2011. *J Am Board Fam Med* 2012;25(5):565–71. [published online: 08 September 2012].
24. Bass MJ. Office-based research: The antidote to learned helplessness. *Can Fam Physician* 1987;33:1987–92.
25. Burkhalter S, Gastil J, Kelshaw T. A conceptual definition and theoretical model of public deliberation in small face–to–face groups. *Commun Theory* 2002;12(4):398–422.

CHAPTER 34

Including primary care research in clinical practice

Chris van Weel

INTRODUCTION

We have now come to the end of this book on primary care research. The book is intended to be a resource for the novice or emerging researcher in the primary care context and to guide them in the identification of a research question, development of their research proposal, use of different methods, reporting on their research and ensuring that it has an impact. Many readers may be pursuing a career as a primary care researcher or obligated to conduct research as part of a degree; some readers, however, will be full-time family doctors or primary care providers in clinical practice who would like to include practical research as a part of their work. This last chapter returns to the heart of primary care and discusses how the busy clinician can engage with primary care research.

THE CLINICAL CHALLENGES OF PRIMARY HEALTH CARE AND FAMILY MEDICINE

The function of primary health care (PHC) and family medicine is to respond to all health problems, in all stages, in all people, without preselection or restriction. This function is captured in the 'ecology of medical care' model[1] that illustrates the position of PHC as the connection between a population or community and the health system. Of all the individuals in the population who experience an episode of poor health, a minority will contact health professionals – in most cases, a family physician (FP) or other PHC professional, who practices in that community. Most problems that present in PHC are completely dealt with there. The hospital sector plays, in terms of the volume of contacts, only a limited role.

The ecology of medical care clarifies four key elements of PHC:

1. A perspective of the community or population served
2. The broad 'clinical field' of health problems and health risks that is covered
3. The individual variation in health needs that should be responded to
4. The importance of coordination of health care from self-care through primary health care to hospital care

The community perspective stresses the specific status of the population in which FPs are practising, in terms of the health needs and risks, demographics, socioeconomic levels and cultural and religious backgrounds, as well as social determinants of health.[2] Populations will consequently differ not only between countries, but also within countries and even within different regions of the same country. PHC has to relate to *its* population.[3]

The clinical domain is that of *all* possible health problems: Mental, social as well as physical, from self-limiting to life threatening, chronic and acute. Given that PHC is the first point of contact, a broad range of early signs of yet undifferentiated health problems characterise this clinical domain in which FPs and other PHC professionals work.[4] Although FPs will recognise the broadness of their field without any problem, this is only scantily documented in textbooks and other literature.

According to the 'ecology model,'[1] most patients take care of their own health most of the time. When someone consults, this may point not only to the severity of the illness, but also to the potential anxiety that the illness generates in that person and their personal need for support. Individual variation stresses the importance of understanding the person with the health problem as much as the health problem as such. Individuals with identical health problems may access care for distinctly different reasons,[5] and this will likewise require distinctly different approaches to care, in other words person-centred medicine.[6]

A majority of patients with chronic health problems suffer from two or more different conditions at the same time.[7] Depending on the health problem, either support, treatment and/or preventive measures may be indicated, and can involve different professionals from PHC or the hospital sector. It is essential that all these interventions contribute in a harmonious way to the health and well-being of the patient and are coordinated. Coordination of care that requires an overview of all health problems in combination with a knowledge of the individual and the community that he or she comes from, befalls the generalist FP.

FROM CLINICAL CHALLENGES TO RESEARCH AND RESEARCHABLE QUESTIONS

These four key elements highlight the complex nature of PHC and family medicine which in turn signals an equally broad need for clinical research to support professional performance. Yet, despite investment in research in the PHC setting, substantial aspects have not been researched, or insufficiently in the specific context in which PHC has to operate. It remains true that 'what is most common has been researched the least,'[8] and as a consequence, FPs in the absence of scientific evidence have to rely on empirical knowledge as a basis for decision making.

This is as much a problem as an opportunity for research. Generating more in-depth knowledge of the key elements of PHC and family medicine can substantially strengthen professional performance and foster the effectiveness and safety of care. As FPs and other PHC professionals have often never been trained in research, research may be considered beyond their professional scope. It is important that professionals in PHC also realise their strengths in the research exercise and what they have to offer that no one else can. This is essential, as the only purpose of research in PHC is to improve the health and health care of individuals and populations.[9] Three reasons why FPs are able to make a singular contribution from their practice to research are

1. PHC professionals are uniquely positioned to critically appraise research proposals to ensure relevance to PHC.
2. PHC professionals possess a wealth of experience and empirical knowledge of responding to health issues in the PHC setting, which also leads to the development of relevant research questions and hypotheses.
3. PHC is in the possession of or has direct access to essential data on populations, individuals' health and health problems (primary health care epidemiology), patients' experiences, expectations and needs, and on the processes and outcomes of clinical care in this context.

This makes FPs and other PHC professionals indispensable partners in PHC research. Coming back to the four key elements of PHC, examples of relevant questions to answer could be

1. The community or population perspective
   a. What is the health status of the community served by the practice?
   b. What are the most important health problems encountered?
   c. Which social determinants have in impact on the health status of this population? Are there barriers to accessing health care?

2. The broad 'clinical field' of health problems and health risks that is covered
   a. What are the most frequent health problems encountered?
   b. To what extent are the possibilities of prevention used?
   c. Do the practices provide the interventions needed to cope with the most important health problems?
3. The individual variation in health needs to respond to
   a. Who are the most frequent users of the practices?
   b. Who should be, due to their health needs, the most frequent users of the practices?
   c. What strategy could be successful to make sure that those in highest need actually use the practice facilities?
4. The importance of coordination of health care
   a. Which patients have chronic health problems and who of them is under treatment of hospital specialists?
   b. Of those under treatment from hospital specialists, is there information available on the care prescribed there?
   c. How often does care prescribed in hospital and PHC contradict each other?

It is important to realise that research often evolves incrementally, from basic questions to more complex studies. Insight in the health status of a population could lead to a randomised trial testing the effectiveness of novel interventions for important health problems. An understanding of why groups with significant health needs seldom visit the practices could trigger participatory research to co-design pathways to care that better suit these groups' needs and perspectives.

FROM THEORY TO PRACTICE: HOW CAN FPS AND THEIR PRACTICES CONTRIBUTE TO RESEARCH?

There are at least three practical ways in which FPs (and other members of their PHC team) can contribute to research.

1. *Critically appraise research proposals and programmes*: One of the recurrent experiences is that most biomedical research does not address problems of patients in the PHC setting and as a consequence fails to support FPs in their clinical decisions. The reason for this is that researchers, academics and those who design research policy may have knowledge of science, but lack an intimate understanding of PHC.

   What you can do as FP: In fact, this is an essential contribution only FPs and other PHC professionals can make. The critical reading or appraisal of research proposals, guidelines under development or published research and giving feedback from a PHC perspective can help improve the relevance and applicability of research to the PHC context.

How you can make this contribution: Ways to organise this can be through membership of a scientific organisation – college, university department – or as a reviewer of research proposals and scientific articles.

What this requires from you: Reading from your perspective as a PHC professional is the key skill, although some ability to read critically or appraise research may also be useful. It also asks for leadership skills, as you may have to stand up to authority and vested interest. It is important to realise is that this is a way to protect the long-term health interest of patients – 'our' patients, communities and populations.

2. *Document the complex nature of primary health care and the health needs of patients:* Related to the previous point, policy makers and experts from science and research often have no insight in the actual problems encountered in PHC. This is one of the reasons why health policy is often less effective than it could be.

What you can do as FP: FPs hold the key to this and are able to provide detailed information on the health problems, health risks and social and environmental determinants of health encountered in the primary care setting.

How you can make this contribution: A critical objective for FPs in this role is to provide information on the realities of PHC to guide political and management decisions.

What this requires from you: Possible methods could be to document your experience, for example, with overviews of the most important health problems identified in daily patient care. The main skills required for this is that of a FP – the ability to diagnose health problems and understand patients and their needs. Robust documentation of what comes up during a clinic or a certain period of time in the practice can be an important way of starting to address this issue. Analysing and reporting on information that is derived from households in a defined community, often collected by community health workers, can also be useful to define local health needs and priorities.

3. *Create access for researchers to essential data of patients and populations:* The only way researchers, policy makers and educators can integrate the role and function of PHC in their missions, is through access to the field of PHC. In other words, by understanding your community, your patients, your work, your clinical and organisational decisions.

What you can do as FP: This stresses the need to open up the interactions between FPs or other PHC professionals and patients for research and other academic tasks. This is a responsibility only you, the FP, can take for your own practice, a responsibility of protecting the safety and privacy of the patients involved and a responsibility to provide data robust enough to meet the criteria for research.

How you can make this contribution: The best way to develop this, is to seek collaboration and support at two levels: (1) collaboration with research institutes and universities can help generate high quality data and (2) collaboration with other practices is helpful to support and secure the leadership role that is required from FPs through networking of practices as Practice-Based Research Networks (PBRN); see Chapter 7. This is generally seen as a key infrastructure of PHC research in many countries, as it makes it possible to share experiences, provide mutual support and enlarge the numbers of patients to recruit for studies.

What this requires from you: In a structured PBRN with collaboration between research and practice, there will be more and more asked of participating FPs in terms of research skills. But at the same time, PBRNs provide a nurturing environment in which it is possible to support FPs – to support you! – in developing research skills. The bottom line, though, is that these research skills are relevant, but only in addition to the clinical and leadership skills you as FP already have.

CONCLUSION

FPs and other PHC professionals can make an essential contribution to primary care research. Even when not specifically trained or experienced in research, they can bring to the research process their in-depth understanding of the PHC context and communities that they serve. This will help to make sure that research will support important decisions in the daily care of patients in the PHC context and help to improve the health of communities.

REFERENCES

1. Green LA, Fryer GE, Yawn BP, Lanier D, Dovey SM. The ecology of medical care revisited. *N Engl J Med* 2001;344:2021–5.
2. Commission on Social Determinants of Health. *Closing the Gap in a Generation.* Geneva: World Health Organization; 2008. Available from: http://www.who.int/social_ determinants/ thecommission/finalreport/en/.
3. Maeseneer J de, Weel C van, Daeren L, Leyns C, Decat P, Boeckxstaens P, Avonts D, Willems S. From 'patient' to 'person' to 'people': The need for integrated, people centered health care. *Int J Person Centered Medicine* 2012;2:601–14.
4. Knottnerus JA. Between iatrotropic stimulus and interiatric referral: The domain of primary care research. *J Clin Epidemiol* 2002;55:1201e6.
5. Olde Hartman TC, Ravesteijn H van, Lucassen P, Boven K van, Weel-Baumgarten E van, Weel C van. Why the 'reason for encounter' should be incorporated in the analysis of outcome of care. *Br J Gen Pract* 2011;61:750–1.
6. Mezzich J, Snaedal J, van Weel C, Heath I. Toward person-centered medicine: From disease to patient toperson. *Mt Sinai J Med* 2010;77:304–6.
7. Fortin M, Bravo G, Hudon C, Vanasse A, Lapointe L. Prevalence of multimorbidity among adults seen in family practice. *Ann Fam Med* 2005;3:223–228.
8. Melker RA de. Diseases: The more common the less studied. *Fam Pract* 1995;12:84e7.
9. Rosser WW, Weel C van. Research in family/general practice is essential for improving health globally. *Ann Fam Med* 2004;2:S2–S4.

Index

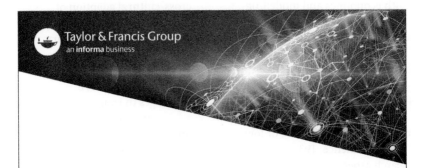

Printed and bound by CPI Group (UK) Ltd, Croydon, CR0 4YY

22/10/2024

01777603-0007